Sexual Aggression

Sexual Aggression

Edited by

Jon A. Shaw, M.D.

Professor of Psychiatry and Pediatrics and
Director, Division of Child and Adolescent Psychiatry,
Department of Psychiatry and Behavioral Sciences,
University of Miami School of Medicine/
Jackson Memorial Medical Center, Miami, Florida

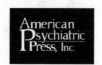

Washington, DC
London, England

Copyright © 1999 American Psychiatric Press, Inc.
ALL RIGHTS RESERVED
Manufactured in the United States of America on acid-free paper
02 01 00 99   4 3 2 1
First Edition

American Psychiatric Press, Inc.
1400 K Street, N.W., Washington, DC   20005
www.appi.org

Library of Congress Cataloging-in-Publication Data
Sexual aggression / edited by Jon A. Shaw. — 1st ed.
       p.   cm.
     Includes bibliographical references and index.
     ISBN 0-88048-757-7
     1. Sex crimes. 2. Sex offenders. 3. Child sexual abuse. I. Shaw, Jon A.
     [DNLM: 1. Sex Offenses—psychology. 2. Violence. 3. Child Abuse,
Sexual—psychology. 4. Sex Behavior—psychology. W 795 S5182
1998]
RC560.S47S488 1998
616.85′82—dc21
DNLM/DLC
for Library of Congress   98-17929
                                                                           CIP

British Library Cataloguing in Publication Data
A CIP record is available from the British Library.

To the children who are
the continuing victims of
emotional neglect and
physical and sexual aggression.

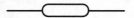

Contents

Section I
Overview of Sexually Aggressive Behavior and Its Psychological Consequences

Section II
Phenomenology and Assessment of
Sexually Aggressive Behavior and Treatment Considerations

Contributors

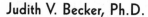

Judith V. Becker, Ph.D.
Associate Dean for Academic Affairs, College of Social and
Behavioral Sciences, University of Arizona, Tucson, Arizona

Toni Cavanagh Johnson, Ph.D.
Private Practice, South Pasadena, California

Jamie R. Funderburk, Ph.D.
Assistant Clinical Professor, University of Florida Counseling
Center, Gainesville, Florida

Arthur H. Green, M.D.
Clinical Professor of Psychiatry, Columbia University College of
Physicians and Surgeons; Medical Director, Therapeutic Nursery;
and Senior Consultant to the Family Center at Presbyterian
Hospital, New York, New York

John A. Hunter, Jr., Ph.D.
Associate Professor of Health Evaluation Sciences and Research
Fellow, Institute of Law, Psychiatry and Public Policy, University
of Virginia, Charlottesville

Robin Jones, M.A.
Project Director (RAP), Center for Community Alternatives,
New York, New York

Debra A. Katz, M.D.
Assistant Professor of Clinical Psychiatry and Neurology, University of Kentucky College of Medicine, Lexington, Kentucky

Harriet P. Lefley, Ph.D.
Professor of Psychiatry and Behavioral Sciences, Department of
Psychiatry and Behavioral Sciences, University of Miami School
of Medicine, Miami, Florida

Louis LeGum, Ph.D.
Private Practice, Gainesville, Florida

Diane H. Schetky, M.D.
Private Practice, Rockport, Maine; Associate Clinical Professor of
Psychiatry, University of Vermont College of Medicine at Maine
Medical Center, Portland, Maine

Anita M. Schlank, Ph.D.
Clinical Director, Minnesota Sex Offender Program, Mooselake,
Minnesota

Linda D. Schwoeri, Ph.D.
Clinical Assistant Professor of Clinical Psychiatry, Robert Wood
Johnson Medical School, University of Medicine and Dentistry
of New Jersey, Piscataway, New Jersey

Jon A. Shaw, M.D.
Professor of Psychiatry and Pediatrics and Director, Division of
Child and Adolescent Psychiatry, Department of Psychiatry and
Behavioral Sciences, University of Miami School of Medicine/
Jackson Memorial Medical Center, Miami, Florida

Ted Shaw, Ph.D.
Private Practice, North Florida Psychological Services; Director,
Adolescents Who Sexually Offend, Gainesville, Florida

G. Pirooz Sholevar, M.D.
Clinical Professor, Department of Psychiatry, Robert Wood
Johnson Medical School, University of Medicine and Dentistry
of New Jersey, Piscataway, New Jersey

Introduction

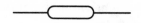

American society has become increasingly preoccupied with themes of violence and sexual aggression. Sexual assault is one of the fastest growing violent crimes in the United States. Of particular importance is the dramatic increase in sexual aggressive and violent crimes committed by juveniles. Terms such as *sexual aggression, sexual abuse, sexual assault,* and *rape* refer to acts of sexual exploitation without consent, without equality, and with the use of coercion. *Sexual aggression* invariably involves the use of threat, intimidation, and exploitation of authority or force with the aim of imposing one's sexual will on a nonconsenting person for personal gratification that may or may not be predominantly sexual in nature. There is a lack of sensitivity to the other, as self-proclaimed entitlement leads not only men but increasing numbers of women to sexually exploit others. The perpetrator's motives and sources of gratification are often an admixture of sexual, narcissistic, and aggressive aims to manipulate, dominate, and control.

This volume attempts to bring together the best current theoretical and clinical thinking on the subject of sexual aggression as it is currently being experienced in our culture. The chapters are divided into two sections.

Section I: Overview of Sexually Aggressive Behavior and Its Psychological Consequences

In Chapter 1, I present an overview of the problem of sexual aggression, focusing on the scope, definition, categories of victims, and dimensional nature of aggression and sexual aggression. I also discuss developmental, biological, ethological, behavioral, psychodynamic, and sociocultural influences. Emphasis is placed on the "cycle of violence": the role of childhood victimization and the history of sexual abuse in the lives of sexual offenders. Three explanatory points of view are discussed: a developmental behavioral model, a social-learning viewpoint, and a psychodynamic perspective. Illustrative clinical cases are presented.

In Chapter 2, Dr. Cavanagh Johnson provides an idiographic perspective on the child's emerging sexual knowledge and sexual behavior within the context of his or her maturational and developmental experiences. Children's sexualized behavior is conceptualized along a continuum from natural to very disturbed. She describes those nonnormative sexual behaviors that should alert the clinician to the need for further investigation.

In Chapter 3, Dr. Sholevar and Ms. Schwoeri examine the multiple forms of inappropriate sexual involvement and sexual aggression that may occur within the context of the family. The authors discuss the incidence and prevalence of incest, review incest from a historical perspective, and examine types of incest patterns, families at risk, family configurations, assessment techniques, and intervention strategies.

In Chapter 4, Dr. Schetky discusses the acute and enduring effects of child sexual abuse, with emphasis on the cognitive, psychobiological, and psychodynamic features associated with sexual victimization. The author presents several clinical vignettes depicting the derivative effects of sexual abuse, as the victims attempt to accommodate to the pattern of betrayal through denial, suppression, dissociation, and disturbances in the sense of self with subsequent changes in attitudes about self, others, and the world at large.

In Chapter 5, Dr. Lefley provides a comprehensive review of the transcultural dimensions of sexual victimization, paying special attention to "examining culturally relative versus universally absolute ideas about morality and appropriateness in gender and adult-child relationships." Ethnic and cultural dimensions affecting definition and interpretation of sexual abuse, disclosure, psychosocial sequelae, and victimization patterns are addressed, as are treatment implications.

Section II: Phenomenology and Assessment of Sexually Aggressive Behavior and Treatment Considerations

In Chapter 6, I describe the male adolescent sex offender, delineating the heterogeneity of sexual offenses, psychiatric comorbidity, character pathology, and the role of sexual victimization and psychosocial factors frequently found in the histories of adolescent sex offenders. Several clinical vignettes are presented along with a discussion of treatment considerations.

In Chapter 7, Dr. Green presents the emerging findings on females who commit sexual offenses against children. It is estimated that 14%–24% of boys and 6%–14% of girls are sexually abused by women and that about 20% of male adolescent sex offenders have been sexually abused by women. Demographic, psychiatric morbidity, and characterological and psychodynamic issues regarding female sex offenders are presented, as well as case illustrations, and treatment strategies are discussed.

In Chapter 8, Drs. Hunter and Becker examine the patterns and determinants of adolescent sexual offending behavior—specifically the role of child maltreatment and the role of exposure to pornography—with the authors particularly focusing on the cycle of violence, social learning, and modeling behavior. Family characteristics, clinical findings, and treatment approaches are discussed. The authors rightfully stress that there is a subset of sex offenders who are not amenable to treatment because of the high level of character pathology.

In Chapter 9, Dr. LeGum and coauthors comprehensively describe the multifaceted and complex process of assessing and evaluating the adolescent sex offender. Such assessment requires multiple informants, a sexual developmental history, and examination of patterns of child maltreatment, school adjustment, nonsexual delinquent behavior, and family and peer influences. The authors discuss recommended diagnostic and evaluative psychological measures as well as provide a general description of how to approach the adolescent sex offender.

In Chapter 10, Dr. Shaw and coauthors address the importance of multidisciplinary, multimodality, and multisystemic therapeutic approaches to the adolescent sex offender, with an emphasis on an integrated model for the treatment of the individual sexual offender that centers on cognitive-behavioral intervention strategies.

In Chapter 11, Dr. Katz notes the emerging importance of the use of psychopharmacological interventions with adolescent and adult sex offenders. Specific attention is given to the role of antiandrogen and hormonal medications and the increasing use of selective serotonin reuptake inhibitors in the management of intense and recurrent sexual preoccupations.

The above selected writings provide a comprehensive introduction to the complex issues associated with sexual aggression in our society. It is apparent that despite increased reports of sexual aggression throughout our society, and particularly among our youth, we are not helpless. We can marshal our understanding of the societal and cultural forces and of the family and individual developmental dimensions that contribute to this experience. There is an emerging scientific knowledge that increasingly will allow us to intervene more effectively not only with the victims of sexual aggression but also with the perpetrators of sexual violence.

Jon A. Shaw, M.D.

Acknowledgments

To my wife, Seana, for her continuing support, patience, and collegiality and her enduring capacity for good will; the faculty and staff of the Elaine Gordon Treatment Center, a residential treatment center for adolescent sex offenders, for their dedicated services and perseverance in the face of many difficult clinical situations; and the authors who contributed so much of their time, patience, and their own understanding of sexual aggression to this monograph. In editing the manuscripts I have been assisted by Marge Watt, who was an incisive critic. I would like to reserve special thanks for Mayra Santos-Tuch, of the University of Miami, for her editing and formatting of the manuscript of the monograph into its final form.

Section I

Overview of Sexually Aggressive Behavior and Its Psychological Consequences

1

Sexually Aggressive Behavior

Jon A. Shaw, M.D.

This overview of sexually aggressive behavior focuses on a number of issues central to an understanding of sexual aggression. The following themes are discussed: scope of sexual aggression; categories of victims; sexual aggression as a dimensional concept; sexual aggression and dating behavior; the nature of aggression, including biological, ethological, developmental, psychodynamic, familial, and sociocultural considerations; the relationship between sexual aggression and narcissism; and the role of sexual trauma in the etiology of sexually abusive behavior.

Sexually Abusive Behavior and Aggression

Terms such as *sexual aggression, sexual abuse, sexual assault*, and *rape* refer to sexual exploitation. To develop a more operational definition of sexual aggression, the National Task Force on Juvenile Sex Offending (1993, pp. 8, 9, 11), in the revised report on the National Adolescent Perpetrator Network, used the term "sexually abusive behavior." Sexually abusive behavior is defined as "any sexual behavior which occurs: 1) without consent, 2) without equality, or 3) as a result of coercion." In this context the following clarifications were offered: *Consent* is defined as implying agreement encompassing "1) an understanding of what is proposed, 2) knowledge of societal standards for what is being proposed, 3) awareness of potential consequences and alternatives, 4) assumption that agreement or disagreement will be respected equally, 5) voluntary decision, and 6) mental competence." *Equality* is when "two participants [are] operating with [the] same level of power in a relationship, neither being controlled or coerced by the other." Finally, *coercion* is defined as "exploitation of authority, use of bribes, threats of force, or intimidation to gain cooperation or compliance."

Any understanding of sexually abusive behavior requires that we understand the nature of aggression, which is the matrix within which the sexually abusive behaviors occur. Sexual offending behavior is frequently perpetrated by individuals with a history of aggressive and antisocial transgressions. Elliott (1994a) documented that rape is usually the final phase in a developmental pathway of unfolding violent and criminal behavior.

A number of observers have commented on the ubiquity of aggression in nature in general and in humans specifically (Freud 1930/1961; Hobbes 1651/1962; Wilson 1975). Much of the confusion in any discussion of aggression is the lack of an agreed-upon definition. Joseph (1973) observed that the term *aggression* is derived from the Latin *aggredi* (to attack, to go to) and *gradi* (to step) and has generally been ascribed the meaning to go forward with the intent of inflicting harm. Sociobiologist E. O. Wilson (1975) defined aggression as "the abridgement of the rights of others, forcing him to surrender something he owns or might otherwise have attained, either by a physical act or by the threat of action" (p. 242).

Sexual aggression invariably involves the use of threat, intimidation, exploitation of authority, or force with the aim of imposing one's sexual will on a nonconsenting person for the purpose of personal gratification that may or may not be predominantly sexual in nature. This gratification is often an admixture of satisfactions associated with sexual, narcissistic, and aggressive motivations.

Perspectives on sexually aggressive behavior necessarily focus on a complex array of biological, developmental, and psychosocial considerations.

Scope of Sexual Aggression

In recent years, our society has witnessed a sharp increase in violent, abusive, and sexually aggressive behavior. Richters (1993) suggested that the United States is the "most violent country in the industrialized world" (p. 3). Cicchetti and Lynch (1993) assert that violence has become the "defining characteristic of American Society" (p. 96). Acts of violence result in the deaths of more than 2,000 children and adolescents under 19 years of age each year (Cicchetti and Lynch 1993). Homicide is the second leading cause of death among those between 15 and 24 years of age and is the primary cause of death for Black males and females between ages 15 and 24 years (Bell and Jenkins 1993). Homicides committed by adolescents have reached the highest levels in history (Elliott 1994b). It has become evident that "sexual assault is one of the fastest growing violent crimes in the United States" (Hampton 1995), with the annual incidence of sexual assault now accounting for 7% of all violent crimes (Hampton 1995).

Paradoxically, there is evidence that the number of criminal acts, arrests, and sexually aggressive crimes by adults has actually decreased since the 1980s (Breiling 1994). This decrease in crime has been related to the "graying of America" and the increased incarceration of criminals. The percentage of total crimes committed by adolescents has decreased as the "baby boomers" have moved through the life cycle.

There is also evidence, however, of a dramatic increase in *violent* crimes committed by juveniles (Office of Juvenile Justice and Delinquency Prevention 1994b). Although adolescents (aged 15 to 18 years) make up only 6% of the population, they commit 25% of the "index crimes" (e.g., arson, homicide, manslaughter, robbery, aggravated assault, burglary, larceny, and forcible rape) (Siegel and Senna 1988). Krisberg (1992) observed that between 1984 and 1989 the juvenile arrest rates for crimes such as homicide, rape, robbery, aggravated assault, auto theft, burglary, theft, and arson increased by 18% and that the arrest rate for violent crimes rose 39%. Elliott (1994c) noted that the national self-report studies indicate that the highest risk for the initiation of serious violent behavior occurs between ages 15 and 16 years and that the risk of initiating violence after age 20 years is measurably lower. From 1983 to 1992 there was a reported 8% to 10% increase in the proportion of adolescents involved in some type of serious violent offenses (Elliott 1994a).

In addition to the increase in violent juvenile crimes, there has been a dramatic and comparable rise in sexually aggressive crimes perpetrated by adolescents. A virtual epidemic of child-on-child sexual victimization is taking place. Forcible rape arrests by juveniles increased 20% nationally between 1983 and 1992 (Office of Juvenile Justice and Delinquency Prevention 1994a). Representative of the increasing scope of sexually aggressive behavior perpetrated by juveniles are statistics from the state of Florida.

There is evidence of an increase in reporting of both sexual abuse and sexual harassment in the community (Charney and Russell 1994; Russell 1986; Wyatt 1985). Demause (1991) suggests four reasons why even these more recent statistics on sexual abuse are underestimates:

1. The reports did not include subjects with known high rates of being sexually abused, such as institutionalized criminals, juveniles in shelters, and individuals with psychoses.
2. The reports were predicated on conscious recall.
3. The subjects who refused to participate were the ones most likely to have a history of abuse.
4. It is likely that some subjects suppressed and therefore failed to report conscious memories of abuse.

Sexual harassment is defined as "attempts to extort sexual cooperation by means of subtle or explicit threats" and sex-related "verbal or physical conduct that is unwelcome or offensive" (Equal Employment Opportunity Commission 1980). It has been reported that approximately 50% of women experience sexual harassment during their working lives (Fitzgerald 1993). Charney and Russell

(1994) note that sexual harassment is widespread, affecting 42% of women and 15% of men in occupational settings. Even more evident is that sexual harassment among children and adolescents is increasing in frequency and severity.

Women as Victims

Sexually aggressive and violent acts against women are common (Biden 1993). It is generally estimated that 6% to 45% of women and 3% to 30% of men have been sexually abused. Two studies of women that used face-to-face interviews revealed that a large number of the women in the studies had a history of having been the victim of contact sexual abuse (Russell 1986; Wyatt 1985). Russell (1986) interviewed a community-based sample of 930 women aged 18 years and older and found that 38% had been subjected to some form of direct physical sexual abuse before 18 years of age. She noted that most of the perpetrators lived under the same roof and that 85% of the abusers were at least 5 years older than the victims. Uncles accounted for 25% and fathers for 15% of the perpetrators. In 80% of the cases, the perpetrator was a parent or guardian. Wyatt (1985) studied 248 women aged 18 to 36 years. In this study, sexual abuse was characterized as involving at least a "five year discrepancy in age, [and] the sexual experience was not wanted and involved some degree of coercion" (p. 511). She found that 45% of women in her sample had a history of "contact sexual abuse." Finkelhor and colleagues (1989) surveyed a representative sample of adult males and females and found that 27% of the women and 16% of the men had experienced childhood sexual abuse.

The increasing societal and scientific interest in sexual aggression developed out of the social revolution ushered in by the women's movement, which recognized and resonated with several major issues in modern American society: 1) the failure of society to protect women from sexual aggression, 2) demands for redefinition of gender roles and of the relationship between the sexes, and 3) increasing concerns with violent crimes and justice (Knopp 1994). The feminists focused our attention on sexual harassment, sexual aggression, and sexual assault. They spoke out against rape, established consciousness-raising groups, and pressed for wider recognition and more generic definitions of rape.

Historically, rape has been defined as the "illicit carnal knowledge of a woman, forcibly and against her will," with "knowledge" generally meaning vaginal penetration (McConaghy 1993, p. 269). In recent years, clinicians have broadened the concept of rape to encompass a more generic sexual assault against others. The National Task Force on Juvenile Sex Offending (1993), in their revised report on the National Adolescent Perpetrator Network, defined rape as an act "to seize or take by force for sexual gratification" (p. 11). In this context, rape may include any criminal sexual assault, heterosexual or homosexual, that involves the use of force. With this enlarged definition has come increasing recognition that sexual aggression is perpetrated not only against women and girls but also against men and boys. This expanded definition of rape has resulted in widening of our conceptual understanding of sexual aggression.

Koss and colleagues (1987), in a national survey of 18- to 24-year-old postadolescents, noted that 53.7% of the women reported some form of sexual victimization. More than 15% of the women reported having been raped, and 12.1% admitted to having been victims of attempted rape. Twenty-five percent of the men admitted to having perpetrated some form of sexual aggression. Approximately 3% admitted to a history of having attempted rape, and 4.4% admitted to having a history of rape. The National Victims Center and Crime Victims Research and Treatment Center (1992) reported that 12.9% of women (12 million) have been raped at least once during their lives. We know that many rapes go unreported.

Children as Victims

The history of society throughout the ages is replete with the multiplicity of ways in which children have been sexually traumatized (Demause 1991). Finkelhor (1991) commented on the "universality of sexual maltreatment of children." Sexual maltreatment of children generally takes three forms: 1) the sexual exploitation of children to gratify one's direct sexual needs, 2) the excessive erotization of children through inappropriate sexual stimulation, and 3) the mortification, vilification, and suppression of the child's emerging sexuality (Finkelhor 1991).

Christoffel (1990) suggested that each year 1.5 million children and adolescents are abused by their adult caretakers. The rise in the reporting of sexual abuse has outpaced the rate of reporting of other forms of child maltreatment. Since 1976, when an estimated 7,000 incidents of child sexual abuse occurred, there has been a dramatic increase in the reporting of sexual abuse of children. The National Committee to Prevent Child Abuse (1998) estimates that of the one million cases of confirmed child maltreatment documented in 1997, approximately 8% involved sexual victimization. Approximately half of female rape victims are under 18 years of age, and one out of six rape victims is a girl under 12 years of age (Office of Juvenile Justice and Delinquency Prevention 1994b).

Ageton (1983) studied a representative sample of adolescents ranging from 13 to 21 years of age from three consecutive birth cohorts. She estimated that each year in the United States 10% of adolescent female teenagers were sexually assaulted. Once a female adolescent had been sexually assaulted, the risk of that person being assaulted in the following year increased by three to four times over the annual probability figures for all female adolescents. One-third of those assaulted indicated that they had been sexually assaulted a second time in the 2-year period after the initial assault. Ageton defined sexual assault as involving the use of force, which ranged from verbal pressure to physical beatings. The offenders in this study were usually boyfriends or dates of comparable age. In only 8% to 17% of the cases was the perpetrator unknown to the victim. Although most of the pressure was verbal (55%–65%), Ageton noted that physical force occurred in 27%–40% of the incidents and usually involved "pushing, slapping and mild roughness." Interestingly, the victims were overrepresented by young women who associated with delinquent peers and received support from these friends for unconventional delinquent acts.

There is a paucity of data on sexual aggression against males. Finkelhor (1984) suggested that the prevalence of sexual abuse against boys under aged 13 years was 2.5% to 5%, and the rate against boys aged 13 to 18 years was 2.5% to 9%. Most reports suggest that the rate of sexual abuse of males is about one-third that of women. A survey of University of California students revealed that 30% of males had had experiences with "sexual deviates" (Landis 1956). Increasing attention is being given to the sexual abuse of boys by women. Among boys who have been sexually victimized, the proportion of cases in which the abuse was perpetrated by a female varied from 2% to 60%, depending on the report (Bolton et al. 1989). Some of the disparity among estimates has been explained by women disguising sexual exploitation as activities of child care (e.g., fondling, washing, exposure, caressing). Knopp and Lackey (1987), in a survey of female sex offenders, found that more than 50% of the victims were male. Fehrenbach (1988), in an early study of female sex offenders, found that 35.7% had abused male children. A more recent study (Matthews et al. 1997) found that juvenile female sex offenders were more likely to choose opposite-gender and younger children as victims. Seventy-five percent of the sample had abused boys, the great majority of whom were under 8 years of age. The abuse of males by females often occurs in the presence of another male. Finkelhor, after reviewing the 1984 American Humane Association data, suggested that only 14% of the sexually abused males had been abused by a lone female perpetrator.

Hunter (1991) studied males who had been sexually abused and found that in 87.5% of the incidents the perpetrator was male. A number of observations have been made about male victims of sexual aggression. Compared with female victims of abuse, males 1) are more reluctant to disclose sexual molestation, 2) are younger at the time of sexual abuse, 3) are more likely to experience sexual arousal, 4) are more likely to be abused by perpetrators outside of the family, 5) are frequently ashamed to confess to their damaged masculinity, and 6) demonstrate more heightened anxiety, worry, and rumination, with male victims focusing on identity issues and conflicts. Identity confusion was evidenced by a greater readiness to display opposite-sex trait identification than was found in the control group. Merry and Andrews (1994) reported on 95 sexually abused children aged 4 to 12 years and found that boys had a higher rate of psychiatric diagnoses than did girls 12 months after disclosure. Eighty-two percent of the boys warranted at least one psychiatric diagnosis, and 73% had two or more diagnoses. The two most common diagnoses found among boys were oppositional defiant disorder and attention-deficit/hyperactivity disorder. Black and De-Blassie (1993), in a review of men who had been sexually abused as children, found that they suffered from sexual preoccupation, gender identity and sexual orientation confusion, depression, substance abuse, difficulties with relationships, posttramatic stress disorder (PTSD), and disturbances in self-esteem and body image.

Sexual Aggression and Dating Behavior

One of the intriguing questions is, when does normal sexual activity become sexually aggressive behavior? Sexual aggression is a dimensional concept: the transgression of the threshold is defined somewhat arbitrarily by the participants and determined by the perceptions, values, mores, and standards of the legal and social community.

There is evidence that dating men and women frequently lose control of their sexual impulses and proceed sexually in spite of their partner's protestations. Muehlenhard and Cook (1988), in a study of psychology students, found that 63% of the males and 46% of the women had experienced unwanted sexual intercourse and that 93% of the women and 94% of the men had experienced unwanted sexual activities. McConaghy (1993) noted that 14% of female and 13% of male medical students in one sample reported sexual experiences in which their partners were so aroused that they could not stop them, even though they did not want sexual intercourse. Fourteen percent of the women and 20% of the men reported sexual experiences in which they made persistent and continuous efforts to have sexual activity with a member of the opposite sex in spite of protests. Koss and Oros (1982) found that in a sample of students at Kent State University, 32.8% of the female students and 23% of the male students reported having had sexual experiences because their partners were so sexually aroused that they felt it was useless to try to stop the sexual experience from occurring even though they did not want to have sex. Twenty-one percent of the female students and 15% of the male students reported having had sex when they did not want to consent because they felt pressured by continuous arguments.

Both men and women frequently feel coerced into sexual experiences against their wishes. Sexually aggressive behavior in dating situations is characterized by a continuum of coercive behaviors ranging from verbal persuasion, verbal arguments, and verbal threats to persistent advances, intimidation, physical threats, and the use of physical force.

Sexually coercive acts of women against men have been generally ignored because there is rarely the use of physical force. Sarrel and Masters (1982) reported on 19 men with sexual dysfunction related to forced sex perpetrated by a woman or a group of women and men. Nonforceful sexual coercion of men has received increasing attention. It is estimated that one-fourth to one-third of the victims of sexual harassment are men (McConaghy 1993). Struckman-Johnson (1988) reported that sexual victimization of men has been on the rise since the late 1970s. She surveyed students at the University of South Dakota and found that 16% of males and 22% of females reported at least one episode in which they were forced to engage in sexual intercourse on a date. Ten percent of the males and 2% of the females admitted to having forced sex on their date at least once in their lives. Most of the males were coerced by psychological pressure, and most of the females were coerced by force. Struckman-Johnson concluded that both men and women engage in a continuum of sexually exploitative behaviors ranging from verbal pressure to the use of physical force and restraint. When men engaged in unwanted sexual intercourse, it was generally because of peer pressure and concerns with sex role expectations and popularity.

Biological and Ethological Perspectives

Durant and Durant (1968), historians of philosophy, contend that the "laws of biology are the fundamental lessons of history" (p. 18). Konner (1993) notes that "every living creature exists in a natural state of conflict with every other creature in its environment" and that in every known human society "males exhibit more aggression than females" (p. 177). He observes that the tendency to do bodily harm to others is found to be greater in males than in females. It has also been noted that rough-and-tumble play, play fighting, threats of fights, serious fights with infliction of damage, and establishment of dominant hierarchies with stable social patterns of behavior are more common in male behavior (Zucker and Green 1993). The best predictor of aggressive behavior in human relationships is the XY chromosome dyad. It is not surprising, therefore, that sexually aggressive behaviors are more characteristically exhibited by males than by females.

Some feminist authors have suggested that man's hormonal biological heritage compels him to be sexually aggressive and exploitative of women. The evolutionary theory of rape assumes that genetic factors underlie male tendencies to rape and that the frequency of these genetic dispositions varies within a species (Ellis 1993). The view that male sexuality is inherently sadistic and exploitative has been seriously questioned by Person (1993), who suggests that more emphasis be placed on developmental determinants of sexually aggressive behavior. Humans are unique in their relative independence from their biological endowment. Although powerful sexual and aggressive drives may, at times, hold sway over judgment and cognitive capacities, it is well to remember that individuals come into the world as children who are absolutely helpless and require many years of nurturance, protection, and education. Dependence on learning and the social milieu for the elaboration of personality structure ensures that sexual and aggressive motivational structures will be profoundly influenced by developmental, family, and social determinants.

Developmental, Familial, and Social Influences

Ethology and evolution provide some understanding of the biological determinants of aggressive behavior, but they do not entirely explain sexually aggressive behavior in man. The lack of a set goal or aim toward which males' aggression is directed makes the concept of an aggressive instinct, with its implication of an organically driven impulse to attack, virtually meaningless (Shaw 1978; Shaw and Campo-

Bowen 1995). Although there are biological systems that, when activated, can result in aggressive and attacking behavior with sexual intent, the general impression is that sexual aggression in males is the result of developmental and social-learning experiences.

Parens (1993) observed that infants at about 6 months of age begin to exhibit directed anger and hostility. When the child is about age 18 months, one can begin to observe rage and hate. Parens suggests that the intensity, duration, and frequency of unpleasure experiences may lead to a "cumulative intrapsychic structuring" (p. 132) in which rage "becomes structured into a constant source of inner pressure to inflict pain and destroy the source of pain" (p. 134).

Aggressive acts associated with the intent to do harm or physical injury become evident only with the achievement of intentionality, around the second half of the first year of life (Landy and Peters 1992; Parens 1989). Individual differences in social behavior related to aggression are apparent before 2 years of age (Kagan et al. 1988). In this context aggressive behavior is frequently in the service of other needs such as seeking out or holding on to material possessions. Olweus (1979) observed that marked individual differences in habitual aggression levels become manifest during early childhood and are evident by 3 years of age. Manifest aggressive behavior accelerates in the second year of life, between the ages of 18 and 24 months, and seems to peak at about 30 to 36 months of age, with subsequent mitigation (Landy and Peters 1992). The child's capacity to regulate intense emotions and impulses is gradually enhanced by the modulating effects associated with the development of language, sublimation, and parental interventions. Aggressive behavior is a measurable behavior trait that stabilizes in the early preschool years and predicts aggressive and disruptive behaviors in adult life.

There is persuasive evidence that aggressive behaviors are transmitted from one generation to the next (Fry 1988; Hall and Cairns 1984; McCord 1988; West and Farrington 1977). Olweus (1980) found that three family variables were associated with childhood aggression: 1) mother's negativism, demonstrated as hostility, coldness, rejection, and indifference; 2) mother's permissiveness toward aggression; and 3) parental use of power-assertive discipline technique. Patterson and colleagues (1989) attributed childhood aggressive behavior in large part to inept parental management techniques in which parents ignore or permit aggressive behavior or, alternatively, respond inconsistently with either explosive-aggressive behavior or indifference. Elliott (1994c) suggested that violence is related to early childhood and family experiences in which there is weak family bonding, ineffective monitoring and supervision, exposure to violence, reinforcement of violent behavior, and acquisition of attitudes and beliefs that support or tolerate the use of violence.

Aggressive behaviors are learned from interaction and exposure to socializing influences in the home, with the peer group, and in school. We know that when the infant's early attachment and bonding to the caretaking object is insecure, avoidant, or disorganized, increased aggressive behaviors may result. Bandura (1973) observed that aggressive behavior is socially learned and maintained through contingencies of reward and punishment. Olweus (1979) reviewed 16 studies on the stability of aggressive reaction patterns in males from early childhood to early adulthood and concluded that the degree of stability of aggression is substantial and approaches that found for intelligence.

A number of longitudinal studies have investigated the relationship between early childhood aggression and subsequent aggressive, antisocial, and delinquent behavior (Campbell and Ewing 1990; Campbell et al. 1986; Cummings et al. 1989; Gersten et al. 1976; Havighurst et al. 1962; Richman et al. 1982). The evidence suggests that antisocial behavior in childhood, particularly when some estimates of frequency, diversity, and age at onset are taken into account, is the single most powerful predictor of later adjustment problems (Kohlberg et al. 1984; Loeber 1982; Robbins 1979). For example, it is known that peer-rated aggression at age 8 years predicts spouse abuse among males at 30 years of age (Eron and Huesmann 1990).

Cultural Influences on Gender and Sexuality

Traditionally, our culture has placed restraining influences on childhood sexuality. There has been a tendency to avoid sexual stimulation, to inhibit sexual impulses, to prohibit erotic play, and to reduce or forbid sexual self-stimulation (Rosenfeld and Wasserman 1993). With the advent of television and videos, current popular culture has assumed an increasing role in the socialization and enculturation of sexual behaviors, with a dramatic shift in the transmission of what is permissible sexually in our culture.

The child learns the rules of behavior in different social contexts. He or she learns what is permissible and allowable and with whom. Sexuality, as well as aggressive behavior, is defined by the cultural, moral, and value systems vis-à-vis the processes of socialization and enculturation governing the delineation of gender roles and the defining attributes of gender identity.

Although we prefer to think that early development is the crucible for the development of morality, it is apparent that moral sexual development is greatly contingent on the middle school years, when the child internalizes the instrumentalities of our culture. It is then that he or she is the most vulnerable to the permeation of popular culture. Postman (1994) states that "it is with television that we can see most clearly how and why the historic basis for a dividing line between childhood and adulthood is being unmistakably eroded" (p. 75). In present society the child and the adult have universal accessibility to the same information. The age of "electronic information" has, in many instances, resulted in popular culture superseding the family as the source of information about what is acceptable sexual behavior. Emde (1993) expressed his concerns about the interrelationship between culture and development. What effect does a culture of violence and sexual aggression have on the internalization of social rules for children?

The development of aggressive behaviors has more recently been conceptualized as evolving subsequent to information processing in which various "scripts," or programmatic repertories, are derived from experience with others and internalized. Huesmann and Eron (1984) suggested that aggressive behaviors as social strategies evolve and are learned through observations, social reinforcement, and modeling. These aggressive "scripts" become "encoded, rehearsed, stored, and retrieved in much the same way as other strategies for intellectual development" (p. 244).

The difference between adult and children's sexuality is disappearing. In commercials we are asked to guess which is the mother and which is the daughter as they apply their skin lotion. Sexual stereotypes of femininity have become more childlike. For example, one clothing manufacturer has run a series of advertisements with adult models depicting what appear to be young adolescent girls and boys scantily clad in jeans in varying sexually suggestive poses.

Television promotes access to all adult sexual secrets, undermines family sources of authority, and promotes other sources of authority (Postman 1994). Television, as a present-centered medium, diminishes the importance of the past and the future. Everything is happening right now. The importance of delayed gratification is denied.

Currently, society, with its diverse cultures, is struggling to define what sexual mores and sexual behaviors are permissible not only for adults but also for children. How do we titrate sexual information to children in such a way that it can be assimilated and mastered consonant with developmental processes so that the traumatic effects of early exposure to violent sexual schemas can be avoided?

Psychodynamic Perspectives

Psychoanalysts are well aware of the problem of aggression as it is manifested in all its variable complexity in the analytic situation and in the observable world. Sigmund Freud developed three distinct aggressive drive theories. In his first two theories there was recognition that aggression may be associated with sexual frustration. In the first drive theory, aggressive impulses were postulated to represent the component of the sexual forces necessary to overcome the resistance of the sexual object. Freud continued to adhere to this conceptualization of aggressive drives as an admixture of aggression and sexual drives until the publication of "Instincts and Their Vicissitudes" (Freud 1915/1957), in which he outlined his second drive theory. In this theory, Freud established a dualistic model in which sexual instincts were separated from self-preservative instincts. The aggressive trends were seen as one of the components of the self-preservative instincts and therefore were given a status independent of the sexual instincts. Loving was related to the sexual drives, and hating was related to the ego drives. Freud wrote, "[T]he ego hates, abhors and pursues with intent to destroy all objects which are a source of unpleasurable feeling for it. . . . whether they mean a frustration of sexual satisfaction or of the satisfaction of self-preservative needs" (Freud 1915/1957, p. 138). In this context, aggression is considered secondary to the frustration associated with failure to get one's needs satisfied.

The increasing importance given to development in psychoanalytic psychology has resulted in a gradual but progressive modification in Freud's theory of aggression. A developmental perspective emerges in which psychological structure and function are viewed as the product of interactions among the biological substrate, maturational processes, and the psychosocial environment.

In the theory of aggression that has been slowly elaborated with the advent of psychoanalytic developmental psychology, it has been increasingly recognized that although instinctive components have a biological basis, their particular expression is modulated by early relationships with primary caretakers and the affective experience of that relationship along the continuum of pleasure and unpleasure. Thus, the quantitative view of the instincts has slowly given way to a qualitative one. The psychoanalytic theory of aggression has moved from a concern with instinct and drives to an interest in the development of emotions, cognitions, and instrumental behaviors and the elaboration of the spectrum of affects such as irritability, anger, hostility, rage, and hate, which may or may not be associated with aggressive behavior.

Marcovitz (1982) notes that there are four types of behaviors that have to be explained in a theory of aggression: 1) activities toward an object, such as assertiveness, exploration, and dominance; 2) instrumental aggression to accomplish a goal or aggressive behavior that occurs as a reaction to frustration or in response to an attack; 3) hatred, in which the aim is the destruction or humiliation of the object; and 4) sadism, the infliction of pain or humiliation on an object for the purpose of sexual excitement and gratification.

As the theory of aggression has progressed from an instinct-based model to an adaptational/developmental perspective, the affects have been given an increasingly central role in our understanding of aggressive behavior (Person 1993). An *affect*, as defined by Kernberg (1992), comprises a number of factors, including an emotional experience along a continuum of pleasure and unpleasure, a specific cognitive component, and a specific expressive facial pattern with both muscular and neurovegetative discharge patterns.

Affects emerge out of developmental experiences. Parens (1993) speculates that there is a spectrum of hostile destructive affects and that the degree of unpleasure determines the range and quality of affect experienced and the adaptive behavior instigated. He postulates that the experience of mild unpleasure stimulates assertive or withdrawn behavior. With increasing intensity of unpleasure, affects of irritability, anger, hostility, rage, and hate will be seen. Parens describes several characteristics of rage:

1. Rage is a complex affect occurring secondarily to intense unpleasure.
2. Rage as a psychic structure has its own configuration and temporal sequence.
3. The rage reaction, depending on its intensity, may involve psychological disorganization, altered states of consciousness, impaired reality testing, regression in ego functions, loss of boundaries between self and object, and perceived helplessness.
4. The intensity, duration, and frequency of unpleasure experiences may lead to a "cumulative intrapsychic structuring" (p. 132)—for example, the rage "becomes structured into a constant source of inner pressure to inflict pain and destroy the source of pain" (p. 134).
5. Rage may become a powerful motivator of behavior.

The central question confronting those interested in the problem of aggression is how the affects associated with aggression become transduced into an enduring pattern of aggressive behavior woven into the tapestry of character structure, or, more important for our consideration, how they become woven into the pattern of sexual-aggressive behavior characteristic of sex offenders.

Narcissism and Aggression

A number of authors have explored the concept of aggression as it relates more specifically to the self and the vicissitudes of narcissism. *Narcissism* is defined as the concentration of psychological interest on the self.

The attempt to understand aggression vis-à-vis a theory of narcissism by necessity places greater emphasis on the psychological and developmental determinants influencing aggressive behavior. Rochlin (1973, 1982) suggests that human aggression is different from animal aggression in that it cannot be explained by ethological considerations, the classical theory of instincts, and that it is peculiarly related to narcissism. Rochlin (1973) notes that "[t]he conventional notion of a human 'appetite' for aggression has obscured the fact that it is narcissism which is insatiable. To satisfy its needs, aggression is commissioned. It is in the service of the self that aggression has its natural task" (p. 257). He believes that narcissism is the "great menace" and that it is only the lifelong dynamic presence of narcissism, and the corresponding difficulty in giving up egocentric aims, that can account for the anatomy of aggression in humans. According to Rochlin, it is when narcissism is damaged and self-esteem is compromised that aggression arises to redress the balance.

Eissler (1971) also observes that humankind's problem is not the aggressive drive as such, but that the aggression is steered by narcissism and ambivalence rather than self-preservation. E. Becker (1975) believes that aggression in humans is related to their efforts to deny their mortality and to secure victory over their limitations. Man yearns for a fate beyond that of an animal, and in his striving to be unique, especially deserving, and above other men, he makes the earth more of a graveyard. The narcissistic aims are associated with the search for perfectibility, omnipotent control, and a sense of specialness that one is entitled to have whatever one wants. Narcissistic rage becomes mobilized when others attempt to thwart the narcissistic aim. It is apparent that aggressive discharge is associated with enhancement of narcissistic gratification and that narcissism in humans frequently leads to aggression.

Kohut (1972) likewise noted the relationship between aggression and narcissism, observing that aggression arises when the self or object fails to live up to the absolutarian expectations expected of them. Noting that "[d]estructive rage is always motivated by an injury to the self," Kohut proposes a two-factor theory of aggression (Kohut 1977, pp. 120–121). Primary aggression is present at birth as a natural endowment and refers to assertive behavior that becomes mobilized whenever frustration is experienced. Secondary aggression, including destructiveness and rage, Kohut (1977) suggests, emanates from failures in early relationships with significant others. He contends that a propensity toward rage and destructive aggression can arise only when the self has been seriously damaged from prolonged failures in the self-object environment.

Fonagy and colleagues (1993) suggest that a child's exposure to aggressive, abusive, and unpredictable parental figures results in a failure of self in which there is a fusion of self-expression with aggression.

Developmental and Traumatic Influences on Sexual Behaviors

Children, from the very beginning of life, are sexual doers, thinkers, and explorers. Before 2 years of age, both girls and boys engage in focused genital exploratory behavior with the apparent purpose of experiencing sexual pleasure (Galenson 1993). It is estimated that approximately 30% of 2- to 7-year-old children systematically masturbate (Langfeldt 1981). By age 3–4 years, children engage in flirtatious sexual play (Araji 1997). The child is constantly experimenting through sexual information-processing behaviors to define the self, gender identity, gender role, and sexual orientation. The child slowly begins to elaborate an evolving definition of a sexual self and a sexual life through a repertoire of behaviors that includes touching the sexual parts of self and others, exhibiting sexual parts and sexual viewing of others, observing what goes on between males and females, and having erotized interactions with others. It is estimated that 30% to 60% of preadolescent children have engaged in exhibiting genitalia or mutual genital play with nonsiblings (Rosenfeld and Wasserman 1993).

In current society, acts of sexually abusive behavior are no longer restricted predominantly to adolescent and adult populations. We now see acts of sexual victimization committed by children. Young children who commit sexual offenses are often referred to as "sexually abusive reactive," because their sexual offenses are thought to be reactive to their own history of sexual victimization or exposure to coercive sexuality.

Sexual aggression is not a rare happening among the adolescent population. Studies of adult sex offenders have consistently demonstrated that the majority begin their sexual offending behavior before 18 years of age (Abel et al. 1985; Longo and Groth 1983). It is estimated that 20% of all rapes and 30% to 50% of all child molestations are committed by juveniles under 18 years of age (Fehrenbach et al. 1986; National Task Force on Juvenile Sexual Offending 1993).

Ageton (1983), in her study of a probability sample of 863 male adolescents aged 13 to 19 years, concluded that the rate of sexual assault per 100,000 adolescent males ranged from 5,000 to 16,000. She also found that the sexual assault was most often a "date rape" in which excessive utilization of alcohol or drugs was associated with verbal pressure and manipulation rather than the use of serious physical violence. More than 70% of the sexual assaults were spontaneous and opportunistic. The offenders, compared with the control subjects, were more likely to be involved in a peer group that endorsed delinquent behavior and was less disapproving of forced sex.

The evidence of psychosocial adversity in the lives of adolescent sex offenders has been well documented. Family violence, physical abuse, and sexual abuse are thought to contribute to the development of aggressive behavior. It is known that in one sample 69% of the youths who had been maltreated as children, compared with 56% of those who had not been maltreated, reported committing acts of violence (Office of Juvenile Justice and Delinquency Prevention 1994a). Although exposure to physical violence and abuse is high among juvenile sex offenders, it is comparable to that generally found among juveniles who exhibit other, nonsexual delinquent behavior (Lewis et al. 1979). Greater emphasis has been placed on the role of sexual victimization in the history of sex offenders.

A cycle of violence and sexual aggression is perpetuated from one generation to the next. Groth (1979), in an early study, found that 31% of 106 rapists had a history of sexual victimization and that their sexual assaults replicated their own victimization. The proportion of adolescent sex offenders with a history of sexual victimization varies from 19% to 82%, depending on the report (J. V. Becker et al. 1986; Knight and Prentky 1993; Longo 1982; Ryan et al. 1996; Shaw et al. 1993). Ryan and colleagues (1996) found that 22% of sexually abusive youths who had been victims of sexual abuse reported that the perpetrator of their own sexual abuse was a female. There is evidence that the earlier the onset of sexual offending behavior, the more likely it is that the child has been sexually victimized (Cavanagh Johnson 1988). Cavanagh Johnson (1988) found that, on average, 72% of child sex offenders aged 6 years and younger, 42% of those aged 7 to 10 years, and 35% of those aged 11 to 12 years had been sexually victimized.

Shaw and colleagues (1994) demonstrated the important role of sexual victimization in the history of adolescent sex offenders committed to a residential center. Of those offenders, 67.3% (37) had a history of being sexually abused; 27.0% (10) of these individuals had a history of being sexually abused by women, and only 10.8% (4) had been victimized by a lone female perpetrator. Although the remaining adolescents had not been directly sexually abused, they invariably came from homes in which they were prematurely exposed to sexual violence, promiscuity, and pornography. Of the adolescent offenders who had been sexually victimized, 52% had been abused by family members. The mean age at sexual victimization was 6 years, with 35% of this group having been sexually abused before age 5 years. There was no statistical relationship between the age at sexual victimization and the onset of sexual offending behavior. There was a substantial trend indicating that those sex offenders who had been abused by women had more psychiatric diagnoses.

Longo (1982) found in his sample of adolescent sex offenders a higher-than-expected number of individuals with a history of direct consenting sexual contact with older males and females. These adolescents reported feeling uncomfortable, insecure, unexperienced, inferior, and unable to satisfy their older sex partners. The author rightfully notes that these sexual experiences were, in and of themselves, traumatic. J. V. Becker and colleagues (1989) found that adolescents who had been sexually victimized manifested more deviant erectile responses than adolescents who had not been sexually abused. The authors raised the possibility that adolescent sex offenders were modeling their own sexual victimization.

Person (1993) observed that the prevailing belief that "male sexuality is innately aggressive and sadistic has persisted with minimal questioning" (p. 29). The view that male sexuality is innately aggressive and sadistic is surprisingly prevalent. For example, a group of female mental health workers at a seminar on sexual abuse unanimously agreed that the "penis is a weapon." Person rightfully asks, "Is the domination and sadistic fantasies in male sexuality primary? Is male sexuality inherently aggressive, or are the aggressive feelings a reaction to life experiences?" (p. 31).

The intertwining of narcissism and aggression is particularly apparent in those sex offenders who were sexually traumatized in childhood. They have transformed the childhood trauma—the helplessness, terror, and frequent sexual arousal—into an identification with the perpetrator. The sexual offense represents a means of turning a childhood trauma into an triumph. It is the means by which the victim symbolically achieves mastery over his or her own sexual abuse and gains revenge. The unconscious wish is to demean and to degrade through the exercise of power and control. As one victim–perpetrator noted, "I am the one who overpowers, rapes and hurts."

Clinical Vignettes

The following clinical vignettes graphically portray the relationship between a history of sexual victimization and subsequent fantasies of sexual aggression.

A., a 13-year-old boy, described his masturbatory fantasy: "I walk into a small room, where there is a girl, 10 or 11 years of age. She is sitting and writing at a desk. I look around to see if there is anybody around. I look twice. I scream at her to stand up. She looks scared and helpless. She is terrified. I tear off her dress. I begin to fondle her. She fights back. I overpower her. I feel strong. I force her to suck my penis. I stick my penis in her vagina. I interrupt the fantasy. I try to [intervene]. Suddenly the image turns into my father. I remember my father coming into my room. It is a small room. He begins to fondle me, touching my penis. I remember he tore off my clothes and made me suck his penis and he stuck his penis into my [anus]. I felt powerless and afraid. I don't like to feel powerless. It's when I feel powerless that I begin to imagine raping a girl. When I tear off her dress, I feel in control." He defines being powerless as meaning, "I can't control other people." Further discussion led to his remembering the sexual excitation, the erection he felt when his father abused him. He had two feelings. He felt scared, helpless, and terrified, but he also had the feeling of sexual excitement. He doesn't understand why he was sexually aroused. He feels guilty about the sexual excitement.

B., a 13-year-old boy, had been sexually abused by his father "so many times I can't remember," starting at 4 years of age. He recounted, in treatment, a recent experience. He had been told to take a "sit out" after he "went off" after a larger boy who had called him a "girl." He described feeling victimized. He experienced a powerful wish to touch the other boy's "ass." He explained that when he gets angry "I want to touch." When asked to elaborate, he noted that "I want him to feel confused and scared." When the therapist wondered if that is what he had experienced with his father, he mumbled a quiet yes. Elaborating further on his fantasy, he noted that he wanted to make the other boy "suck my penis" and to stick "my penis in his [anus]." When the therapist wondered what that would be like for him, he described "feeling powerful." He noted that the best feeling he had ever had was the feeling of power in "overruling" somebody and being sexually in control. It is evident that the aggressive revenge fantasy mobilized by his victimization incorporates not only aggression but sexual domination as well as a powerful sense of narcissistic triumph compensating for his sense of helplessness and powerlessness.

C., a 14-year-old boy, was brought in for treatment after anally sodomizing two younger boys and tying one up with ropes and holding a knife to his throat. He showed little remorse, regret, or victim empathy. He had a history of sexually victimizing other boys. In his therapy he would reveal and openly acknowledge "violent sexual fantasies." He described how he "seeks out" little boys, wishes to "trap them," and wants "to have control over them." He spoke of the pleasure "in having the power to make anybody I want to do anything I want." He enjoys his victims being "scared, shaking and cooperative." He coerced them by threatening to cut off their penises or to shoot them in the head.

He recalled how when he was a young boy, from 3 to 7 years of age, his mother would come home drunk and make him sleep with her, forcing him down on her, coercing him to have oral sex with her, or laying on top of him, trying to get him to stick his penis into her. He described these experiences without affect, minimizing their importance. He spoke of "enjoying the scary moment." It is only with continuing therapy that he began to talk about feeling trapped, his repugnance for her drunken breath, her threats to not feed him, her slapping him, and her vague threats of castration.

D., a 14-year-old boy with a history of abusing little boys and girls, described a repetitive rape fantasy focusing on a mental health worker who is tall and blond and has large, prominent breasts. He tangentially referred to a pinup in his room, describing the model as a beautiful, tall blond with large breasts and comparing her to the mental health worker. He subsequently recounted his own history of victimization by a 13-year-old female baby-sitter. She undressed him and made him lie on top of her. He was scared. He had never seen a girl naked before and was surprised and horrified by the pubic hair. He was surprised that she didn't have a penis. He had only a vague memory of what happened. He only remembered feeling helpless as she tried to put his penis into her. The baby-sitter was described as a large blond woman with big breasts. We can see how the gradual elaboration of D.'s sexual life emanated from his sexual victimization and how that experience became woven into a sexual-aggressive rape fantasy in which he imagined dominating a powerful blond woman, a reenactment, in a reversal of his own sexual victimization.

These vignettes illustrate the intertwining of the experience of sexual victimization; the peculiar encoding of the affective experience of helplessness, terror, shame, and sexual excitement; and its transduction into a pattern of sexual aggression infused with narcissism.

Sexual Victim to Perpetrator

What is the process by which children who have been sexually victimized become adolescent sex offenders? Essentially, the explanatory models that have been proposed are based on one of three perspectives: developmental behavioral, social-learning, and psychoanalytic. These perspectives, as we will see, are synergistic rather than mutually exclusive.

Developmental Behavioral Perspective

The developmental behavioral model suggests that early sexual sensitizing experiences determine deviant patterns of erotization. Money (1986) introduced the concept of the "lovemap" as a way of conceptualizing this process. He postulates that falling in love is the projection of an idealized and unique love imago onto another. He suggests that each one of us creates an internalized image of the idealized love object and the pattern of sexual behaviors that would be associated with the highest intensification of the sense of loving and being loved out of our early developmental experiences. The lovemap is conceptualized as a developmental representation in the mind. It is a schema depicting the idealized lover and the idealized pattern of sexual-erotic behavior one would like to experience with the lover (Money 1986). It is this wish, intrinsic to the fantasy, that becomes the driving force in sexual-erotic life. Thus, developmental experiences with significant others are crucial to the elaboration of a sexual life.

We know that the sexual life of children begins to configure shortly after birth and becomes patterned on the bases of early sensitizing experiences. In the first year of life, children discover the pleasure of genital sensations, which may become associated with "other" experiences. Money (1986) suggested that a relatively stable configuration of one's pathways for sexual gratification and imagery of erotic attraction can occur by 8 years of age. It is clear that children may be exposed to animate or inanimate non–sexually arousing stimuli that, through their pairing with sexually arousing stimuli, may acquire a conditioned sexually evocative status.

For example, in our culture silk and lace have acquired a sexually evocative and arousing capacity through their pairing with images of scantily clad voluptuous women. When silk and lace become paired with animate sexual releasers, they take on sexual releasing properties. We know that some boys and men have been sensitized to silk and lace as sexually arousing stimuli—a phenomenon that has been successfully exploited by lingerie companies.

Early aberrant sexual experiences can result in deviant imagery of sexual-erotic gratification. Sexual arousal may occur in association with aggressive sexuality, enemas, corporal punishment, abusive discipline, or other arbitrary and sometimes terrifying experiences. We know that boys who have been sexually victimized may experience their first sexual arousal associated with an erection during the victimization, an experience that is often confusing and terrifying because the child feels betrayed by his own body. These early experiences of sexual arousal and sexual excitement may become consolidated in the central masturbatory fantasy.

Social-Learning Perspective

The social-learning perspective is predicated on a model associated with a pattern of maladaptive learning. Exposure to coercive sexuality, pornography, imitation, modeling, and identification with sexually aggressive significant others may socially legitimize a spectrum of sexually aggressive behaviors.

Psychoanalytic Perspective

The psychoanalytic perspective is predicated on the assumption that the sexual victimization is experienced as a narcissistic wound exposing the limitations and powerlessness of the self. From a developmental point of view, the narcissistic defenses have been defined as those processes whereby the idealized aspects of the self are preserved and the limitations of the self and others are denied. Narcissistic defenses ensure that the individual keeps imminent knowledge of his or her own limitations out of conscious awareness. The child elaborates an illusion of safety and a sense of certainty that he or she will prevail, denying his or her sense of helplessness before the laws of biology. The cloak of narcissistic perfectibility is often extended to parents, to whom one attributes powerful and loving protection.

A number of developmental theorists have described the process by which this sense of narcissism becomes elaborated and then slowly titrated away by painful reality. Winnicott (1953) speaks of the illusion–disillusion process in early development. In the early practicing subphase of Mahler's separation-individuation phase (Mahler et al. 1975), the young toddler is reportedly oblivious to danger or real threats of bodily injury. The emerging child has no awareness of the limitations of the self and/or the object. It is only with further psychological development that the sense of infantile omnipotence, with its protective shell of narcissistic invulnerability, slowly becomes eroded by doses of painful reality. If the child is fortunate, the dawning awareness of reality will be imposed on him or her in small quantities so that he or she can assimilate such awareness piecemeal with an increasing sense of mastery, autonomy, and self-direction. Thus, the child's illusion of safety is gradually modified through the developmental experience by an increasing appreciation of reality (Shaw 1989).

The sudden and unexpected experience of sexual victimization prematurely shatters the narcissistic defenses, and this exposes the child to the horrific experience of terror, helplessness, and profound betrayal. The sense of helplessness may lead to a powerful narcissistic wish to restore the sense of limitless power and invulnerability to injury through the mobilization of sexual aggression as a way to triumph over the images of the self that are helpless and damaged.

The psychoanalytic explanation of how the experience of sexual victimization may lead to sexual offending behavior rests on two basic conceptualizations. One way to conceptualize this pathway is that the central matrix of the sexual victimization, with its array of affects, possibly sexual excitement, arousal, and sadomasochistic features, may become organized and consolidated into the central masturbatory fantasy and result in a preferred pattern of sexual arousal and gratification. The affective experience of sexual victimization becomes integrated into the libidinal drive structure. Kernberg (1992) states that the affects are the primary psychobiological building blocks of drives. The sexual and aggressive drive structures are products of development that are elaborated out of the centrality of affective relationships with significant others. These affects are invariably woven into a motivational structure intertwined with other elements to include a cognitive appraisal, a wish, and self and object representations bridged by a particular pattern of relatedness as well as an action tendency. It is in this context that we can begin to understand how the intense affective memory of sexual victimization may become ingrained into a pattern of sexual aggression. The affective experiences of sexual excitement, sexual aggression, pleasure and unpleasure, domination and helplessness, rage, sadism-masochism, and perpetrator-victim are assimilated and integrated into the libidinal drive structure and crystallize as the pathway for sexual gratification. Analogous to Freud's (1905/1953) metaphor of the "stream bed," once sexuality has found a channel of expression, there is a tendency for it to remain in that channel and thus for the sexual behavior to be repeated.

The second way to conceptualize this pathway within a psychoanalytic framework rests on the observation that sexually aggressive behavior may come to serve narcissistic aims in which the wish is to master a traumatic experience, seek reparation and restoration of an omnipotent self, and split off self representations of a damaged and emasculated self. This perspective defines the sexual offending behavior as a behavioral reenactment in which the compelling motivation is to achieve mastery over a traumatic experience. The compelling need to repeat and to reenact the past—to turn passive into active and to actualize the unsatisfied wish intrinsic to fantasy—is invariably intertwined with memory. As Schur (1966) observed, the wish is always associated with a memory of a past gratification and the perceptual experience of that gratification. In "Beyond the Pleasure Principle," Sigmund Freud (1920/1955) suggested that behavior not only is determined by the motivation to gratify instinctual wishes but also may be determined by the wish to achieve mastery over a traumatic experience by repeating the experience. Through such repetition the individual hopes to achieve the mastery that was denied him or her on first exposure. Intrinsic to the psychodynamics of sexually aggressive offenders whose behavior is a reaction to their own victimization may be the wish to obliterate the memory of helplessness by turning the experience into a sexually aggressive narcissistic triumph in which the perpetrator achieves mastery over the memory of his or her helplessness.

Ferenczi (1932/1980) described the psychological effects of sexual attacks. He explained the child's sense of "physical and moral helplessness" when confronted with the "overpowering force and the authority" of the perpetrator (p. 228). He described the child's loss of executive capacities, his being "paralyzed by enormous anxiety," and his being compelled "to subordinate the self like an automaton to the will of the aggressor, to divine each one of his desires and to gratify them" (p. 228). Ferenczi noted that "the most important change, produced in the mind" is the "anxiety-fear ridden identification" with the perpetrator. The child feels "enormously confused, in fact, split, innocent and culpable, and his confidence in the testimony of his own senses is broken" (p. 228). The child identifies with the self-object experience and its emotional bridge of sexual excitement, aggression, intimacy, blurring of boundaries, and sadomasochistic relatedness.

One is repeatedly impressed with the profound narcissistic investment in the perpetrator's need to control, dominate, and subject the victim completely to his or her will. Sexual aggression becomes reparative, a split-off defensive structure to counteract the unbearable and unacceptable affective states of helplessness, betrayal, and powerlessness. Thus, a reversal of the victimization occurs. The representation of the aggressive object is destroyed, the self-image of helplessness and inadequacy is obliterated, and the victim recaptures the sexually aggressive excitement now within the context of a powerful, omnipotent, dominant self in which one is invulnerable and triumphant. In the internalization of the affective relationship of the victim–perpetrator dyad, there is an identification with "suffering self and sadistic object" (Kernberg 1993). The subject is swallowed up by the all-encompassing aggression in the victimization experience. Fonagy and colleagues (1993) suggest that a child's exposure to aggressive, abusive, and unpredictable parental figures results in a failure of self in which there is a fusion of self-expression with aggression. Goldberg (1995) believes that the sexual behavior intrinsic to the perversions serves the purpose of warding off self-fragmentation and is a result of a developmental failure.

Sensitized to sexual excitement and sexual arousal as passive victims, the boys described in the clinical vignettes in this chapter internalized the erotized, aggressivized experience in a distorted internalized representation. This representation then became incorporated into a wish that involves a compulsion to repeat the experience in the service of mastery.

Stoller (1991) has suggested that "[p]erversion is the erotic form of hatred" (p. 37). The perverse act is a reenactment in which the perpetrator seeks to convert a childhood tragedy into an adult triumph. Such an act is motivated by a revengeful wish to humiliate as one was once humiliated. Stoller (1991) suggests that it is the dynamics of humiliation that are the basis of perversions. The sexually traumatized child anesthetizes the humiliation and transforms it into a narcissistic victory. The spectrum of intense affects—such as sexual excitement and sexual arousal, helplessness and rage, sadism and masochism, love and betrayal, and pleasure and unpleasure—may be woven into one's central masturbatory fantasy and become a motivational structure. It is evident that sexually aggressive behavior serves not only a sexual aim but also the narcissistic aim to split off the damaged and emasculated self and to restore an earlier narcissistic state of limitless power and control. The childhood tragedy is thereby turned into a triumph, but at great psychic cost. Bach (1994) notes that the narcissistic transformation results in an impaired capacity for love and in human relationships in which others are treated as things rather than human beings.

Conclusion

Sexually aggressive behavior is understood as a multidetermined and complex array of phenomenon. It is apparent that aggression is intrinsic to its manifestation and, along with narcissistic entitlement and sexual urges, provides the impetus for sexually abusive behavior. Sexually aggressive behavior can be conceptualized as a dimensional construct representing various degrees of coercion and aggression, different patterns of expression, and a range of victim profiles. It is the product of development and arises from learned social experiences with family, significant others, and the larger culture. The increasing exposure of youth to violence and violent sexual behavior, whether through coercive family experiences, sexual victimization, media portrayal of explicit sexual aggression, or the increased cultural tolerance of sexually aggressive behavior, has resulted in children who are at increased risk of becoming sexually aggressive.

References

Abel GG, Mittelman M, Becker JV: Sex offenders: results of assessment and recommendations for treatment, in Clinical Criminology: The Assessment and Treatment of Criminal Behavior. Edited by Ben-Aron M, Hucker SJ, Webster CD. Toronto, M & M Graphics, 1985, pp 191–205

Ageton SS: Sexual Assault Among Adolescents. Lexington, MA, Lexington Books/DC Heath, 1983

Araji SK: Sexually Aggressive Children. Thousand Oaks, CA, Sage Publications, 1997

Bach S: The Language of Perversion and the Language of Love. Northvale, NJ, Jason Aronson, 1994

Bandura A: Aggression: A Social Learning Analysis. Englewood Cliffs, NJ, Prentice-Hall, 1973

Becker E: Escape From Evil. New York, Free Press, 1975

Becker JV, Cunningham-Rathner J, Kaplan MG: Adolescent sex offenders. Journal of Interpersonal Violence 1:431–445, 1986

Becker JV, Hunter JA, Stein RM, et al: Factors associated with erection in adolescent sex offenders. Journal of Psychopathology and Behavioral Assessment 11 (suppl 4):353–362, 1989

Bell CC, Jenkins EJ: Community violence and children on Chicago's South Side, in Children and Violence. Edited by Reiss D, Richters JE, Radke-Yarrow M, et al. New York, Guilford, 1993, pp 46–54

Biden JC: Violence against women. Am Psychol 48:1059–1061, 1993

Black CA, DeBlassie RR: Sexual abuse in male children and adolescents: indicators, effects and treatments. Adolescence 28:123–133, 1993

Bolton FG, Morris LA, MacEachron AE: Males at Risk. Newbury Park, CA, Sage Publications, 1989

Breiling J: A model for preventing sexual offenses. Paper presented at the annual meeting of the American Association for the Treatment of Sexual Abusers, San Francisco, CA, November 1994

Campbell SB, Ewing LJ: Follow-up of hard to manage preschooler: adjustment at age 9 and predictors of continuing symptoms. J Child Psychol Psychiatry 31:871–889, 1990

Campbell SB, Ewing LJ, Breaux AM, et al: Parent-referred problem three-year-olds: follow-up at school entry. J Child Psychol Psychiatry 27:473–488, 1986

Cavanagh Johnson T: Child perpetrators—children who molest other children: preliminary findings. Child Abuse Negl 12:219–229, 1988

Charney DA, Russell RC: An overview of sexual harassment. Am J Psychiatry 151 (suppl 1):10–17, 1994

Christoffel KK: Violent death and injury in U.S. children and adolescents. American Journal of Disease Control 144:697–706, 1990

Cicchetti D, Lynch M: Toward an ecological/transactional model of community violence and child maltreatment: consequences for children's development, in Children and Violence. Edited by Reiss D, Richters JE, Radke-Yarrow M, et al. New York, Guilford, 1993, pp 96–110

Cummings EM, Iannotti RJ, Zahn-Waxler C: Aggression between peer in early childhood: individual continuity and developmental change. Child Dev 60:887–895, 1989

Demause L: The universality of incest. Journal of Psychohistory 19:123–164, 1991

Durant W, Durant A: The Lessons of History. New York, Simon & Schuster, 1968

Eissler KR: Death drive, ambivalence, and narcissism. Psychoanal Study Child 26:25–78, 1971

Elliott DS: The developmental course of sexual and non-sexual violence: results from a national longitudinal study. Paper presented at the annual meeting of the American Association for the Treatment of Sexual Abusers, San Francisco, CA, November 1994a

Elliott DS: Serious violent offenders: onset, developmental course, and termination: the American Society of Criminology 1993 Presidential Address. Criminology 32 (suppl 1):1–21, 1994b

Elliott DS: Youth Violence: An Overview (F-693). Boulder, CO, Center for the Study and Prevention of Violence, Boulder Institute for Behavioral Sciences, University of Colorado, March 1994c

Ellis L: Rape as a biosocial phenomenon, in Sexual Aggression. Edited by Nagayama Hall GC, Hirschman R, Graham JR, et al. Washington, DC, Taylor & Francis, 1993, pp 17–42

Emde R: The horror! the horror! Reflections on our culture of violence and its implications for early development and morality, in Children and Violence. Edited by Reiss D, Richters JE, Radke-Yarrow M, et al. New York, Guilford, 1993, pp 119–123

Equal Employment Opportunity Commission: Title VII: Guidelines on Sexual Harassment. Federal Register 45:219. Rules and Regulations 74676–74677, November 10, 1980

Eron LD, Huesmann LR: The stability of aggressive behavior—even unto the third generation, in Handbook of Developmental Psychopathology. Edited by Lewis M, Miller SM. New York, Plenum, 1990, pp 147–156

Fehrenbach PA: Characteristics of female adolescent sex offenders. Am J Orthopsychiatry 58:148–151, 1988

Fehrenbach PA, Smith W, Monastersky C, et al: Adolescent sexual offenders: offender and offense characteristics. Am J Orthopsychiatry 56 (suppl 2):225–233, 1986

Ferenczi S: Confusion of tongues between adult and child (1932), in Final Contributions to the Problems and Methods of Psychoanalysis. New York, Brunner/Mazel, 1980, pp 225–230

Finkelhor D: Child Sexual Abuse: New Theory and Research. New York, Free Press, 1984

Finkelhor D: Commentary on the universality of incest. Journal of Psychohistory 19:218–219, 1991

Finkelhor D, Hotaling G, Lewis I, et al: Sexual abuse and its relationship to later sexual satisfaction, marital status, religion and attitudes. Journal of Interpersonal Violence 4:379–399, 1989

Fitzgerald LF: Sexual harassment. Am Psychol 48:1070–1076, 1993

Fonagy P, Moran GS, Target M: Aggression and the psychological self. Int J Psychoanal 74:471–485, 1993

Freud S: Three essays on the theory of sexuality (1905), in The Standard Edition of the Complete Psychological Works of Sigmund Freud, Vol 7. Translated and edited by Strachey J. London, Hogarth Press, 1953, pp 125–245

Freud S: Instincts and their vicissitudes (1915), in The Standard Edition of the Complete Psychological Works of Sigmund Freud, Vol 14. Translated and edited by Strachey J. London, Hogarth Press, 1957, pp 109–140

Freud S: Beyond the pleasure principle (1920), in The Standard Edition of the Complete Psychological Works of Sigmund Freud, Vol 18. Translated and edited by Strachey J. London, Hogarth Press, 1955, pp 7–64

Freud S: Civilization and its discontents (1930), in The Standard Edition of the Complete Psychological Works of Sigmund Freud, Vol 21. Translated and edited by Strachey J. London, Hogarth Press, 1961, pp 61–145

Fry DP: Intercommunity differences in aggression among Zapotee children. Child Dev 59:1008–1019, 1988

Galenson E: Sexuality in infancy and preschool children. Child Adolesc Psychiatr Clin North Am 2:385–392, 1993

Gersten JC, Langner TS, Eisenberg JG, et al: Stability and change in types of behavioral disturbances of children and adolescents. J Abnorm Child Psychol 4:111–127, 1976

Goldberg A: The Problem of Perversion: The View From Self-Psychology. New Haven, CT, Yale University Press, 1995

Groth AN: Sexual trauma in the life histories of rapists and child molesters, Victimology: An International Journal 4:10–16, 1979

Hall WM, Cairns RB: Aggressive behavior in children: an outcome of modeling or social reciprocity. Dev Psychol 20:739–745, 1984

Hampton HL: Care of the woman who has been raped. N Engl J Med 332:234–237, 1995

Havighurst RJ, Bowman PH, Liddle GP, et al: Growing Up in River City. New York, Wiley, 1962

Huesmann LR, Eron LD: Cognitive processes and the persistence of aggressive behavior. Aggressive Behavior 10:243–251, 1984

Hobbes T: Leviathan (1651). New York, Collier Press, 1962

Hunter JA: A comparison of the psychosocial maladjustment of adult males and females sexually molested as children. Journal of Interpersonal Violence 6:205–217, 1991

Joseph E: Aggression redefined: its adaptational aspects. Psychoanal Q 42:197–213, 1973

Kagan J, Reznick S, Snidman N: Biological bases of childhood shyness. Science 240:167–171, 1988

Kernberg O: Aggression in Personality Disorders and Perversions. New Haven, CT, Yale University Press, 1992

Kernberg O: The psychopathology of hatred, in Rage, Power and Aggression. Edited by Glick RA, Roose SP. New Haven, CT, Yale University Press, 1993, pp 61–79

Knight RA, Prentky RA: Exploring characteristics for classifying juvenile sex offenders, in The Juvenile Sex Offender. Edited by Barbaree HE, Marshall WL, Hudson SM. New York, Guilford, 1993, pp 45–83

Knopp F: Building bridges: working together to understand and prevent sexual abuse. Paper presented at the annual meeting of the American Association for the Treatment of Sexual Abusers, San Francisco, CA, November 1994

Knopp F, Lackey LB: Female Sexual Abusers: A Summary of Data From 44 Treatment Providers. Orwell, VT, Safer Society Program, 1987

Kohlberg L, Ricks D, Snarey J: Childhood development as a predictor of adaptation in adulthood. Genetic Psychology Monographs 110:91–172, 1984

Kohut H: Thoughts on narcissism and narcissistic rage. Psychoanal Study Child 27:360–400, 1972

Kohut H: The Restoration of the Self. New York, International Universities Press, 1977

Konner MJ: Do we need enemies? The origins and consequences of rage, in Rage, Power and Aggression. Edited by Glick RA, Roose SP. New Haven, CT, Yale University Press, 1993, pp 173–193

Koss MP, Oros C: Sexual Experiences Survey: a research instrument investigating sexual aggression and victimization. J Consult Clin Psychol 50:455–457, 1982

Koss MP, Gidyez CA, Wisniewski N: The scope of rape: incidence and prevalence of sexual aggression and victimization in a national sample of higher education students. J Consult Clin Psychol 55:162–170, 1987

Krisberg BI: Youth crime and its prevention: a research agenda, in Juvenile Justice and Public Policy. Edited by Schwartz I. New York, Lexington Books, 1992, pp 1–19

Landis JT: Experiences of 500 children with adult sexual deviance. Psychiatr Q 30:91–109, 1956

Landy S, Peters RD: Toward an understanding of a developmental paradigm for aggressive conduct problems during the preschool years, in Aggression and Violence Throughout the Life Span. Edited by Peters RD, McMahon RJ, Quinsey VL. Newbury, CA, Sage Publications, 1992, pp 1–30

Langfeldt T: Sexual development in children, in Adult Sexual Interest in Children. Edited by Cook M, Howells K. New York, Academic Press, 1981

Lewis DO, Shankok SS, Pincus JH: Juvenile male sexual assaulters. Am J Psychiatry 136 (suppl 9):1194–1196, 1979

Loeber R: The stability of antisocial and delinquent child behavior: a review. Child Dev 53:1431–1446, 1982

Longo RE: Sexual learning and experiences among adolescent sexual offenders. International Journal of Offender Therapy and Comparative Criminology 26:235–241, 1982

Longo RE, Groth AN: Juvenile sex offenses in the history of adult rapists and child molesters. International Journal of Offender Therapy and Comparative Criminology 17:151–155, 1983

Mahler MS, Pine F, Bergman A: The Psychological Birth of the Human Infant: Symbiosis and Individuation. New York, Basic Books, 1975

Marcovitz E: Aggression: an overview. Psychoanalytic Inquiry 2 (suppl 1): 11–19, 1982

Matthews R, Hunter JA, Vuz J: Juvenile female sexual offenders: clinical characteristics and treatment issues. Sexual Abuse: A Journal of Research and Treatment 9:187–199, 1997

McConaghy N: Sexual Behavior. New York, Plenum, 1993

McCord J: Parental behavior in the cycle of aggression. Psychiatry 51:14–23, 1988

Merry SN, Andrews LK: Psychiatric status of sexually abused children 12 months after disclosure of abuse. J Am Acad Child Adolesc Psychiatry 33:939–944, 1994

Money J: Lovemaps. New York, Irvington Publishers, 1986

Muehlenhard CL, Cook SW: Men's self-report of unwanted sexual activity. Journal of Sex Research 24:58–72, 1988

National Committee to Prevent Child Abuse: Current Trends in Child Abuse Reporting and Fatalities: The Results of the 1997 Annual Fifty State Survey. Chicago, IL, National Committee to Prevent Child Abuse, 1998 [Available from NCPCA, 332 S. Michigan Ave., Ste. 1600, Chicago, IL 60604]

National Task Force on Juvenile Sexual Offending: National Adolescent Perpetrator Network Revised Report. Juvenile and Family Court Journal 44 (suppl 4):3–108, 1993

National Victims Center and the Crime Victims Research and Treatment Center: Rape in America: A Report to the Nation. Charleston, SC, Medical University of South Carolina, 1992

Office of Juvenile Justice and Delinquency Prevention: Juveniles and Violence (Fact Sheet 19). Washington, DC, U.S. Department of Justice, Office of Justice Programs, November 1994a

Office of Juvenile Justice and Delinquency Prevention: Violent Families and Youth Violence (Fact Sheet 21). Washington, DC, U.S. Department of Justice, Office of Justice Programs, December 1994b

Olweus D: Stability of aggressive reaction patterns in males: a review. Psychol Bull 86:852–875, 1979

Olweus D: Familial and temperamental determinants of aggressive behavior in adolescent boys: a causal analysis. Dev Psychol 16:644–660, 1980

Parens H: Toward a reformulation of the psychoanalytic theory of aggression, in The Course of Life, Vol 2: Early Childhood. Edited by Greenspan S, Pollock G. Madison, CT, International Universities Press, 1989, pp 83–121.

Parens H: Rage toward self and others in early childhood, in Rage, Power and Aggression. Edited by Glick RA, Roose SP. New Haven, CT, Yale University Press, 1993, pp 123–147

Patterson GR, DeBaryshe BD, Ramsey E: A developmental perspective on antisocial behavior. Am Psychol 44:329–335, 1989

Person ES: Male sexuality and power, in Rage, Power and Aggression. Edited by Glick RA, Roose SP. New Haven, CT, Yale University Press, 1993, pp 29–44

Postman N: The Disappearance of Childhood. New York, Vintage Books, 1994

Richman N, Stevenson J, Graham PJ: Preschool to School: A Behavioral Study. London, Academic Press, 1982

Richters JE: Community violence and children's development: toward a research agenda for the 1990s, in Children and Violence. Edited by Reiss D, Richters JE, Radke-Yarrow M, et al. New York, Guilford, 1993, pp 3–5

Robbins L: Sturdy childhood predictors of adult outcomes: replications from longitudinal studies, in Stress and Mental Disorder. Edited by Barrett et al. New York, Raven, 1979, pp 219–233

Rochlin G: Man's Aggression: The Defense of the Self. Boston, MA, Gambit Press, 1973

Rochlin G: Aggression reconsidered: a critique of psychoanalysis. Psychoanalytic Inquiry 2:121–132, 1982

Rosenfeld AA, Wasserman S: Sexual development in the early school-aged child. Child Adolesc Psychiatr Clin North Am 2:393–406, 1993

Russell D: The Secret Trauma: Incest in the Lives of Girls and Women. New York, Basic Books, 1986

Ryan G, Miyoshi TJ, Metzner JL, et al: Trends in a national sample of sexually abusive youths. J Am Acad Child Adolesc Psychiatry 35 (suppl 1): 17–25, 1996

Sarrel PM, Masters WH: Sexual molestation of men by women. Arch Sex Behav 11:117–131, 1982

Schur M: The Id and the Regulatory Principles of Mental Functioning. New York, International Universities Press, 1966

Shaw J: Man and the problem of aggression. Journal of the Philadelphia Association for Psychoanalysis 5 (suppl 1):41–53, 1978

Shaw J: Unmasking of the illusion of safety. Bull Menninger Clin 51:49–63, 1989

Shaw J, Campo-Bowen A: Aggression, in Conduct Disorders in Children and Adolescents. Edited by Sholevar GP. Washington, DC, American Psychiatric Press, 1995, pp 45–57

Shaw J, Campo-Bowen A, Applegate B, et al: Young boys who commit serious sexual offenses: demographics, psychometrics and phenomenology. Bulletin of the American Academy of Psychiatry and the Law 21:399–408, 1993

Siegel LJ, Senna JJ: Juvenile Delinquency. New York, West Publishing, 1988, p 51

State of Florida, Department of Health and Rehabilitation Services: Juvenile sexual offenders in Florida: a profile, a description of sexual offenders and their juvenile justice experience. Tallahassee, FL, State of Florida Department of Health and Rehabilitation Services, July 1994

Stoller RJ: The term perversion, in Perversions, Near Perversions in Clinical Practice. Edited by Fogel GI, Myers WA. New Haven, CT, Yale University Press, 1991, pp 36–58

Struckman-Johnson C: Forced sex on dates: it happens to men too. Journal of Sex Research 24:234–241, 1988

West DJ, Farrington DP: The Delinquent Way of Life. London, Heinemann, 1977

Wilson EO: Sociobiology: The New Synthesis. Cambridge, MA, Harvard University Press, 1975

Winnicott DW: Transitional objects and transitional phenomena: a study of the first not-me possession. Int Psychoanal 34:89–97, 1953

Wyatt G: The sexual abuse of African-American and white women in childhood. Child Abuse Negl 9:507–519, 1985

Zucker KJ, Green R: Psychological and familial aspects of gender identity disorder. Child Adolesc Psychiatr Clin North Am 2 (suppl 3):513–542, 1993

2

Development of Sexual Behavior Problems in Childhood

Toni Cavanagh Johnson, Ph.D.

Child development is the study of the organism from its inception in utero to its gradual movement into puberty. Books on child development frequently do not separate out sexual development from other areas of development, but instead incorporate it under biological, social, and personality development.

The development of sexuality during childhood is far too complex to conceptualize as a single entity. Toni Cavanagh Johnson, in the book she coauthored with Eliana Gil (Gil and Johnson 1993), outlined seven lines of sexual development in children:

- The biological
- The change from sensual to erotic
- The behavioral
- Gender role and gender object-choice

- Cognitive understanding
- Sexual relationships
- Sexual socialization

These lines of development can be plotted separately in order to determine which area or areas of the child's sexual development may be more advanced or regressed than others. Johnson described the expected progress within each line and how development along each of the lines may be disrupted.

This chapter takes the behavioral line of children's sexual development as its focus. (For purposes of this chapter, the term *children* refers to prepubertal children.) First, a definition of natural and healthy sexuality in childhood is provided and functions as a baseline for understanding children's sexual behaviors. Then, 21 characteristics of problematic sexual behavior are presented. From the continuum of sexual behaviors in children, three groups, or patterns, of problematic behaviors are delineated. Case examples involving children in each of these three groups are provided.

Natural and Healthy Sexual Behaviors

It is expected that 40% to 85% of children will engage in at least some natural and expected sexual behaviors before age 13 years (Friedrich et al. 1992; Goldman and Goldman 1988; Johnson 1995; Kilpatrick 1992; Wyatt et al. 1993).

Natural and expected sexual exploration during childhood is an information-gathering process by which children explore each other's bodies, visually and tactually (e.g., "playing doctor"), as well as explore gender roles and behaviors (e.g., "playing house"). Children involved in natural and expected sexual play are of similar age, size, and developmental status and participate on a voluntary basis. Although siblings engage in mutual sexual exploration, most sexual play is between children who have an ongoing mutually enjoyable play and/or school friendship. The sexual behaviors are limited in type and frequency and occur in several periods of the child's life. The child's interest in sex and sexuality is balanced by curiosity about other aspects of his or her life. Natural and expected sexual exploration may result in embarrassment but does not usually leave children with deep feelings of anger, shame, fear, or anxiety. If the children are discovered in sexual exploration and instructed to stop, the behavior generally diminishes, at least in the view of adults. The affect of the children regarding the sexual behavior is generally characterized by lightheartedness and spontaneity. Sexual arousal, and sometimes orgasm, occur in some prepubertal children.

The type and frequency of behaviors in which children engage vary a great deal from child to child. Some of this variation can be attributed to the particular child's sexual interest and curiosity as well as the amount of sexual drive and sexual feelings the child has. The child's age, family stress, family violence, family sexuality, and time spent in day care also influence the type and frequency of sexual behavior (Friedrich et al. 1998). Children's sexual behaviors, as well as their level of comfort with sexuality, may be affected by family living space, the child's neighborhood, his or her level of sexual interest, and parental and religious attitudes and values. Society and culture also appear to influence children's sexual behaviors.

Problematic Characteristics of Children's Sexual Behavior

Sexual development in childhood can be negatively impacted by living in a sexually charged environment in which the adults do not shield the children from pornography and/or R-rated and X-rated movies, in which sex and aggression are paired or sex is used as an exchange commodity. Neglect, abandonment, sexual abuse, and physical and emotional abuse can all have a strong negative impact on the child's overall emotional and physical development, including his or her sexual development. Although for most children, these negative influences do not have a permanent impact on sexual development, they can have serious effects that require intervention.

The following characteristics of children's sexual behavior are indications that their sexual development is going awry.

1. Sexual behaviors engaged in with children with whom there is no ongoing mutual play relationship. In general, children seek out other children with whom they agree to engage in sexual exploration. Because most children are very aware of adult's prohibitions on overt sexual play, friends are sought who will keep the secret. Children do not generally pick someone to engage in sexual behaviors whom they distrust or with whom they have an antagonistic relationship, because that person may tell on them.

2. Sexual behaviors engaged in with children of different ages or at different developmental levels. Unless there are no similar-age children in the neighborhood, most children select playmates of the same age. Although age and developmental level are generally closely related, this is not always true. Developmentally delayed children may choose to play with younger children because their developmental level is more similar to their own. Children with poor social skills may also play with younger children. In some cases, older children may take advantage of the social position that accrues from their age. It is important to assess age, developmental level, and the relationship between the children to determine if sexual behaviors between children of different ages are problematic. In general, the wider the age difference, the greater the concern.

3. Sexual behaviors that are out of balance with other aspects of the child's life and interests. Children are interested in every aspect of their environment, from the sun's rising to how babies are made. Although children may explore some aspects of their world more extensively at certain periods of their young lives, their interests are generally broad and intermittent. Children's sexual behaviors follow the same pattern. During one period they may be very interested in discovering about sexuality, and at another time they may wish to know how the dishwasher works or what makes Mommy mad. Their interest fluctuates often in a day, a week, and a month. When a child is preoccupied with sexuality—for example, when he or she prefers to masturbate rather than to engage in regular childhood activities—there is cause for concern.

4. Seemingly excessive knowledge about sexuality for developmental age and sexual behavior that is more consistent with adult sexual expression. As children develop, they acquire knowledge about sex and sexuality from television, movies, videos, magazines, their parents, relatives, school, and other children. Knowledge gathered in these time-honored and more recent and ubiquitous ways is generally assimilated, without disruption, into the child's developing understanding of sex and sexuality; integration of this knowledge enhances the child's natural and healthy sexual interest. When children have been over-exposed to explicit adult sexuality or have been sexually misused, they may engage in or talk about sexual behaviors that are beyond age-appropriate sexual knowledge and interest.

5. Sexual behaviors that are significantly different from those of other same-age children. The frequency and type of children's sexual behaviors depend, to a certain extent, on the environment (i.e., home, neighborhood, culture, religion) in which the children have been raised, their parent's attitudes and actions related to sex and sexuality, and their peers' behaviors. If a child's sexual behaviors stand out among those of his or her neighborhood peers, there is cause for concern.

6. Sexual behaviors that continue in spite of the child's having been given consistent and clear requests to stop. Most adults are consistent in their admonitions against children's openly engaging in sexual behaviors. Although adults may be inconsistent regarding other behaviors, and children may continue engaging in them, children generally learn very quickly that there is a strong taboo on overt sexual behavior. Children's sexual behaviors that continue in the view of adults despite requests to stop or even punishment may be a conscious or unconscious way of signaling that they need help. When children "cry for help," they may persist in the behavior until adults pay heed, discover, and curtail the antecedents of the sexual behavior.

7. Sexual behavior that appears to be compulsive (the child appears to be unable to stop himself or herself from engaging in the behavior). Most children engage in sexual behaviors when they choose to do so. They become interested or curious and then pursue the activity. At very young ages, children realize they should not engage in sexual behaviors in front of adults, and thus they separate themselves to engage in the behaviors. Some children appear to feel driven to engage in sexual behaviors even though they will be punished or admonished. Generally, this type of sexual behavior is in response to stimuli that reawaken memories that are traumatic, painful, or overly stimulating.

8. Sexual behaviors that occur in public or other places where the child has been told they are not acceptable. When a child has been told not to engage in sexual behaviors or told to do so only in private, he or she generally responds so as not to be reprimanded. A child's inability to conform to these requests may indicate that his or her sexual behavior is driven by anxiety or other discomforting or overwhelming emotions. This type of sexual behavior is generally not within the full conscious control of the child. The child who feels anxious in the presence of certain precipitating stimuli may respond directly by masturbating or engaging in other sexual behaviors. Hiding the sexual behaviors or finding friends to engage in the behaviors in private may not be possible for the child. Anxiety-, guilt-, or fear-driven sexual behavior often does not respond to normal limit setting.

9. Sexual behaviors that elicit complaints from other children and/or that adversely affect other children. Generally, children complain when something is annoying or discomforting to them. When a child complains about another child's sexual behaviors, it is an indication that the behavior is upsetting to the child and should be taken seriously. In natural and healthy sexual play, both children agree, overtly or indirectly, not to tell, and engage in the play willingly. It is quite unlikely that either would tell on the other; therefore, if one child is telling, there is cause for concern.

10. Sexual behaviors that are directed at adults, who feel uncomfortable receiving them. Children hug adults and give them kisses. In general, they do so spontaneously to express affection and caring, or they are complying with the request from a parent to kiss the adult (usually a relative). When a child continues to touch an adult in a manner more akin to adult–adult sexual contact, offers himself or herself as a sexual object, or solicits sexual touch from adults, there is cause for concern.

11. Children (4 years and older) who do not understand their rights or the rights of others in relation to sexual contact. Children who do not understand who has the right to touch their bodies or whose bodies they can touch may themselves have had their own personal boundaries violated. Some children may live with persons who do not respect their emotional, physical, or sexual privacy. These children may not have learned proper boundaries and hence may violate others' boundaries. Sexual abuse often involves teaching children to touch others in a sexual way. Children who have been sexually abused may have been taught how to stimulate adults or other children.

12. Sexual behaviors that increase in frequency, intensity, or intrusiveness over time. Although sexual behavior in children is natural and expected, the frequency is not generally high; such behavior is sporadic and occurs outside the vision and knowledge of others. Concern is raised when a pattern of sexualized behavior develops unabated and the behaviors encroach into others' emotional and physical space.

13. Sexual behavior that is associated with fear, anxiety, deep shame, or intense guilt. Children's affect regarding sexuality is generally lighthearted, spontaneous, giggly, or silly. If a child has been caught engaging in sexual behaviors, the adult's response may, in some cases, generate embarrassed or guilty feelings in the child. Yet, these feelings are qualitatively different from the deep shame and intense guilt, fear, or anxiety experienced by a child who has been fooled, coerced, or threatened into sexual behaviors or overly exposed to adult sexuality.

14. Extensive, persistent, mutually agreed-upon adult-type sexual behaviors with other children. Children generally engage in a variety of spontaneous and sporadic sexual behaviors with other children for purposes of exploration and the satisfaction of curiosity. Some children who feel alone in the world may turn to other children to decrease their loneliness. Children who do so often do not see adults as sources of emotional warmth and caring. If the children have been prematurely sexualized and/or taught that sex equals caring, they may try to use sex as a coping mechanism against their loneliness.

15. Sexual behavior involving manual stimulation of or oral or genital contact with animals. Children in urban and suburban areas rarely have contact with the genitalia of animals. Children on farms might have some sexual contact with animals, but such contact is limited. Children's engaging in repeated sexualized behavior with animals that is known to or observed by others or their harming animals raises concern.

16. Sexualization of nonsexual things or of interactions with others or relationships. For example, an 8-year-old imagines that a girl whom he does not know and has shown no interest in him "wants to have sex with me." Another example is when a child tries to give a hickey to her foster father or says she wants to be his girlfriend to please him. Yet another example is when farmyard animals are discussed as "always" wanting to "hump" each other.

17. Sexual behaviors that, unintentionally or intentionally, cause physical or emotional pain or discomfort to self or others. Children's engaging in any behaviors, including sexual behaviors, that induce pain or discomfort to themselves or others is a cause for concern.

18. Sexual behavior that is intended to hurt others. When sex and pain, sex and disappointment, sex and hurt, or sex and other negative emotions and experiences have been paired, the children may use sex as a weapon. They may use their sexual behavior in much the same way as it has been used against them.

19. Sexual behavior preceded, followed, or accompanied by verbal and/or physical expressions of anger. In healthy development, sexual expression and exploration are accompanied by positive emotions. Verbal or physical aggression that accompanies children's sexual behaviors is a learned response to sexuality. In general, children who repeat this behavior have witnessed repeated instances in which verbally and/or physically aggressive behavior has occurred, often in the context of sex. Children may have witnessed their parents or other adults hitting one another when fighting about sexual matters. Some children may have witnessed a parent being sexually misused. Some parents who verbally assault their partners use highly sexual words. Children who have been sexually abused may feel anger and suspicion about all sexual expression. Children's association of negative and hostile emotions with sexual behavior may be their response to having been coerced, forced, bribed, fooled, manipulated, or threatened into sexual contact or to being aware of this having happened to someone else. When verbal or physical expressions of anger are paired with the child's sexual expression, there is cause for great concern.

20. Use of distorted logic to justify sexual actions ("She didn't say 'no'"). When caught doing something wrong, children often try to make an excuse. When young children use rationalizations about problematic sexual behaviors with others that demonstrate a lack of empathy after hurting someone, disregard others' rights, and deny any responsibility for their own actions, there is cause for concern.

21. Sexual behaviors that are associated with coercion, force, bribery, manipulation, or threats. Healthy sexual exploration may include teasing or daring; unhealthy sexual expression involves the use of emotional or physical force or coercion to engage another child in sexual behavior. Children who engage in coercive sexual behavior may find a child who is emotionally or physically vulnerable so as to coerce him or her into the sexual behavior. Groups of children may use sex to hurt other children, although this occurs only infrequently among young children.

Sexual Behaviors in Children: A Continuum

The sexual behaviors of children can be conceptualized along a continuum from natural and healthy to very disturbed. On one end of the continuum is sexual play (group one). On the other end is molestation of other children (group four). In the middle are sexually reactive behavior (group two) and extensive mutual sexual behavior (group three). Sexual behaviors that fall into groups two, three, and four are considered problematic.

It is important to conceptualize sexual behavior problems as a continuum of behaviors to avoid the misattribution of children as sex offenders. Many professionals, when asked to assess children's sexual behaviors, dichotomize the behaviors into two groups, sexual play and sexual molestation. A very unfortunate consequence of this approach is that it is more likely that children with sexual behavior problems will be overidentified as young sex offenders. Most children with sexual behavior problems fall into the middle two groups—that is, they exhibit sexually reactive behavior or engage in extensive mutual sexual behavior; very few children molest other children (Gil and Johnson 1993).

Not overpathologizing children's sexual behaviors has become even more critical in the 1990s, when many states are registering youths as "sexual predators" regardless of age. For instance, Colorado maintains a database, the Central Registry, in which all persons who have a sustained petition of sexual abuse against them are registered as "sexual predators." During the first 2 years a parent can request that their child's name and record be removed from the registry. Subsequent to that the person's record remains in the registry for life. Children as young as 6 years of age have been listed in the Central Registry (J. Wright, personal communication, July 1995).

The four groups can be better understood by examining the key behaviors that characterize each group (Table 2–1). The child can then be matched to one of the four groups based on his or her pattern of behavior. It is important to realize that the classification of sexual behaviors into four groups is a conceptual model by which children's sexual behaviors can be better understood. The model is intended to apply to prepubertal children, both boys and girls, who have intact reality testing and an IQ over 70. Each child's behaviors may not correspond exactly to all of the characteristic features for a particular group. Yet, overall, the pattern of the child's behaviors should generally correspond to the core features of the group. By determining the group that best describes the child's sexual behavior, one

Table 2–1. Continuum of sexual behaviors in children: key features

	Group One Sexual play	Group Two Sexually reactive behavior	Group Three Extensive mutual sexual behavior	Group Four Molestation
Sexual behaviors	See below and 21 problematic characteristics in text	See below and 21 problematic characteristics in text	See below and 21 problematic characteristics in text	See below and 21 problematic characteristics in text
Scope	Few to many	Several problematic behaviors	Many adult sexual behaviors	Many abusive behaviors
Frequency/Duration	Intermittent, at different ages and different frequency	Intermittent to frequent	Ongoing	Previous, ongoing, and increasing Possibly, compulsive need A pattern of disturbed sexual behavior (not a one-time event)
Intensity	Balanced; can be stopped and started at will	Out of balance with other aspects of life	Pervasive need for reassurance through sexual contact	Preoccupation with sex Sexualization of most contact with people and things
Affect associated with sexuality	Silly, giggly, light-hearted affect Possibly, parent- or religion-induced guilt	Anxiety, shame, guilt, fear, confusion	Neediness, confusion, sneakiness, "What's the big deal" attitude	Anxiety, anger, aggression, rage, confusion

(continued)

Table 2–1. Continuum of sexual behaviors in children: key features (continued)

	Group One Sexual play	Group Two Sexually reactive behavior	Group Three Extensive mutual sexual behavior	Group Four Molestation
Interpersonal relationships	All kinds	Possibly, isolation, uncertainty, wariness	Distrust of adults as caregivers Expectation of being hurt Unattachment Reliance on sexual relationship for emotional strength Prone to victimization by adult who takes advantage of child's neediness and confusion	Antagonism Very limited social skills and relationships with people of any age No reliable way to get approval
Other behaviors to evaluate	School performance Friendships	Family relations Self concept Impulse control	Problem-solving/coping skills Empathy	Relationship to authority figures Peer relations
Age difference	Similar age	Similar age Playmates Living companion	Similar age Living companion	Younger or older (up to 12-year difference)
Level of coercion	Request/teasing Mutual	Generally no discussion prior to behavior; if discussion, no coercion Noncoercive	Agreement at conscious or unconscious level Noncoercive	Threats/bribes/trickery Manipulation Coercion

Degree of secrecy	Secret	May be observable	Secret	Secret
Siblings	Sibling sex play (foster, natural, or step)	Sibling sexual contact (foster, natural, or step)	Mutual sibling incest (foster, natural, or step)	Forced sibling incest (foster, natural, or step)
Relationship to other	Friends	Accessible children May approach adults	Willing children Sex may become a stable aspect of the relationship	Vulnerable children May be directed at adults
Planning?	Spontaneous/planned	Spontaneous/impulsive	Planned	Planned/spontaneous or explosive
Family	All types of families	Possibly, sexual abuse, other abuse Lack of emotional support and cohesion between family members Poor boundaries Sexual confusion	Possible polyabuse in family history Emotional distance and unsupportiveness in parents/caregivers Extramarital affairs Overt and covert sexuality in home Poor boundaries	Possibly, generations of abuse in families Neglect/abandonment Psychiatric disorders Poor boundaries Sexualized environment Criminal justice problems Parental violence Mostly households with mother as single parent
Reaction to discovery	Shyness, embarrassment, running and hiding	Possibly, surprise (if discovery dissociated from time of sexual behavior), upset and confusion, or fear	Denial or blaming of other child involved or inability to see problem with the sexual behavior	Aggressive and angry blaming of the other child involved and/or person who discovered the abuse, or denial of the behavior

(continued)

Table 2–1. Continuum of sexual behaviors in children: key features (continued)

	Group One Sexual play	Group Two Sexually reactive behavior	Group Three Extensive mutual sexual behavior	Group Four Molestation
Sexual arousal	Arousal No arousal	Arousal No arousal	Arousal No arousal	Arousal No arousal
Motivation	Curiosity/exploration To be like friends Mimicking of what has been seen in real life or on television Sexual stimulation	Anxiety reduction Posttraumatic stress reaction To reduce confusion Making sense of sexual misuse or victimization Recapitulation of previous, unassimilated, uncontainable sexual overstimulation To decrease physiological arousal Sexual stimulation	Coping mechanism to decrease isolation, loneliness, or neediness Reduction in boredom Reduction of depression Way to make life more bearable Stabilization of sense of self Provides an attachment figure Connection to the otherwise hostile world Reduction in physiological arousal Prone to victimization by older person who takes advantage of child's neediness and confusion Sexual stimulation	Reduction in anxiety, fear, loneliness, anger, abandonment fears, or other strong unpleasant internal sensations Reduction in confusion Recapitulation of previous physical, sexual, or emotional overstimulation Reduction in physiological arousal paired with early and/or ongoing stress Desire to hurt others Retaliation Posttraumatic stress reaction Sibling rivalry Compulsive sexual drive Sexual stimulation

Possible etiological factors	Natural and healthy childhood curiosity, exploration, and experimentation Television, videos, printed materials Friends	Recent or ongoing sexual abuse Emotional abuse "Traumatic sexualization"[a] Pornography History of sexual abuse in family Overtly sexual lifestyle in home	Sexual and/or emotional and/or physical abuse Abandonment Neglect Extramarital liaisons of parents Inadequate early bonding to caregiver Physiological/hormonal problems Sexual abuse in a group Lack of adult attachments Continuous out-of-home placement	Intense rivalry for attention between siblings Lack of positive emotional relationships Physiological/hormonal problems Trauma-induced neurobiological changes Pairing of sex with anger/aggression/anxiety Sexual and/or emotional and/or physical abuse Neglect/abandonment Inherited vulnerabilities Violence in family history Sexualized relationships Sexualized environment in family Poor boundaries Caregivers with many unmet needs

(continued)

Table 2–1. Continuum of sexual behaviors in children: key features (*continued*)

	Group One Sexual play	Group Two Sexually reactive behavior	Group Three Extensive mutual sexual behavior	Group Four Molestation
Treatment	Sometimes, education of parents and/or children regarding sex and sexuality Values clarification	Self-understanding Making sense of previous experiences with overwhelming sexuality Sex education Parent support and education in parallel with child's therapy Well-articulated plan to modify sexual behaviors Parallel group therapy for parents and children	Increased attachment to adults to allow child to have emotional and dependency needs met Learning to substitute emotional contact for sexual contact See also treatment of group-two behaviors	Intensive treatment Skills training Ten goals for children who molest Intensive treatment of parents Boundary issues Parallel group therapy for parents and identified children and their siblings Family therapy Intensive prevention work in family Violence reduction

[a]Finkelhor.

should be better able to understand the child's needs for intervention and treatment, as well as the needs of the child's family.

These four groups represent a wide range of sexual behaviors. Within each group, as well as across all four of the groups, the nature of the behaviors lies on a continuum from less to more. For instance, some children whose sexual development corresponds most closely to that in group one do not engage in any sexual play behaviors, whereas others engage in a very large number of such behaviors (Goldman and Goldman 1988; Haugaard and Tilly 1988; Kilpatrick 1992; Wyatt et al. 1993). Some children whose behaviors correspond most closely to those in group two may have touched another child one time, whereas others may have touched a child 30 or more times. For some children whose behaviors correspond most closely to those in group three, their sexual behaviors are a minor, rather than a major, part of the relationships they develop; others with group-three behaviors relate to each other only sexually and in a way that is consuming and compulsive and very difficult for adults to detect or, if they do, stop. Some children whose behaviors correspond most closely to those in group four have just begun to molest children out of disappointment, fear, isolation, and depression, whereas others have developed over time a pervasive, intrusive, and manipulative style of relating to peers and adults.

Group One: Sexual Play

Group-one behaviors involve sexual play. As can be seen in Table 2–1, the characteristics of children with behaviors in this group follow the definition given earlier in this chapter in the discussion of natural and healthy sexual behaviors. By far the largest group of children exhibit behaviors best described by this group. All types of children and families are represented by this category. In fact, the sexual behaviors of most children who have been abused correspond to this category. Most studies of sexually abused children indicate that 35% or fewer of sexually abused children show problematic sexual behaviors (Kendall-Tackett et al. 1993). One study showed that approximately half of sexually abused children show an increase in sexual behaviors (Friedrich et al. 1992).

Kilpatrick (1992) indicates that there has been a trend toward decreased sexual behaviors during childhood over the last six decades. This downward trend was true for all of the cohorts studied except for the 1940–1949 birth-year cohort, in which an increase was found. The sample population consisted of women aged 16 to 60 years in the southern part of the United States. Kilpatrick also found a large difference between Blacks and Whites in childhood sexual behaviors; almost twice as many White women as Black women reported engaging in sexual behaviors as children.

Wyatt and colleagues (1993), in a retrospective study, found some interesting associations between childhood sexual play and later sexual behavior in their sample, which consisted entirely of women. The authors noted that "[c]onsensual childhood sexual behaviors established a trajectory for voluntary sexual involvement in adolescence and a broader range of activities in childhood" (p. 96). They also found that, "[i]n general, earlier consensual sexual involvement and activities had few serious sexual or psychological consequences in adulthood. . . . Women who recalled that both their parents and religious affiliations communicated negative messages about sexual intimacy reported less childhood sexual behavior . . ." (p. 97). Both intra- and extrafamilial sexual abuse were associated with more voluntary childhood sexual activities: "Severe incidents of attempted rapes in adulthood were related to a background of conflicting sexual messages and activities, including no endorsement of sexual intimacy by childhood socialization figures, having mothers with little formal education, and frequent sexual play with others as a child but little masturbatory experience as an adolescent" (p. 98).

Group Two: Sexually Reactive Behaviors

In the natural and healthy course of child development, the developing body and mind of the child interact with other people and the environment in a compatible way that broadens the child's horizons and increases the child's understanding of his or her world in a stepwise fashion. Essential to the natural and healthy development of sexuality in children is the opportunity to be active agents of their own exploration and discovery. If sexual experiences are thrust upon them before they are ready, they will have no way to understand the behaviors. A significant number of the children with behaviors most closely corresponding to those in the sexually reactive group have been sexually, physically, or emotionally abused; abandoned; or neglected. Those who have not have lived in sexually overwhelming environments in which they have not been adequately shielded from disturbed adult sexuality. Poor boundaries in chaotic homes that often have physical battery between the caregivers overwhelm these children's developing sexuality. Their confusion about sex and sexuality manifests in more frequent and more visible sexual behaviors. These sexual behaviors are generally driven by fear or anxiety as well and are frequently precipitated by stimuli in the environment. Most of these sexual behaviors are not under the behavioral control of the child. In many cases, they erupt from the child without conscious awareness.

Piaget's notion of assimilation and accommodation helps us to understand how healthy sexual development can progress and how distressed sexual development can occur (Piaget 1954/1971). Piaget believed that as children explore their world they develop cognitive structures that help organize their experiences so that understanding can take place. New experiences are assimilated into the developing structures. The structures may have to be modified to accommodate new information if it is discrepant or an expansion of previously acquired information. When children are bombarded by intrusive and overwhelming adult sexual behaviors, they cannot assimilate and accommodate these experiences into their developing sexuality. Instead, these experiences can disrupt the child's developing understanding of sexuality. When the child is unable to assimilate a traumatic or confusing recurring sexual experience, an accommodation may occur that is contrary to healthy development. For instance, after a child has been used as a sexual object, he or she may believe that this is the role children assume toward adults. The child may incorporate into his or her developing understanding of sexual relationships the belief that in order to get attention he or she must engage in sexual pleasuring of the other person.

Piaget's concept of assimilation and accommodation, although introduced to describe a component of cognitive development, can also be applied to sexual development to help in understanding how a child's developing sexual feelings can be transposed prematurely into adultlike sexual strivings. From infancy onward, if children experience pleasurable touch, they develop a healthy sensuality. Generally, sensuality—the pleasurable feelings that accompany skin contact—gives way to erotic feelings, sexual excitement, and increased desire for physical and genital contact with others with the influx of the hormones around puberty. When a child's body and genitalia are massaged and used for the purposes of adult erotic pleasure, the child may become prematurely eroticized. The child's body is unable to assimilate and accommodate these sensations and to make meaning of them. The sensations flood the child's sensory structure, and he or she can be bombarded prematurely with adultlike sexual desires and strivings.

Some children who have been sexually abused or prematurely overstimulated act this out in the form of sexual behaviors that are beyond what is natural and healthy, but many do not. For many sexually reactive children, there is no plan to the behaviors. They are reacting to things in the environment or to their thoughts and feelings. Because these behaviors erupt, they are generally much more noticeable than the behaviors characteristic of group one, which the child can plan to do when others are not around. Some children whose behaviors are best described as sexually reactive may attempt to engage in sexual behaviors with children outside the sight of adults. Force or coercion is not involved when a sexually reactive child approaches another child. Because there is no coercion, the recipients of sexually reactive (group-two) behaviors are not generally adversely affected in any significant or long-standing way. Yet some children may feel victimized by the sexual behavior. Sexually reactive children may engage sexually with children in their play group or school. Some children may be sexual with siblings or relatives. Many sexually reactive children engage in solitary sexual behaviors. Among the most frequent are touching and rubbing of their genitals and masturbation.

Some sexually reactive children experience posttraumatic stress reactions. These may precipitate the child into recreating sexually traumatic events with other children or adults. Sometimes the child will try to replicate previously experienced confusing sexuality in an attempt at understanding what happened to him or her. Much sexually reactive behavior is an attempt to decrease anxiety, shame, guilt, or fear that the child feels. Some of the behaviors in which these children engage are driven by the desire for sexual stimulation.

Children who exhibit sexually reactive behavior need a coordinated educational and behavioral plan to assist them to decrease problematic sexual behavior. Depending on the severity of the problem, these children will also benefit from individual or group counseling so that they can develop an understanding of the precipitating reasons for the behavior and learn ways to be with children and not engage in sexual behaviors. If the child has been abused, an understanding and resolution of the abuse should be sought. In some cases the sexual behaviors will remit within weeks; in other cases it takes longer. Parents need education and support to assist their child in decreasing the behaviors and to deal with the abuse to the child (Johnson 1998).

Children who engage in group-two, or sexually reactive, behaviors exhibit characteristic problematic behaviors 2, 3, 4, 5, 6, 7, 8, 9, 10, 11, 13, 15, and 16 (see section on problematic characteristics of children's sexual behaviors earlier in chapter).

Group Three: Extensive Mutual Sexual Behaviors

Children who do not feel a connection to their parents or other adults who have been charged with their care may move toward peers for their emotional comfort. Some children lose all faith in adults and feel awash in a hostile environment. If their experiences have included sexual, physical, or emotional abuse, abandonment, or neglect and they have lived in environments that were suffused with intrusive sexuality, some of these children move toward peers in a sexual way to feel safe and to find an anchor in the chaos of their lives.

The behaviors exhibited by these children can be understood as belonging to group three, which is characterized by extensive mutual sexual behaviors. These children often have no model for a healthy parent–child relationship built on trust and caring. Many of these

children have been repeatedly physically and emotionally abandoned by their parents and feel little or no connection or comfort
with any adult. As their sexuality was developing, they generally
saw and heard sexually charged events and were sexually intruded
upon. Frequently, children whose behavior most closely corresponds
to this group confuse sex with caring, believing that someone will
care about them if they have sex with them or that someone who
has sex with them cares about them. Because of their young age,
many of these children do not associate sex with sexual pleasure or
excitement, but instead view it as a sustaining life force. Some of
these children are simply engaging in extensive sexual behaviors
without thinking. Many of the behaviors may be almost mechanical,
constituting a vain attempt at emotional equilibrium.

These children may be easy prey to adults or adolescents who
take advantage of their sexual confusion and neediness. Some of
these children without treatment may grow up to have multiple
partners, engage in prostitution, or confuse their sexual needs for
their sexual rights.

Although a substantial number of children with extensive mutual sexual behaviors live in out-of-home care or have been taken
out of and returned to their own homes, some of them are birth
siblings. In the mutual sibling incest home, the parents are often
very sexual in their interactions with each other and with other
family members. Many of these parents are having extramarital affairs and are not available to meet the physical and emotional needs
of their children. The sexual, physical, and emotional boundaries in
the home are generally very loose. The children's world is sexualized
and diffuse and lacks containing and caring adults. Some of these
siblings sexualize their own relationships and engage in extensive
mutually agreed-upon sexual behaviors. The children seek comfort
in each other in the face of the parental void and chaos of the sexualized home environment.

Children who engage in group-three, or extensive mutual sexual, behaviors exhibit characteristic problematic sexual behaviors
2, 3, 4, 5, 6, 7, 8, 10, 11, 13, 15, 16, and 20 (see section on problematic characteristics of children's sexual behaviors earlier in
chapter).

Group Four: Molestation

Children who have experienced the most disruption in their sexual development are those who engage in sexually abusive behaviors. Most of these behaviors are engaged in with other children. A few children engage in these behaviors with adolescents and adults. The sexual disturbance cuts across these children's thinking, affect, behavior, and attitude. In the most severe cases, the sexual disturbance is seemingly intertwined with the child's overall manner of relating to others. Their sexual behaviors are abrasive, abusive, and intrusive. There is a fundamental lack of respect and appreciation of others' rights. Boundary violations are frequent, with invasion into the emotional, physical, and sexual space of others.

The child's sexual problems have a discernible history. One sexual behavior does not constitute a child's being a molester; rather, a history of sexual problems precedes the abusive behavior. There are many concomitant intrusive and disruptive sexual behaviors that are part of the current behavior of the child.

Children who engage in sexually abusive behaviors lack an understanding of the meaning of sex. The underlying feelings regarding sex are often anger and aggression, and sometimes rage is connected to sexual expression. Many are preoccupied with sex and sexualize relationships with peers, adolescents, and adults. The vast majority of these children have conduct disorder and have very poor interpersonal relationships with peers, adults, and authority figures. Some of the children threaten violence to other children if they tell anyone about the sexual behaviors. Victims of these children may be older or younger. Sometimes children whose behavior most closely corresponds to this group molest infants. They generally seek out vulnerable children and use many of the standard childhood threats, bribes, and coercive techniques such as "I won't be your best friend" or "I'll give you candy if you . . ." Most do not use physical violence, although some do. Some of these children cause physical damage to their victims. Whereas in some of these children the molestation is planned, in others it occurs spontaneously or explosively. Some of the offensive behavior of these children can be seen in their sexually explosive and vulgar language, taunts, and intrusive, sneaky touching and hugging. Some of these children, if they are tall enough, engage in sexual nuzzling of the breasts of adults with their faces.

Some of the physical feelings these children experience are associated with anger, fear, and residual trauma- or stress-related sensations rather than sexual feelings. Sexual arousal may or may not be part of the behaviors of these children. The closer the children are to puberty, the higher the probability that sexual arousal is involved. Children who have been sexually abused may experience sexual arousal more often than those who have not. Children's sexually abusive behavior may have the aim of alleviating negative feelings that overwhelm them. Sometimes the abuse is intended as retaliation against the victim. Generally, a chaining of feelings, sensations, and environmental cues precipitates the sexual behaviors in these children; the behaviors are generally not solely for sexual satisfaction or pleasure.

Children who engage in group-four, or sexually abusive, behaviors exhibit characteristic problematic sexual behaviors 1, 3, 4, 5, 6, 7, 8, 10, 11, 12, 13, 15, 16, 17, 18, 19, 20, and 21 (see section on problematic characteristics of children's sexual behaviors earlier in chapter).

All children are born and begin their sexual behaviors in a natural and healthy manner (group-one behaviors). Because of disruptions from their environment, some children move to group-two behaviors, which are the behaviors exhibited by the largest number of children with sexual behavior problems. Some children move from group-two to group-three behaviors, the next largest group. Some may move from group-two to group-four behavior, the smallest group by far. Other children may progress from group-one behaviors, to group-two, group-three, and group-four behaviors in succession.

Case Examples

Case 1

A., aged 10, and B., aged 11, are both boys at a residential treatment facility. Prior to entering the facility, A. lived with his mother and stepfather. A.'s mother had been physically, emotionally, and sexually abused as a child and had given birth to A. when she was 17 and unmarried. She worked hard to keep A. and his sister at home and safe but fell prey to men who took advantage of her and her children. She was physically and emotionally abused by A.'s stepfather, who also emotionally and sexually abused A. and his sister. A. was also physically abused on a regular basis by his stepfather, who frequently accused him of having sexual thoughts about his mother.

Child protective services removed A. and his sister from their home because they were engaging in sexual behavior with each other. The emotional, sexual, and physical abuse to the children was unknown at the time of their removal. A.'s sister was placed in a separate institution for fear that he would continue to engage in sexual behavior with her. He was very depressed, anxious, and fearful when he entered the residential center. His acting-out behavior took the form of angry outbursts that resulted in broken furniture and loss of status on the residential unit. He missed his sister and frequently asked to see her, but his request was denied. He did not ask about his mother or stepfather. He was not actively aggressive toward staff or other children, and although superficially compliant, he was at most times distrustful and emotionally disconnected from staff.

B. was brought to the residential center after being hospitalized for severe depression and suicidal ideation. He alternated between being physically aggressive with peers and at home and being totally withdrawn. As a young child, B. was abandoned by his mother and father and lived on and off in foster care for many years. On several occasions he was returned to his mother, only to be removed because of her drug and alcohol problems. He was emotionally neglected by his mother and frequently left alone for long periods when his mother went on a binge. While in foster care B. was sexually abused by an adult male neighbor. B. did not tell anyone about this. When he was returned home he missed the neighbor and tried to go to see him. In the last four foster homes, B. had engaged in sexually reactive behaviors with other foster children. When the children were caught, they were punished. In one foster home, B.'s hands had been tied to the sides of his bed to stop him from masturbating as he was falling asleep. One foster parent told the social worker that B., who was 4 years old at the time, must have the devil in him to be doing sexual behaviors at his age.

Late one night a residential staff caught B. and A. in the bathroom with B. applying petroleum jelly to his penis while standing behind A. B. and A. were friends as much as any of the children on the unit. Both were emotionally needy and confused. But B., who was a year older than A., was much bigger and more aggressive, and he was standing in a position to insert his penis in A.'s rectum. Because of these characteristics it was decided that B. was an offender and A. was the intended victim. When interviewed, both boys said it was the other one's idea; both said they wanted to do it and denied being forced, and both said it made them feel better. B. was not believed, and it was felt that A. was intimidated into silence. B. was removed to a sex offender treatment program.

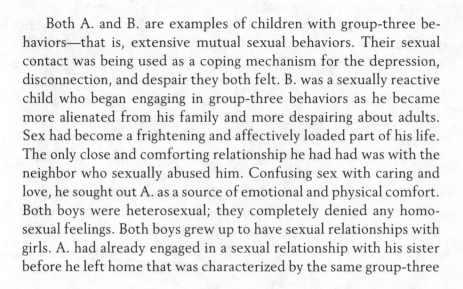

Both A. and B. are examples of children with group-three behaviors—that is, extensive mutual sexual behaviors. Their sexual contact was being used as a coping mechanism for the depression, disconnection, and despair they both felt. B. was a sexually reactive child who began engaging in group-three behaviors as he became more alienated from his family and more despairing about adults. Sex had become a frightening and affectively loaded part of his life. The only close and comforting relationship he had had was with the neighbor who sexually abused him. Confusing sex with caring and love, he sought out A. as a source of emotional and physical comfort. Both boys were heterosexual; they completely denied any homosexual feelings. Both boys grew up to have sexual relationships with girls. A. had already engaged in a sexual relationship with his sister before he left home that was characterized by the same group-three dynamics. He and his sister had clung to each other in a sexual way to overcome the abandonment feelings in the highly charged sexual environment of their home. Both children had engaged in many problematic sexual behaviors alone and with other children who engaged in sexually reactive (group-two) behaviors prior to seeking each other out and engaging in extensive mutual sexual behaviors.

Since few children molest other children, it is possible that neither A. nor B. will progress into more disturbed sexuality. However, either A. or B. could become a child who molests given further alienation from parents, family, and adults and the use of acting out to express loss, depression, and anger. Being returned to the abusive and sexually chaotic home could also be a factor in the development of molestation behavior. Because most children who molest come from a home where physical violence and sexuality are frequently paired, there is a higher chance that A. might molest someone. When puberty begins, with the rush of hormones and the confusion of the sexual urges, and if there is a complete lack of role models for positive and mutually satisfying relationships, either boy may engage in erratic and emotionally hurtful sexual relationships.

Case 2

C., aged 9, is in the third grade. At age 3 years, he was sodomized one time by his father, who had been physically abusive to him throughout the first 3 years of his life. The sodomy was discovered because C. was bleeding quite profusely from his rectum when his mother came home one day. C.'s father was physically and emotionally abusive to C.'s mother, who was also very aggressive toward the father. Life in the home was very confrontative and combative. (C.'s mother lifted weights and was an exceptional athlete.) After discovering the sodomy, she would have stayed in the marriage, but C.'s father disappeared because the police were notified by the hospital when C. disclosed the sodomy during the medical examination. C.'s mother felt it was an invasion of the privacy of her home when the authorities were brought into the situation. Although she felt that C.'s father was wrong to sodomize their son, she said that she could handle the father and that he would never do it again. She blamed the police and social services for destroying her marriage to the "son of a bitch."

Before entering the third grade at the neighborhood school, C. had been expelled from four private schools because of his threatening, coercive, and assaultive physical behaviors toward teachers and children and the sexual behaviors in which he engaged. The sexual behaviors included masturbation in public, genital touching of self and other children, exposing his genitals on the playground and in the classroom, and disruptive and assaultive sexual language toward teachers and students. This behavior had been continuous since the age of 5 years.

His third-grade experience in the neighborhood public school began the day after he was expelled from his fourth private school. C.'s mother was so mad at him that she "didn't want to see his face." On C.'s enrolling at the school, C.'s mother was forthright with the information that C. was a "pain in the neck," had no friends, hit kids, and had been expelled for sexual behaviors. The school officials took no special precautions, did not speak to the other schools, and did not ask for a transfer of records regarding C.

C. sexually and physically abused four of his classmates. The boys, D., E., F., and G., ranged in age from 8 to 9 years.

D. was young for his grade. His home life was very disrupted by a physically abusive father who drank too much. D. always struggled academically, but he tried very hard. His only friend was E., with whom he played much of the time. E. had been sexually abused by an uncle when he was 5 years old. Neither D. nor E. was a leader in the class. They were somewhat isolated from the other children. Their home lives were similar, and they lived on the same block. Their mothers were friends. Both mothers were struggling with the current abusive men in their lives (one of the mothers was married, and the other had a boyfriend) and their own family history, which was replete with alcohol, abuse, frustration, low income, and multiple incarcerations of family members. They cared a lot for their children but were consumed by the task of keeping the family together. Daily life was a struggle for both women.

F. was an average to low-average student who excelled in sports. He was bigger than most of the other third-graders and had status in the group because of his prowess in athletics. He was a good-look-ing boy to whom the third-grade girls were attracted. He was well liked by his teachers, who felt that, despite his low-average grades, he put much effort into his school subjects. F.'s parents were con-sistent in their parenting of F., although their own relationship was somewhat strained at times. All of F.'s siblings did well in school.

G. was a fairly good student and had many friends. He was a rela-tively good athlete and had a cheery and bright disposition. His family was intact, although there were many squabbles between his parents. His father had left his mother several times but had always returned. The parents were emotionally abusive toward each other, but when dealing with G. and his five siblings they were loving.

C.'s problems with assaultive and physically aggressive behavior became evident within several weeks of his entering school. The first incident was when C. put his hands around G.'s neck and tried to strangle him. Several children stopped C. G. had handprints on his neck when he arrived at the nurse's office after the assault. C. punched D. several times on the playground and wrestled E. to the floor in the classroom. Several other boys and girls were hurt by C. when he pushed them down stairs and hit them with balls on the playground. G. and F. were grabbed by the hair several times and pinched on their arms and bottoms. The entire classroom of children was privy to his sexual comments and scatological language. His class-room behavior was very disruptive. His teacher had C. sit next to her and rewarded any positive behavior, but little progress was made. C.'s disruptive behavior lasted throughout the school year. He was suspended several times but was always returned to his classroom. There was no recommendation for special education services.

C. had oral–genital contact with each of the four boys 25 or more times throughout the school year. These behaviors occurred in the school bathroom, behind the building on the elementary school playground, and on the school bus that they all rode together. The children had told the teacher about the hitting, pinching, and other physical behaviors but not the sexual touching.

D., E., F., and G. were supposed to go to summer school but refused. Their parents called the school, saying their children were afraid to attend school but they did not know why. After extensive interviews by the school psychologist, each of the boys told of the oral–genital contact by C. to them. They were all made to suck C.'s penis also. The boys did not want to do this with C. anymore and so refused to go back to school. Each of them was fearful of the hitting, pinching, and shoving.

Evaluations of the children showed that each of the boys had different reactions to the sexual and physical assaults by C. Emotionally, D. and E. were the most troubled by the behaviors, becoming more fearful, anxious, and distant. It was hard to comfort them, and they cried easily. Developmental milestones that previously had been met were lost. Both were having nightmares, wetting their pants in the day, and having frequent nighttime accidents. G. was more easily intimidated by people and events and was less gregarious. Whereas he had previously had an interest in everything and showed a voracious appetite for exploring his environment, he was less willing to leave his parents' side. Nevertheless, he continued to do well in his daily life. F. was the least affected and did not show any behavioral changes. Neither G.'s nor F.'s parents had noticed any behavioral or emotional changes in their sons that concerned them prior to the boys' refusing to go to summer school.

The Child Sexual Behavior Checklist (Johnson 1998), a list of 150 sexual and other related behaviors that is filled out by the parents or caretakers, was used to assess these children's sexual behaviors. The children most affected in the sexual realm, as in the emotional realm, were D. and E. Both children were engaged in multiple sexual behaviors. They touched their genitals frequently in public and seemed unable to stop. Their use of sexual language had increased. D. had been caught peeking at others in the bathroom and writing a note about sex to a girl at school. E. had tried to touch his mother's breast; he also had been caught pulling back the foreskin of a dog's penis. D. and E. were both very anxious about sexual topics. G. showed some sexual behaviors of concern such as entering the bathroom at home when he knew someone else was using it, showing his genitals at home by walking nude in the house, and asking innumerable questions about AIDS and other sexually transmitted diseases. He had not tried to engage any other children in sexual behavior. F. showed no sexual behaviors of concern except for a greater-than-usual amount of sexual talk and jokes.

During the interviews it was disclosed that D. and E. had engaged each other in mutually agreed-upon oral–genital contact on four occasions. Also D. and E. had separately asked another child to engage in oral–genital contact. Both had been rebuffed and had not pursued it any further. Their anxiety about sexuality was coupled with intense shame and guilt about their sexual behavior with each other. Both children wanted to stop the behavior but described "just doing it." Of the four children, only G. described pleasurable or erotic sensations from the sexual behaviors. He said his penis felt "kind of tingly" when he touched it and let it wiggle freely when he walked around. D. and E. said it felt mostly bad when they touched each other. F. said he did not engage in any sexual behaviors. All four victims said they did not experience any good feelings when C. made them engage in oral-genital contact.

The four boys abused by C. were, in general, exposed to the same or similar sexually and physically abusive behaviors. However, the abuse affected them differently, both emotionally and in terms of their sexual development.

C. engaged in sexually abusive behaviors represented by group four (i.e., molestation). D. and E. engaged in sexually reactive (group-two) behaviors, and there is the possibility of their moving to engaging in extensive mutual sexual (group-three) behaviors if their life circumstances were to change. When questioned, the teacher of the third-grade classroom said that the children most vulnerable that year were D. and E. Even before C. entered the classroom these boys were more likely to be bossed around and teased by the other children. These vulnerable children, of the four children abused by C., experienced the worst emotional aftereffects and were more affected in the realm of sexuality. They showed the most problematic sexual behaviors, were the most confused about sex, and had begun to repeat the oral–genital contact performed on them with each other, and each had tried to engage another child in sexual behaviors. D. and E. are examples of children with behaviors toward the more disturbed end of the group-two group. If they were to be separated from their families or there were to be more intense disruption and lack of parental and family support, these children might begin engaging in group-three behaviors. They are emotionally needy and neglected children who might try to use sexual behavior to cope with their feelings.

Both boys need help to comprehend the sexual and physical abuse by C. (group therapy will be helpful for this), understand about sex and sexuality, learn to modify their sexual behaviors, and become more attached to healthy adults. Their parents need help to work out the family situations and to provide for the emotional needs of the children. Sex education will be important. The parents will need guidance to help the boys modify their sexual behaviors and assistance in dealing with their feelings related to C.'s abuse of their children. The children need to be taught about their rights and how to access adults when they need help.

G. is engaging in sexually reactive (group-two) behavior, and F. is at the far end of group-one behavior (sexual play). G. and F. will both need help in understanding the abusive behavior toward them by C. and prevention work to ensure that any further attempts at abusing them will be disclosed to adults who can help them. G. will need sex education and time to have all of his questions answered. His concern about AIDS needs to be explored thoroughly. He will need to understand his rights and the rights of others related to sex and sexuality, as he is abrogating people's rights by his sexual behavior. G.'s parents will need help with their relationship to ensure that they are available to him emotionally.

All of the parents need help to sort through their feelings about the abuse to their children and why the children did not tell them. They will need education and support regarding how to modify any problematic sexual behaviors of their children (Johnson 1998). They will also need to understand behavioral signs to look out for that may indicate ongoing emotional trauma to their children. Furthermore, they will need to know how to talk to their children about sex and, perhaps, sex education and values clarification about sex (Johnson 1995). It will be helpful to stress the love, support, and containment children need from their parents.

It is important to remember the varying response of children to abuse when evaluating children who have been victimized. Not all children respond the same; nor do they need the same interventions, support, and information or the same length of treatment. In some cases, the parents may need to receive treatment and support longer than do the children.

Attempting to classify children's sexual behaviors along a continuum is also important to reduce the possibility of mislabeling. In some cases an attempt is made to determine if the child is involved in sexual play or molestation behavior as if there were only these two diagnostic groups. When a problem is noted with the sexual behavior of a child, there are three groups—sexually reactive behaviors, extensive mutual behaviors, and molestation. This can result in overpathologizing the child's behavior.

Summary

Children's sexual development starts in utero and continues through puberty and into adulthood. This chapter discusses one of seven lines of sexual development in children, sexual behavior. The sexual behavior of children is affected both positively and negatively by the child's environment and the specific experiences and the context of those experiences. There are 21 indications that children's sexual behaviors are deviating from natural and healthy sexual development. Children's sexual behaviors can be categorized in one of four groups—sexual play, sexually reactive behavior, extensive mutual sexual behaviors, and sexually abusive behavior (molestation)—with a range of behaviors within each group.

References

Friedrich W, Gramsch P, Damon L, et al: The Child Sexual Behavior Inventory: normative and clinical comparisons. Psychological Assessment 4 (suppl 3):303–311, 1992

Friedrich W, Fisher J, Broughton D, et al: Normative sexual behavior in children: a contemporary sample. Pediatrics 101(4):E9, 1998

Gil E, Johnson TC: Sexualized Children: Assessment and Treatment of Sexualized Children and Children Who Molest. Rockville, MD, Launch Press, 1993

Goldman R, Goldman J: Show Me Yours: Understanding Children's Sexuality. New York, Penguin Books, 1988

Haugaard J, Tilly C: Characteristics predicting children's responses to sexual encounters with other children. Child Abuse Negl 12:209–218, 1988

Johnson TC: Child Sexuality Curriculum for Abuse Victims and Their Parents. South Pasadena, CA, Author, 1995

Johnson TC: Sexuality Curriculum for Children and Young Adolescents and Their Parents. South Pasadena, CA, Author, 1998

Kendall-Tackett KA, Williams LM, Finkelhor D: Impact of sexual abuse on children: a review and synthesis of recent empirical studies. Psychol Bull 113 (suppl 1):164–180, 1993

Kilpatrick A: Long-Range Effects of Child and Adolescent Sexual Experiences. Hillsdale, NJ, Lawrence Erlbaum, 1992

Piaget J: The Construction of Reality by the Child (1954). New York, Ballantine, 1971

Wyatt GE, Newcomb MD, Riederle MH: Sexual Abuse and Consensual Sex. Newbury Park, CA, Sage Publications, 1993

3

Sexual Aggression Within the Family

G. Pirooz Sholevar, M.D., and
Linda D. Schwoeri, Ph.D.

Sexual aggression within the family takes many forms. The sexual aggression may be overt and coercive and directed toward a family member, usually a female. A child, a wife, a sibling, or another relative may be victimized. More frequently, the sexual aggression, particularly that directed toward a child, may appear to be erotic, with the aggressive nature of the act concealed by the use of material or psychological reward to induce compliance. A more subtle form is when the victim appears outwardly to consent to the sexual act. Yet another form is when the parents fail to protect the child when she is faced with sexual dangers.[1] Such

---

[1]To enhance readability, and because the majority of victims are female, we use the feminine pronoun (except when discussing specifically cases of mother–son incest and female molestation of male children). It should be noted, however, that males also are victims of aggression against family members.

dangers may be omnipresent in the family.

Although overt sexual aggression in the family is the most readily apparent, the other forms also occur quite commonly. All forms have the same effect of victimizing the young child by violating her developmental needs and the right for protection against violent behavior. Noncoercive sexual activities may undermine the development of the child more than coercive ones because the child may blame herself and feel ashamed for "participating" in the act.

The multiple forms of inappropriate sexual involvement in the family described as an incestuous relationship have received considerable attention in the literature. Sexual aggression toward children, once dismissed by some people as a "fact of life" or a part of "normal child rearing," is now recognized as a significant phenomenon that undermines the psychological stability of the family and makes the victims vulnerable to a range of psychological disorders. The sexual abuse of young girls and wives has become particularly recognized since the women's movement has sensitized society to the oppression of females. The sexual abuse of young boys remains significantly underreported because of the low level of social consciousness in this area and the intensity of the shame experienced by those boys who have been victimized or raped.

The misuse of the child in the incestuous relationship is a manifestation of the breakdown in the family's ability to regulate the needs and rights of different family members. One misconception in the professional and lay literature is to view the nature of the incest as a *sexual* act. In reality, incest is a complex phenomenon, with aggression, dependency, and the fear of abandonment being central to the behavior. Sexuality is only a means for the expression of family disturbances. The action is usually set in motion by a range of psychological mechanisms the aim of which is to protect the perpetrator's self-image and self-esteem.

This chapter reviews the occurrence of sexual aggression and incest in families, taking into consideration both individual psychopathology and family dysfunction. Some of the literature on the prevalence and incidence rates of incest is reviewed, and a variety of assessment and treatment considerations are discussed.

Definition of Incest

The definition of incest is at once simple and complex (Sholevar 1978). When an act is being defined as incest, the following factors must be considered: 1) the nature of the act, 2) the degree of relationship between the parties, and 3) the ages of the parties involved. Narrowly defined, incest is intimate sexual genital contact between close relatives. However, this definition overlooks the sexual activity with younger children that can include obviously sexual acts such as oral-genital contact, fondling of the genitals, "dry" intercourse, frottage (Faller 1988), and mutual masturbation (Meiselman 1978). Openly seductive behavior by a relative may be included in a definition of incest, but unless there is involvement of the genitalia or anus of one of the partners, the act cannot be *legally* defined as incest. Therefore, what constitutes incest in a *legal* definition may be too restrictive clinically, because incestuous behavior can include gestures, looks, and touching of a sexually explicit nature. For example, a father's fondling of the breasts of his pubertal daughter is an invasive act and can lead to sexual excitation and even orgasm in one or both of the participants.

The relationship of the parties is too narrowly specified in the definition of incest and should be expanded to include reconstituted and foster families. Few disagree with the incestual nature of the interaction when close relatives in biologically related families are involved. However, children, adult stepchildren, and foster and stepchildren are not uniformly or adequately protected by law in all states. This poses a serious clinical problem, especially when a stepparent's unconscious or even conscious sexual attraction for a stepchild may have been from the beginning a major factor in the decision to marry.

The age of the partners involved is also relevant. Sexual contact between younger children (prepubescent) may be considered *sexual play*. Sexual play may also occur between an older and younger adolescent as a result of impulsiveness, sexual anxiety, or age-related fears about moving into the adult world. Sexual play, however, is not characterized by the use of force and is usually entered into with some level of *mutual agreement*. The age difference between the parties should be less than 4 or 5 years.

Incidence and Prevalence of Incest

Incest is perhaps one of the most emotionally charged words in the literature on child abuse and neglect. Incidence rates (i.e., the number of new cases occurring in a specified time period) rarely reflect the true number of children victimized. Furthermore, the total incidence of child sexual abuse known to authorities, whether reports are "validated" or not, is undoubtedly significantly higher than that reported in studies.

In 1991 there were 375,000 reports of children who had been sexually abused. In 85% of these cases, the abuser was a family member or someone close to the family. Sexual activities included genital exposure, intimate kissing, fondling, masturbation, fellatio, cunnilingus, or digital or penile penetration (National Resource Center on Child Sexual Abuse 1992).

There is widespread agreement that each year at least one million children are victims of child abuse, with many cases either never reported or simply dismissed with no further inquiry. There are many discrepancies in the numbers reported, however, because child abuse itself comprises several types of maltreatment. Sexual abuse is a part of a spectrum of maltreatments that includes physical abuse, neglect, and emotional maltreatment. The nature of the sexual act in the sexual abuse further complicates the reporting. An interdisciplinary task force, Project on Child Abuse and Neglect, which studied approximately 200 cases in Michigan, found that 41.2% of the cases involved sexual contact, 19.3% oral sex, and 15.7% genital intercourse. In the largest number of cases, the victims reported forced sexual contact but no injury. The largest number of offenders were biological fathers, and the next largest group was stepfathers. Biological fathers represented 35.7% of the cases when those still married (28.1%) and no longer married (7.6%) to the mother were combined. Stepfathers and mother's boyfriends accounted for 17.3% and 9.2% of the cases, respectively.

The National Institute of Mental Health funded a data-gathering project to study the incidence and prevalence of intrafamilial and extrafamilial child sexual abuse in women aged 18 years and older. In a sample of 930 women in San Francisco, 16% reported having experienced at least one incident of intrafamilial sexual abuse prior to age 18 years. Twelve percent had been sexually abused by a *relative* before age 14. Thirty-one percent reported having experienced at least one incident of sexual abuse by a *nonrelative* before age 18, and 20% reported having been subjected to sexual abuse by a non-relative before age 14.

The first national prevalence study found that 27% of the women and 16% of the men in the sample had experienced some form of child sexual victimization (National Resource Center on Child Sexual Abuse 1992). A study by Finkelhor (1990) determined that the median age at abuse was 9.6 years for girls. Large-scale community surveys indicate that 1 in 4 girls and 1 in 10 boys have been sexually abused before age 18 (Finkelhor 1979, 1984, 1990; Russell 1986).

In summary, no figures can accurately reflect the incest problem, and the National Resource Center on Child Sexual Abuse (1992) notes that, despite numerous studies, they simply do not know for certain how many children are sexually abused each year. One restriction to obtaining an accurate estimate of the prevalence of child sexual abuse is that children do not readily disclose their victimization because of fear, shame, or lack of understanding of its wrongfulness, among other explanations. The lack of a mandated reporting system to a national central authority imposes another restriction.

Differences in study samples and methodology, such as those that follow, are further indications of underreporting:

1. There is no uniform definition of terms across studies. For example, some studies include adolescents up to the age of 18 years, whereas other studies exclude children over age 12 years.
2. Some studies include intrafamilial sexual abuse as well as sexual abuse by unrelated adults.
3. Studies are generally retrospective and depend on the ability and willingness of adults to recall events that may have been repressed from consciousness.
4. Research methodologies for data collection vary considerably. (Telephone calls, personal interviews, and written questionnaires will provide different estimates.)

5. Sampling methods, including recruitment methods, vary, and this results in large differences in findings.

Historical Perspective on Incest

Incest is a familiar theme in mythology, history, and religion. Greek mythology abounded with accounts of incest among close relatives. Zeus, born of the union between a brother and sister, raped his mother, Rhea, and married his sister Hera. He produced many children through incestuous relationships, including a child with his daughter Persephone, who herself was the offspring of incest between Zeus and his sister. Oedipus is the most celebrated case of incest in the psychiatric literature.

Brother–sister incest was common among the Egyptian deities. In ancient Egypt, the practice of incest was well celebrated. Cleopatra was the product of many generations of incestuous relationships and married one of her siblings. The conservation of wealth and power seemed to be an important motive for the Egyptians as well as other ancient groups.

Since the early seventeenth and eighteenth centuries, parent–child incest has been viewed as inappropriate sexual intimacy that disrupts the developmental needs of the child (Aries and Duby 1989). The incestuous relationship is illegal throughout the United States. The last group to practice incest or marry their close relatives were the Mormons. The practice of marriage between cousins, a common practice in Middle Eastern countries, has been abandoned in the Western world.

The incest taboo has been supported by psychological and sociological, as well as sociobiological, theories and serves the function of protecting the human species. Freud (1913/1953) proposed the theory of the "primal herd," in which was described the killing of the tyrannical father by his sons to gain access to the women in the herd. The incest taboo in this view was a way of regulating rivalry between the sons and fathers for the women. Malinowski (1927), providing an anthropological explanation, described the incest taboo as a method of regulating the balance of power in the family. Mead (1935) hypothesized that the function of the incest taboo was to minimize the jealousy and rivalry between the children and the parents of the same sex while maintaining family cohesiveness and integrity.

Causality

Different theories of causality of incest have been proposed; however, one of the primary factors is the *sexual attraction of the offender to children*. This attraction can be *situational* and the result of arousal by pornography or physical contact, or the result of some regressed, psychological state in the offender. It can be more *characterological*, as in the case of the pedophile, who engages in a compulsive pattern of sexual attraction and victimization of children. A second factor is the *willingness to act on the sexual attraction*. This will depend in part on the intensity of the feeling, the character of the offender, and his or her overcoming physical or environmental constraints on this behavior. The final, and most important, factor is the *child's participation*, which is brought about through conscious manipulation, coercion, or unconscious projective identification.

The closeness of the relationship between victim and offender plays a significant role in the initiation, duration, and frequency of the behavior, as well as the nature of the act; the child's reaction to it; the parent's reaction upon discovery; and the psychological damage to the child. In the case of father–daughter incest, it is not uncommon for the father to progress from appropriate affectionate behavior to more intrusive sexual behavior, including mutual masturbation, oral or anal sex, and then intercourse. Given the closeness of the biological relationship, there is more access to the child, less need for persuasion, and ultimately more harm because of the misuse of the child's affection and trust.

Children with mental retardation or physical disability are 4 to 10 times more vulnerable to victimization than nondisabled children (National Resource Center on Child Sexual Abuse 1992). In about 2% of cases, mental retardation of victim or offender or of both is a causative factor (G. Goff and D. Demetral, personal communication to K. C. Faller, cited in Faller 1983, p. 79). Lacking positive and gratifying experiences at school or with peers because of their disabilities, children with mental retardation or physical disability are prone to accept the sexual attention of the offender regardless of his or her relationship to them. Furthermore, these children may be more compliant or lack ability to assert their rights or complain and may even believe they are a burden to family members.

Risks to Individuals and Families

At-Risk Families

A review of the research by Finkelhor and colleagues (Browne and Finkelhor 1986; Finkelhor 1987, 1990, 1995; Finkelhor and Baron 1986; Finkelhor and Berliner 1995) has indicated that certain family contexts place the child at greater risk for sexual and physically aggressive behavior than do others:

1. Single-parent homes
2. Child's having a poor relationship with parents or being subjected to very punitive discipline practices
3. Presence of a stepfather in the child's home
4. Absence of the mother from the home because she is working outside the home, is ill, or has a disability
5. Presence in the home of a sexual abuser who reveals high arousal to children or has history of sexual deviance and deviant fantasies that date back to his or her adolescence
6. Conflict or disruption in the normal adult heterosexual relationship in the home
7. Alcohol use at the time of sexual abuse (typically not a causative factor in the abuse)
8. A history of sexual and physical abuse in one or both parents' family history

Violence can be readily manifested as a response to the cumulative stress that occurs when too many of these contexts are present in the family.

Psychological Impact of Incest

The long-term effect of incest may include disturbances in object relations manifested by an inability to form trusting relationships, withdrawal, depression, and various disturbances in social behavior. It is not uncommon for victims of incest to display dissociative symptomatology. They may present as stoically accepting psychological manipulation of themselves, an abuse of their person, or even sexual harassment. They simply seem to "take it" and not express indignation. Helping them to face the insult to themselves is one of the most difficult parts of treatment because of the shame and guilt they experience. Sexuality becomes disturbed, and its expression may run the gamut from lack of sexual interest to excessive or impulsive sexual activity. Greenacre (1950/1969) noted that the traumatized child often acts out or "plays out" the trauma in an attempt at mastery of the event. Sexually abused children (not only incest victims) tend to repeat trauma-related patterns of sexual behavior. Rasmussen and colleagues (1992) suggest three outcomes for these children: 1) they can express and then work through their feelings, 2) they can develop self-destructive behavior such as self-victimization, or 3) they can identify with the aggressor and abuse others.

Triangulation

Triangulation of the children into the marital problems and the use of the child as a scapegoat is a common observation (Rist 1979). Intergenerational patterns of shame in families contribute to psychiatric disturbances such as addictive behavior or compulsion and sexual, physical, or emotional abuse. Friedrich and colleagues (Friedrich et al. 1988, 1993) found that sexually abused children display more behavior problems than nonabused children in a nonpsychiatric population. Sexually abused girls tend to have more *externalizing* psychopathology than do nonpsychiatric control subjects. Their sexual behavior problems are associated with higher levels of aggression, acting-out behavior, and conduct problems (Costentino et al. 1995).

Incestuous families use major shared intrapsychic defenses—denial, dissociation, and projective identification—which contribute to the intergenerational abuse. *Denial* is a shared family defense that keeps the incest secret while protecting the family's appearance as a normally functioning family. The *dissociative process*, which is part of the victim's defenses, prevents the feelings and impulses attached to the incestuous relationship from reaching awareness. It also dilutes the anxiety that can erupt through the patient's fears of losing the security and approval needed to establish and maintain a sense of self in the family. *Projective identification* is both an interactional and an intrapsychic defense that is pervasive in incestuous families. Projective identification defends against the sexual deficiencies in both mother and father, serves to reduce the fear of separation and the dissolution of the marriage, and further maintains the family-of-origin integrity. The victim of sexual abuse becomes a collaborator in both father's and mother's unacceptable impulses. There is a reciprocal unconscious collusion between child and family in this projection process. The child becomes a caretaker of the father's sexual and functional role in the family, possibly protecting him from further acting-out beyond the family. She also protects the mother's fragile view of herself as a competent wife and mother. Through this unmanageable dual role, the child keeps the family together.

Posttraumatic Stress Disorder

Child sexual abuse is one of the major contributors to posttraumatic stress disorder (PTSD) and dissociative disorders. PTSD symptoms, which include intrusive, distressing dreams and recollections, avoidant behaviors, a numbing of general responsiveness, and symptoms of increased arousal and dissociative behavior (American Psychiatric Association 1994), are manifested in the behavior of most incest victims. Dissociative features are quite common in victims of abuse and often are part of the borderline syndrome exhibited. "Sleeper effects" have been found, whereby children's problems do not surface until many years later and are often triggered by developmental challenges (Briere 1992; Finkelhor and Berliner 1995).

Types of Incest

Incest is a defensive function that aims to maintain family homeostasis while attempting to contain the anxieties and conflicts about abandonment, aggression, and sexuality. Sholevar (1978) has proposed a comprehensive view that incestuous behavior may develop when the coping mechanisms in the family can no longer manage family conflicts without violating the integrity of the system. Thus, in one sense, the incestuous behavior is an expression of the family's efforts to solve its problems and create a new equilibrium with a more manageable level of dissonance. However, like all primarily defensive behavior, incest does not achieve an enduring pattern of wholesome social balance in the family. The family continues with its defective relationship, further burdened by the consequences of the incestuous behavior.

Father–Daughter Incest

▶ Prevalence and Disclosure

The literature on father–daughter incest is more available and well documented than that on other types of incest. Available figures indicate that 70% to 80% of *reported* incest cases occur between daughters and their natural father or father-figure (Green 1988; Swanson and Biaggio 1985). In about 50% of cases of father–daughter incest, it is the natural father who is the perpetrator (Brant and Tisva 1977; DeFrancis 1965).

Sgroi (1988) notes that the abuse moves in a predictable pattern from one of an engagement phase to sexual interaction, secrecy, disclosure, and, often, suppression following disclosure. The behaviors progress from less to more sexual forms and are maintained by the powerful reinforcement provided by the inequities in the parent–child relationship. The victim makes few sexual demands, and the offender experiences intense pleasure based on his power and dominance.

The secrecy required to protect the relationship, as well as to maintain family cohesion, becomes a powerful reinforcer. Summit (1983) has called this an "accommodation." Here the victim who feels helpless and entrapped accommodates through secrecy, helplessness, and entrapment, which is followed by an unconvincing disclosure by the victim and then retraction. It is very common for a victim to recant and deny that the abuse ever occurred.

Sexually abused children also tend to repeat trauma-related patterns of sexual behavior. They may move from a passive to a more active and sexually aggressive mode as a way of gaining temporary relief from the experienced trauma and its memory (Costentino et al. 1995).

▶ Paternal Characteristics and Risk Factors

Finkelhor (1990) reviewed 29 studies of paternal sexual abuse that discussed paternal characteristics, patterns of behavior, and dynamics. These studies reported that fathers who abused their daughters did not exhibit one particular psychological profile. Some fathers presented with personality disorders characterized by a tendency to exhibit intense involvement and overcontrolling attitudes toward their daughters bordering on paranoid thinking. They were heavily dependent on the family for emotional and social relationships. Others presented with pedophilic sexual preferences (Abel et al. 1983), a sexual orientation characterized by disinterest in, disgust with, or conflict over sexual relations with adults (Baker 1985; Marshall et al. 1986). Faller (1988) has disputed the more classical incest pattern in which incest becomes a family defense against disintegration or further disruption. She found paternal preferences for children to be just as potent as the wife's lack of desire or desirability and other more structural problems in the family. Based on the early work by the Kinsey Institute, it was believed that alcohol consumption weakened inhibitions and allowed for the initiation of the incestuous behavior. In subsequent studies, however, drug and alcohol abuse has *not* been found to be a major factor (Herman 1981; Mandel 1986; Parker and Parker 1986).

Finkelhor and Baron (1986) and Russell (1984) note that daughters are at greater risk for sexual abuse by *stepfathers* than by natural fathers because of the weakened bond created by the absence of an early caretaking relationship. Russell (1984), in fact, states that a stepdaughter is *seven* times more likely to suffer abuse than is a natural daughter. One factor contributing to this increased risk is that the role of the stepfather may be unclear, in which case the relationship between the child and parent is further complicated. If the mother does not attempt to clarify the stepfather's role, the incest taboo is further diluted. This is especially problematic when the adult has the psychological and sexual readiness to become aggressive and abusive toward children. Another factor is that in some cases the mother's own psychopathology can contribute to the violence and sexual abuse. The coercive cycle can manifest itself as a type of jealousy over the stepfather's attention to the daughter.

Social isolation, poor social skills, and a limited social network also have been noted among fathers who sexually abuse their daughters (Araji and Finkelhor 1986; Kirkland and Bauer 1982; Panton 1979; Parker 1984; Scott and Stone 1986). Lacking more appropriate sexual partners, the father or stepfather may turn to the daughter, especially if the marital relationship becomes problematic.

It has been suggested that more than half of incestuous fathers studied have a family background of physical, though not necessarily sexual, abuse (Brandon 1985; Mandel 1986; Parker and Parker 1986). Reports of previous incest involving other family members in the families of origin as victims have been confirmed (Bennett 1985; Brandon 1985). Results from the Minnesota Multiphasic Personality Inventory (MMPI) and projective instruments demonstrate that one-quarter to one-third of incestuous fathers are *not* psychiatrically ill. They have elevated scores for aggressiveness/ rebelliousness factors indicative of persons who show a disregard for the rights of others and violate social norms while experiencing minimal feelings of guilt. These factors are suggestive of sociopathic tendencies. Some of the findings regarding dominance–dependency and abusiveness–passivity have been contradictory. Victims report a history of aggressiveness and abusiveness among these men. Faller (1988) has found that the initiation of a divorce often opens the way for these aggressive and abusive behaviors. Very often following a divorce, the noncustodial father with sexual and aggressive tendencies that he concealed during the marriage acts out those tendencies.

Sibling Incest

Although father–daughter incest is the most frequently discussed and reported form of incest, sibling incest is believed to be the *most widespread* (Forward and Buck 1979). Sibling incest has been estimated to be at least *five times* more prevalent than parent–child incest (Cole 1982; Smith and Israel 1987). The subject of sibling incest has not been studied or documented as well as have other forms of incest. Therefore, there has been a tendency to group all intrafamilial incest dynamics together rather than to define the different characteristics of each type. Debate continues among different professionals concerning the traumatic effects of sibling incest. Some mutual sexual exploration among same-age children is seen as a normal part of a child's psychosexual development (Bank and Kahn 1982; Courtois 1988; Forward and Buck 1979; Russell 1986).

More frequently, sibling incest can provide a mutual nurturance and acceptance that is missing in the relationship with the parents (Bank and Kahn 1982). Sibling incest more commonly occurs when children live in overcrowded homes, are unsupervised, and are poorly cared for by their parents (Finkelhor 1979; Meiselman 1978; Russell 1986). The playful sexual activities go unrestrained and over time develop into incestuous behavior. Victimization is possible, however, when underlying the incestuous act are violent, coercive, and power-oriented motives. Courtois (1988) suggests three variations of this relationship: 1) a pubescent brother who uses a younger, naive sister for sexual experimentation; 2) a misfit or outcast brother who substitutes a sister for female friends and abuses her affection; and 3) a much older brother who forces sexual activity on a sister through coercive means. Most often, the incest stops once the siblings engage in appropriate peer relationships outside the home. The brother often models his behavior on what was witnessed between the father and daughter in the home. These relationships can develop into an intergenerational pattern in which these brothers continue the pattern with their own children.

Personality factors and characterological disturbances motivate and sustain incestuous behavior between siblings; however, incest between siblings is more likely to occur when indiscriminate sexuality occurs in the family. Physical proximity, such as shared rooms and beds, helps siblings turn to each other for emotional care. This type of incest is underreported because the neglectful parents either do not recognize it or covertly condone it.

In the absence of longitudinal studies, it is difficult to predict the long-term effects of sibling incestuous behavior. However, re-searchers have observed that some of the problems that the sisters in these relationships experience are similar to those experienced by daughters who are victims of father–daughter incest. They are less likely to marry, are more likely to be abused in their marriages if they marry, and continue to fear sexual assault (Courtois 1988; Russell 1986). In addition, they often have more guilt and feelings of complicity (Courtois 1988), experience lowered sexual self-esteem (Finkelhor 1980), have difficulties in sexual and intimate relationships and preorgasmic functioning (Cole 1982; Meiselman 1978; Russell 1986), are at risk for depression and suicide attempts (Cole 1982; Laviola 1989; Loredo 1982), and are often victimized socially and sexually (Cole 1982; Deyoung 1982; Meiselman 1978).

Some general observations have been made above regarding the impact of sibling incest:

1. Children who are denied appropriate parental nurturance may turn to each other and become locked into a physical and emotional bond that ties them to the family through secrecy for protection and security.
2. The guilt attached to the secret is increased if the incestous behavior is a first sexual experience.
3. The incestuous relationship can interfere with the children's ability to establish (more socially appropriate) love relationships because the mutual dependency and sense of acceptance granted by the relationship hinder development.
4. If violence occurs or if the relationship is no longer mutually consensual, the victim feels entitled to repair this harm through exploitation in other relationships, holding those relationships responsible for the abuse inflicted by the past.

Mother–Son Incest

Mother–son incest is estimated to constitute as much as 10% of all cases of incest. Maternal psychosis often has been erroneously impli-cated in the genesis of this relationship; in the cases reported in the literature, however, repeated separation from the mother at significant developmental periods is described. Affected by such extensive separation, the son may see incest as a way of gaining closeness to his mother or as revenge for the separation. This type of incest seldom occurs in intact families because the presence of the father tends to maintain the family structure and bring about the appropriate distance between mother and son. However, some female sex offenders have reported abusing children at the insistence of a man (see Chapter 7, this volume).

Incest With Extended Family Members

Incest with extended family members (between children and, e.g., grandparents, uncles, or aunts) may be discovered by the parents, but they generally do not try to prosecute the perpetrators or obtain treatment for them. Researchers have concluded that there is less psychological harm associated with incest with relatives, especially those distant from the nuclear family, because the family members attach less emotional significance to their relationship with the perpetrator (Landis 1956; Peters 1976).

Detection of Incestuous Behavior

Individual Manifestations

Behaviors of the child or adolescent and conditions that should alert the clinician to the possibility of incestuous behavior include the following:

1. Extreme fear for no apparent reason
2. Severe depression
3. Serious runaway behavior
4. Contracting of venereal disease, but denial of being sexually active or of being a victim of rape
5. Pregnancy, possibly in conjunction with vague stories about the father of the child
6. Inability to trust, as exhibited in poor object relations

7. Sexual precociousness or inhibition
8. Severe conduct disorders and academic failure following a previous history of good adjustment and success in school
9. Acute psychotic breaks or sudden self-destructive behavior
10. Sleep disorder or frequent excessive sleepiness
11. Ongoing school truancy that is often the result of the child's reversed role in the family (the child may refuse to attend school because she or he views school as a child's activity)
12. Pseudo-mature behavior at an early age
13. Depression, guilt, and embarrassment, particularly following sexual behavior
14. Displaced anger toward others
15. Somatic complaints, such as headaches or stomachaches, that have no organic cause
16. Loneliness much of the time and lack of friends
17. Tendency to be angry with the mother for mistreatment of the father or to feel sorry for the father

The individual manifestations of incestuous behavior depend on the child or adolescent's psychological makeup and age and the general environment in the home. These factors influence the course and outcome and must therefore be assessed carefully.

Sexually inappropriate and aggressive behavior is reflected in intergenerational, interpersonal, and intrapsychic disturbances. Characteristics typical of boundary disturbances include

1. Poor body/self image
2. Disturbances among family members in which inappropriate sexual behavior is fostered between members
3. Exploitation and subtle manipulation and coercion through touch and body contact of family members
4. Lack of respect for both physical and emotional privacy as evidenced in, for example, intrusive, overly detailed questioning of the adolescent's sexual behavior
5. Lack of affective communication, misinformation about sex, and the inability to discuss feelings regarding sex
6. Distortions, myths, and stereotypes—stemming from the lack

of knowledge about sex—that very often manifest in the disturbed relationships

In the assessment of the family dynamics, the therapist must especially attend to the patient's presentation. Incestuous behavior can be described as a continuum, with varying degrees of aggressive and coercive behavior being a part of the sexual experience. Questions can be raised about sleeping arrangements, bathroom "rules," attitudes about intercourse and when dating is appropriate, exposure to television shows and movies, and so forth. The therapist should not overlook the possibility of false memory and confusion of memory in which the events of childhood can be mislabeled as being incestuous because of the arousal, fear, or anxiety involved with the entire sexual issue. The family's communication patterns are also observed—for example, do father and mother display a great deal of conflict avoidance while maintaining secretiveness and hostility in their exchanges? Do the children, especially the incest victim, talk to parents and not to each other? Is there a level of discomfort raised in the therapist as she or he explores family interactions? Does the therapist feel a "pressure" exerted by the family to minimize the obvious problems?

In addition, information from collateral sources such as other family members and even the children's friends is important. Assessment can include reports from the school authorities and the legal system, including probation departments. Medical consultation should be considered, particularly if infections, pregnancy, bulimia, and anorexia are part of the incest syndrome.

Detection Through Family Interactions

Incestuous behavior should also be suspected when there is an overly close relationship between a parent and child, particularly of the opposite sex. One child may receive extreme preferential treatment over another child in the family. The father may show extreme jealousy as his daughter reaches puberty. Very often the parents have a background of emotional deprivation, neglect, and/or victimization, sexual or physical.

The Role of Denial

The denial of incest by the family is a general rule rather than an exception. Even when the child repeatedly has informed the health-care professional of incestuous acts, she may retract her statements under parental pressure or because of fear of punishment. Trepper and Barrett (1989) described the many forms that denial takes as occurring in multiple stages. In the first stage, there is denial of the *facts*. Family members simply deny that incest ever occurred. As this phenomenon drops away, there begins a second stage—denial of *awareness*—in which the incest is admitted but blame is projected outward. For example, the father may blame the incestuous behavior on his drinking, or the mother may simply say that she was not at home or was never told about the incident(s). The child may say that she did not realize that what was happening was sexual. In the third stage—denial of *responsibility*—each person involved blames the other or some external factor. After this source of denial is stripped away, there is a fourth stage—denial of *impact*—in which the family denies the immediate and long-term impact of the incest by minimizing its traumatic effects. The family holds back and becomes more protective through obfuscation. The clinician must gradually, progressively, but cautiously confront the denial.

Disclosure

If the clinician is in the position of being the first to learn about the incest, it is best to help the victim prepare for the disclosure to her family because it can result in retaliation, violence, further denial, or additional scapegoating in the family. Courtois (1988) suggests that the motivation behind the disclosure needs to be explored. Is the victim making the disclosure to seek relief from guilt? Is she motivated by anger and the need to retaliate? Does she suspect other incest in the family and want to protect someone in the family? Is she attempting to confront the issue in order to make the incestuous behavior a reality rather than deny it any longer?

The therapist should take time with the patient and be certain that multiple aspects of issues have been explored. Once such exploration has taken place, the therapist can move into family treatment. She or he should recommend a careful assessment of the patient's pretrauma functioning and family history, the traumatic incestuous events, and any other types of trauma that may have occurred. In light of the recent controversy over "false memory," it is imperative that the treating physician or clinician ensure that memories are not the product of suggestion.

Family Configurations and Incest: Structural Considerations

Certain dysfunctional family structures and patterns occur commonly in incestuous families (Alexander 1990; Trepper and Barrett 1986, 1989). These include the following:

1. Weakened generational boundaries cause poor demarcation of roles and responsibility ties among members.
2. The family is isolated from the social community, dependent on itself for most of its emotional needs and perhaps lacking the social skills for engaging in more appropriate peer relationships.
3. Children are triangulated into the emotionally detached parental system.
4. Disturbances in the marital and sexual relationship are exhibited in interactions such as blaming, scapegoating, and "acting-out."
5. Distancing maneuvers, such as provocations, fights without conflict resolution, and abandonment of parental and marital roles, are noted.
6. Family secrets exist regarding sexual matters, including affairs, promiscuity, and abortions in the family. Splits, alliances, and coalitions among members result from this secret keeping.
7. There are disturbances in the sibling subsystem manifested by the siblings' either functioning separately from one another or fusing identities. The children "appear" older than they are but are emotionally quite unsophisticated and immature.
8. Active and intentional encouragement of the denial of feelings creates an atmosphere of constant doubt and questioning of reality.

9. Parent–child disturbances can be seen in the inconsistent, unpredictable, and erratic parenting around discipline and management issues.
10. The children are parentified and remain so throughout their childhood and, possibly, adulthood.
11. Abused children learn a *victim* role that involves helplessness and intimidation against changing or speaking up.

Incest is not simply sexual abuse of a child. It is the abuse of the child's relationship with her parents, with her siblings, and with future generations. Her exploitation leaves her vulnerable, distrustful, and confused because the person on whom she most depends for love, safety, and loyalty has neglected her and abused the parental and family role. The child gets pulled into the family's sexual needs. Furthermore, these relationships may continue for a number of years, with all-too-negative results. The victim of father–daughter incest leaves the relationship in one of four possible ways: 1) the daughter refuses to continue the relationship; 2) the daughter leaves home; 3) the mother, daughter, or another family member becomes involved in fights with the father and reports the incest; or 4) the daughter becomes pregnant (venereal disease rarely provides a similar exit into medical discovery of the incest). Obviously, the more aggressive and coercive the relationship, the more psychologically damaging the relationship is to the victim.

Family and Individual Assessment Techniques

The clinician assessing an incestuous family should be mindful that the family members are deeply fearful of the consequences of revealing their incestuous relationship to the therapist or outsiders and will adhere to denial of any inappropriate, deviant, or exploitative relationships. The nonincestuous family, on the other hand, will exhibit some anxiety but will cooperate with the therapist in the assessment of their family behavior.

The multiple factors that predispose and encourage incestuous behavior necessitate consideration. The family therapist working with the identified patient and family engaged in the incestuous behavior must have adequate assessment measures in order to evaluate the family's structure, defensive style, and coping skills and to design the proper treatment plan.

Assessment Tools

Several assessment tools can be used in the interview:

1. The MMPI can be used both to evaluate possible psychopathology—including sociopathy and depression, which are both relevant in cases of incest—and to identify general personality characteristics.
2. The Thematic Aptitude Test (TAT) can be used to uncover material concerning interpersonal relations and perceptions of roles of individuals in the family as well as to identify defenses and conflicts.
3. Olson's Circumplex Model (Olson 1982) measures the two interacting dimensions of cohesion and adaptability. *Cohesion* assesses the degree to which family members are emotionally connected or distant from one another. *Adaptability* assesses the extent to which the family exhibits flexibility and adaptation to change. Most families involved in incest appear as rigid and enmeshed or as chaotic and enmeshed.
4. The Family Strengths and Family Coping Strategies Inventory (Olson 1982) is an objective measure of those families that are most vulnerable to incest because of a past history of sexual or physical child abuse. Dimensions such as problem-solving ability, extended family and its availability, and utilization of social networks are assessed.
5. The Child Posttraumatic Stress Disorder Reaction Index (Frederick et al. 1992) is a 20-item self-report interview format that addresses the child's symptoms.
6. The DSM-IV criteria for PTSD (American Psychiatric Association 1994) describe the manifestations of PTSD in detail.
7. The Child Behavior Checklist (Achenbach and Edelbrock 1986) is a comprehensive assessment tool for obtaining information from both parents and the child's teacher(s).

Interviewing the Victim

Because talking to the victim can be especially difficult, we suggest contacting the National Clearinghouse on Child Abuse and Neglect Information, at 1-800-394-3366 (http://www.calib.com), for information on special training in this area. The techniques for interviewing should above all place the victim at ease while being objective and clear.

Family Intervention Strategies With Incest

Considering the complexities involved in cases of incest, it is safe to say that no one set of intervention strategies is appropriate for all families. Some guidelines are needed to ensure that all family members' needs are addressed and that the legal, medical, and psychological issues are considered.

Stage One: Early Intervention

Early intervention requires a coordination of services among caseworkers and the juvenile court and probation department; the appropriate services depend on the nature of the act. The first step in intervention is to *report* the suspected incestuous relationship to the local child protection service, which in turn will inform state social services. This reporting is mandated by the National Child Abuse Prevention Act of 1974 and by state laws that cover physical and sexual abuse of children, incest, and child neglect. The law requires physicians, mental health professionals, teachers, and others who come in contact with children to report cases of suspected abuse. The incest victim frequently reveals the incestuous relationship after she has obtained a promise that the secret will be kept. As a result, the mental health professional may consider not reporting the incest. Such a decision would reenact the silent pact between the victim and offender and place the victim at great risk, further undermining her trust in adults or authority figures.

Protection is the primary concern for the victim as well as for other siblings in the home. It may mean that the offender and victim must live apart for a period of time. It may be best to remove the offender, since removing the victim communicates blame and separates her from the family, who will in turn further isolate her in an effort to keep the secret. Removing the offender can actually promote change because it underlines an adult's responsibility for the protection of children, holds the offender accountable, reassigns the child's position as child in the family in which parentification existed, and increases motivation for treatment since the offender will want to return to his home. Because incest violates children's basic right to protection and safety, through removal of the offender, professionals can be recognized as setting appropriate and needed limits and boundaries on family behavior. Notifying child protection agencies and establishing a liaison with the necessary personnel alerts the family to the seriousness of the situation, adds to the child's protection under the law, enlists the protection agency's help in making decisions concerning the conditions of visitation, and places appropriate constraints on supervision of interaction.

Stage Two: Crisis Management

Once the report has been made, *crisis management* is implemented. The family may react to the disclosure or suspicion of incest with different forms of acting-out, including suicide attempts by the mother or the victim; new forms of seductive or even promiscuous behavior and violence; and mimicked incestuous behavior between siblings. Once the offender is removed, the mother may become overwhelmed with the responsibilities for family management and neglect or abandon the children. A characteristic pattern is increased alcohol use, emotional withdrawal, and erratic behavior. The therapist will need to set limits on his or her availability while providing a sense of security for the family during their crisis. This may necessitate the involvement of crisis team members who can respond to different family members as needed. The therapist's ability to maintain objectivity and boundaries is crucial at this time.

Stage Three: Individual and Family Treatment

The third stage is to provide *individual treatment* for the victim, make it available to her mother, and offer *family treatment*. The mother may need to become involved in therapy groups with other mothers or to attend parenting skills classes or stress management programs as part of the total family treatment. The offender will need his own individual treatment. Family intervention/family therapy will develop as the incest pattern is revealed and the patient feels prepared to speak in front of all of the family members. All decisions regarding the return of the offender to the family home should be made only after consideration of the impact that such decisions will have on all family members.

Therapists need to remain alert to the family's style of interaction, which includes secrecy, denial, fusion, and enmeshment. The family members will be especially adept at merging with the therapist if it is allowed, and therefore a firm boundary between clinician and patient/family is vital. Families in which incest is taking place are skilled at engaging the therapist in side-taking strategies. Overly identifying with the victim, feeling sorry for the offender, or simply missing the powerful projections of blame in the family can greatly impede treatment as well as create further distortions in the family's already weakened sense of reality.

Broader Interventions With Incest

Many individual strategies can be applied in treatment that prepare the victim and strengthen her attempt to confront the incest and her victimization.

1. Individual sessions can include a rehearsal of the confrontation prior to the family session. Solution-based techniques (Bass and Davis 1988; de Shazer 1985, 1988; de Shazer et al. 1986; Dolan 1985)—for example, imagining the worst that could happen if the offender is confronted and then role playing this feared confrontational scene with the therapist—are helpful in treatment. Psychotherapy for PTSD symptoms includes supporting adaptive coping skills by positive self-talk and relaxation with visualization; normalizing the symptoms; and decreasing avoidance.
2. The therapist can encourage the patient to write three-part healing letters in which the details of the incest are described, the

feelings and aftermath are outlined, and the responses are pre-dicted. These letters, written *but never mailed*, help prepare the patient for the responses she can expect and give her a sense of power and some control over the encounter. These techniques aim at offering hope to the patient while mobilizing her own internal resources.

3. Another solution-based strategy described by de Shazer (1985, pp. 120–122) is having the patient write down on a small piece of paper her feelings—that it wasn't her fault and she is *not* to blame—and, after the patient reads what she has written, set the paper on fire. This type of ritual is aimed at promoting self-healing through symbolic activity.

4. Associational cues are also part of the repertoire of techniques aimed at providing symbolic sources of comfort and security. In this technique, as described by Dolan (1991), the patient is 1) helped to identify an experience in which "relative" but not total comfort and security was experienced; 2) directed to "no-tice and describe all the details of the experience with special attention to sights, sounds, sensation"; 3) "make adjustments, additions, and subtractions of details to further enhance the comfort and security of the experience," 4) tell the therapist when the experience is "just right," and 5) invite her to "enjoy the experience one more time and while doing so, to select a little symbol that can serve to remind her of the pleasant expe-rience in the future."

5. The therapist encourages the involvement of supportive family members or friends who will listen to the patient's story and help the victim get through discussing the details.

6. In cases of father–daughter incest, sessions should be held be-tween mother and daughter to help heal wounds through un-derstanding and forgiveness. This offers protection and a sense of safety for the victim, as well as making it possible for the mother to assume a parental position in the family. Very often, mothers in this situation are frightened for their physical and financial safety and jeopardize their children's rights rather than risk family integrity.

Conclusion

The phenomenon of incest can be best understood and treated within the context of the family. Incestuous relationships are a sign of disturbances in family relationships in which the family members are unable to negotiate their basic needs for nurturance, trust, affection, sexuality, and aggression. The difficulties with the negotiation of the above functions are the result of the failure of the family and its members to achieve their progressive development in the contemporary and historical spheres. Being unable to pursue a developmental course in a normative fashion, the family will fall back on the defensive maneuver of regulating the aggressive, sexual, dependency, and affectionate needs of its members in an exploitative and socially unacceptable manner. The goal of this behavior is generally to prevent family breakup or abandonment of other family members, which historically is a common fear in incestuous families. However, unlike families with other primarily defensive relational patterns, incestuous families are burdened by further social, clinical, and legal consequences of the behavior.

It has been a major conceptual misperception to treat the incestuous behavior as a manifestation of the perpetrator's personality deficiencies. There is a need to look not only at the perpetrator's role but also at the contributions of the parents and the vulnerabilities in the victim that make her particularly prone to exploitation by the perpetrator. However, even this expanded view does not recognize the powerful impact of family organization and rules in the promotion of incestuous behavior.

References

Abel G, Mittelman M, Becker J, et al: The characteristics of men who molest young children. Paper presented at the World Congress of Behavior Therapy, Washington, DC, December 1983

Achenbach T, Edelbrock C: Manual for the Child Behavior Checklist and Revised Child Behavioral Profile. Burlington, VT, University of Vermont, Department of Psychology, 1986

Alexander PC: The role of the extended family in the evaluation and treatment of incest, in Casebook of Sexual Abuse Treatment. Edited by Friedrich WN. New York, WW Norton, 1990, pp 79–87

American Psychiatric Association: Diagnostic and Statistical Manual of Mental Disorders, 4th Edition. Washington, DC, American Psychiatric Association, 1994

Araji S, Finkelhor D: Abusers: a review of the research, in A Sourcebook on Child Sexual Abuse. Edited by Finkelhor D, and Associates. Newbury Park, CA, Sage Publications, 1986, pp 89–118

Aries P, Duby G: A History of Private Life, Vol 3. Cambridge, MA, Belknap Press/Harvard University Press, 1989

Baker D: Father-daughter incest: a study of the father. Dissertation Abstracts International 46 (suppl 3):951B, 1985

Bank SP, Kahn M: The Sibling Bond. New York, Basic Books, 1982

Bass E, Davis L: The Courage to Heal. New York, Harper & Row, 1988

Bennett SR: Cognitive style of incestuous fathers. Dissertation Abstracts International 42 (suppl 2):778B, 1985

Brandon C: Sex role identification in incest: an empirical analysis of the feminist theories. Dissertation Abstracts International 47 (suppl 7): 3099B, 1985

Brant RST, Tisva VB: Sexually misused child. Am J Orthopsychiatry 47:80–90, 1977

Briere J: Child Abuse Trauma: Theory and Treatment of the Lasting Effects. Newbury Park, CA, Sage Publications, 1992

Browne A, Finkelhor D: Impact of child sexual abuse: a review of the research. Psychol Bull 99 (suppl 1):66–77, 1986

Cole E: Sibling incest: the myth of benign sibling incest. Women and Therapy 5:79–89, 1982

Costentino D, Heino F, Meyer-Bahlburg D: Sexual behavior problems and psychopathology symptoms in sexually abused girls. J Am Acad Child Adolesc Psychiatry 34 (suppl 8):1033–1039, 1995

Courtois C: Healing the Incest Wound: Adult Survivors in Therapy. New York, WW Norton, 1988

DeFrancis V: Protecting the Child Sex Victim. Denver, CO, American Humane Association, 1965

de Shazer S: Keys to Solution in Brief Therapy. New York, WW Norton, 1985

de Shazer S: Clues: Instigating Solutions in Brief Therapy. New York, WW Norton, 1988 de Shazer S, Berg I, Lipchick E, et al: Brief therapy: focused solution development. Fam Process 25:207–222, 1986

Deyoung M: Self-injurious behavior in incest victims: a research note. Child Welfare 62:577–584, 1982

Dolan Y: A Path With a Heart: Ericksonian Utilization With Resistant and Chronic Clients. New York, Brunner/Mazel, 1985

Dolan Y: Resolving Sexual Abuse. New York, WW Norton, 1991

Faller KC (ed): Child Sexual Abuse. New York, Columbia University Press, 1983

Faller KC: Child Sexual Abuse: An Interdisciplinary Manual for Diagnosis, Case Management and Treatment. New York, Columbia University Press, 1988

Finkelhor D: Sexually Victimized Children. New York, Free Press, 1979

Finkelhor D: Sex among siblings: a survey report on its prevalence, variety, and effects. Arch Sex Behav 9:171–194, 1980

Finkelhor D: Child Sexual Abuse: New Theory and Research. New York, Free Press, 1984

Finkelhor D: The sexual abuse of children: current research reviewed. Psychiatric Annals 17 (suppl 4):233–241, 1987

Finkelhor D: Early and long-term effects of clinical sexual abuse. Professional Psychology 5:325–330, 1990

Finkelhor D, Baron L: High-risk children, in A Sourcebook on Child Sexual Abuse. Edited by Finkelhor D, and Associates. Newbury Park, CA, Sage Publications, 1986, pp 60–88

Finkelhor D, Berliner L: Research on the treatment of sexually abused children: a review and recommendations. J Am Acad Child Adolesc Psychiatry 34 (suppl 11):1408–1423, 1995

Forward S, Buck S: Betrayal of Innocence: Incest and Its Devastation. New York, Torcher, 1979

Frederick C, Pynoos R, Nader K: Child Post-Traumatic Stress Disorder Reaction Index, 1992 [Available from R. Pynoos, Adult Psychiatry, 300 UCLA Medical Plaza, Los Angeles, CA, 90024-6968]

Freud S: Totem and taboo (1913[1912–1913]), in Standard Edition of the Complete Psychological Works of Sigmund Freud, Vol 13. Translated and edited by Strachey J. London, Hogarth Press, 1953, pp vii–xv, 1–162

Friedrich WN, Beilke RL, Urquiza AJ: Behavioral comparisons of children from sexually abusive and distressed families. Journal of Interpersonal Violence 2:39–402, 1988

Friedrich WN, Beilke RL, Urquiza AJ: Children from sexually abusive families: a behavior comparison. Journal of Interpersonal Violence 2:391–402, 1993

Green AH: Overview of the literature on child sexual abuse, in Handbook for Health Care and Legal Professionals. Edited by Schetky DH, Green H. New York, Brunner/Mazel, 1988, pp 30–54

Greenacre P: The prepuberty trauma in girls, in Trauma, Growth and Personality (1950). Edited by Greenacre P. New York, International Universities Press, 1969, pp 204–233

Herman JL: Father-Daughter Incest. Cambridge, MA, Harvard University Press, 1981

Kirkland K, Bauer C: MMPI traits of incestuous fathers. Journal of Criminal Psychology 38:645–495, 1982

Landis JT: Experiences of 500 children with adult sexual deviance. Psychiatr Q 30 (suppl):91–109, 1956

Laviola M: Effects of older brother–younger sister incest: a review of five cases. Journal of Family Violence 4 (suppl 3):259–274, 1989

Loredo C: Sibling incest, in Handbook of Clinical Intervention in Child Sexual Abuse. Edited by Sgroi S. Lexington, MA, DC Heath, 1982, pp 181–188

Malinowski B: Sex and Repression in Savage Society. London, Routledge & Kegan, 1927

Mandel MD: An object relation study of sexually abusive fathers. Unpublished doctoral dissertation, California School of Professional Psychology, 1986 [Dissertation Abstracts International 47 (suppl 5):2173B, 1986]

Marshall WL, Barbaree H, Christopher D: Sexual offenders against female children: sexual preferences for age of victims and type of behavior. Canadian Journal of Behavioral Science 18:424–428, 1986

Mead M: Sex Temperament in Three Primitive Societies. New York, Mentor Books, 1935

Meiselman KC: Incest: A Psychological Study of Causes and Effects With Treatment Recommendations. San Francisco, CA, Jossey-Bass, 1978

National Resource Center on Child Sexual Abuse Newsletter 1 (suppl 4), November/December 1992

Olson D: Family Inventories. St Paul, MN, Family Social Service, University of Minnesota, 1982

Panton J: MMPI profile configurations associated with incestuous and nonincestuous child molesting. Psychol Rep 45:335–338, 1979

Parker H: Intrafamilial sexual abuse: a study of the abusive father. Unpublished doctoral dissertation, University of Utah, Salt Lake City, 1984 [Dissertation Abstracts International 45 (suppl 12):3751, 1984]

Parker H, Parker S: Father-daughter abuse: an emerging perspective. Am J Orthopsychiatry 56:531–549, 1986

Peters J: Children who are victims of sexual assault and the psychology of offenders. Am J Psychother 30:398–421, 1976

Rasmussen LA, Burton JE, Christopherson BJ: Precursors to offending and the trauma outcome process in sexually reactive children. Journal of Sexual Abuse 1:33–48, 1992

Rist K: Incest: theoretical and clinical views. Am J Orthopsychiatry 49:680–691, 1979

Russell DEH: The prevalence and seriousness of incestuous abusive stepfathers vs biological fathers. Child Abuse Negl 8:15–22, 1984

Russell DEH: The Secret Trauma: Incest in the Lives of Girls and Women. New York, Basic Books, 1986

Scott R, Stone D: MMPI profile consultation in incest families. J Consult Clin Psychol 54:364–368, 1986

Sgroi S: Vulnerable Population: Sexual Abuse Treatment for Children, Adult Survivors, Offenders and Persons With Mental Retardation, Vol 2. Lexington, MA, DC Heath, 1988

Sholevar GP: A family therapist looks at the problem of incest. Bulletin of the American Academy of Psychiatry and the Law 11:75–79, 1978

Smith H, Israel E: Sibling incest: a study of the dynamics of 25 cases. Child Abuse Negl 11:101–108, 1987

Summit R: The child sexual abuse accommodation syndrome. Child Abuse Negl 7:177–193, 1983

Swanson L, Biaggio M: Therapeutic perspectives on father-daughter incest. Am J Psychiatry 142:667–674, 1985

Trepper TS, Barrett MJ: Treating Incest: A Multiple Systems Perspective. New York, Haworth Press, 1986

Trepper TS, Barrett MJ: Systemic Treatment of Incest. New York, Brunner/Mazel, 1989

4

Sexual Victimization of Children

Diane H. Schetky, M.D.

This chapter discusses the short- and long-term effects of child sexual abuse and reviews the recent research in this area. The cognitive, psychodynamic, and psychobiological changes involved in the process of moving from victim to patient are explored. This knowledge is essential to diagnosing and treating victims of child sexual abuse. It is also important in a forensic context when experts are asked to assess damages and predict treatment needs.

Case Examples

Case 1

A. is a middle-aged college professor who presents with symptoms of panic disorder and depression. He reveals a history of sexual abuse perpetrated by his priest when he was a teenager. He did not dare disclose his abuse at the time for fear he would not be believed, and thus he never received treatment for it. He feels guilty for having allowed the sexual relationship to continue but recognizes how neglect by his parents rendered him vulnerable. He still feels rage at his priest for taking away his youth and innocence and "leaving a big empty space." He no longer trusts the church and eschews organized religion. He is able to effectively use therapy with a female therapist, and his symptoms improve.

Case 2

B. is a tall, macho 22-year-old who was referred by his attorney for a forensic evaluation. B. had been a promising student in junior high school prior to sexual abuse by his scoutmaster. Once the abuse began, his grades plummeted, he lost respect for authorities, and he eventually dropped out of school. Many of his friends and family members refused to believe his allegations of abuse against his scoutmaster, who was a prominent and highly regarded member of the community. After floundering for several years, B. found refuge in the military. He likes the discipline there and, in particular, enjoys giving orders to people under him. His rage with his perpetrator is still seething, and he states, "I want blood." His behavior is quite impulsive and often violent. When approached by a homosexual in a bar, B. severely beat him to the point that he had to be hospitalized. B. rejects therapy because he does not want to think about his abuser and he is not sure he would trust a therapist. When upset, he turns to alcohol. He has decided to sue the Boy Scouts of America, thinking this might make him feel better.

Case 3

C., now aged 18, was repeatedly victimized within her home by both parents, whom she stated were part of a cult. For years she accepted the abuse as normal because she never knew otherwise. As a teen, she was placed in foster care, where she was abused by her foster father. There followed a series of foster home placements that were of brief duration owing to her manipulative, angry behavior and substance abuse. The pattern of victimization continued with boyfriends and culminated in sexual abuse by a female therapist. C. tells her current therapist, "Everybody in my life abused my boundaries, so as a kid I didn't have any sense of what is right and what is wrong." She has no sense of entitlement and has great difficulty setting limits. She is confused about her sexual identity and avoids sex because it brings back too many painful memories. She is mistrustful of her new therapist and fears that she, too, will victimize her. C. now has been diagnosed with borderline personality disorder, bulimia, somatization disorder, and dysthymia.

Case 4

D. was 5 years old when she was brought for evaluation by her mother because of compulsive masturbation and grabbing at her younger brother's genitals. D. frequently displayed dissociative symptoms, and it was difficult to question her about possible sexual abuse. Once in therapy, she gradually disclosed sexual abuse by her father. Her parents separated, and her mother took appropriate steps to protect her.

D. remained terrified that her father would retaliate for her disclosure. She refused to sleep alone and would experience much anxiety when her mother left the house. D. made some strides in therapy and decided she wanted to testify against her father in criminal court. There were numerous postponements in the trial that were very disruptive to her life. By the time the case was heard, she was 7 years old. She testified for over 2 hours, and her father was acquitted. She attempted to blame herself because she had responded affirmatively to leading questions asking whether it was all right to tell a lie sometimes. She explained that she had been afraid of her father's attorney. She knew how the attorney wanted her to answer his question, and she agreed with him because she wanted him to like her.

After 3 years of therapy, she has stopped acting out sexually but still reverts to compulsive masturbation when anxious. She wants nothing to do with her father. She worries that he will be angry about the things she said in court about him and that he will follow through on his threats to harm her if she disclosed. She continues in therapy.

The patients in these cases all share the trauma of sexual abuse during childhood by a loved and trusted person in a position of authority. From this shared experience of trauma their courses diverged. A. was unable to disclose his abuse as a teen, received no therapy, and quietly suffered from depression and posttraumatic stress disorder (PTSD) for many years until the sudden onset of panic attacks brought him into treatment. B. rejected therapy, C. was reabused in therapy, and only D. received immediate intervention. Family support was nonexistent for some of these victims. Two of these victims became involved with the legal system, and their involvement resulted in additional stresses and publicity. C. entered foster care and had to deal with lack of permanency for most of her adolescent years. In spite of seeing many therapists over the years, she continues to be revictimized and exhibits a panoply of psychiatric disorders.

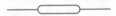

These cases illustrate the variety of patterns sexual abuse may follow, including homosexual, heterosexual, incestuous, and extra-familial abuse and single versus multiple perpetrators. Additional variables include the age of the victim at the time of abuse; the relationship to the perpetrator; the type, extent, and duration of the abuse; and whether there were threats made around disclosure. These patients' cases point to the range of clinical symptoms that may follow sexual abuse, including both internalizing and externalizing behaviors and the tendency to identify with the aggressor. They demonstrate the persistence of some symptoms, with or without therapy, and the many confounding variables that complicate research studies on the long-term effects of sexual abuse.

Accommodating to Abuse:
Cognitive and Emotional Changes

Children who are repeatedly traumatized rely on a variety of defenses and cognitive distortions to make sense of their abuse and to cope with their dysfunctional families. Self-blame is common and allows them to feel as if they have some control over the abuse and their future. It further serves to protect their image of the perpetrator. Shengold (1979) described the splitting that occurs wherein the child needs to see the abusing parent as good because the image of a good parent mitigates the intensity of her or his fear and rage. The very young child cannot exist emotionally without the image of caring parents and so distorts reality to preserve that fantasy. Anger gets suppressed and turned inward into self-loathing or self-destructive behavior. This becomes reinforced when the offender or family members blame the child for the abuse with comments that imply that the child asked for the abuse or could have prevented it.

Herman (1992) has spoken to the difficulty the abused child has in forming inner representations of a safe, consistent caretaker and the fragmented identity that ensues along with difficulty in emotional self-regulation. Herman notes that because the child cannot develop an inner sense of safety, she remains more dependent than other children on external sources of comfort and solace and may be indiscriminate in those she turns to to meet her needs. Paradoxically, this puts her at increased risk for revictimization.

Sexual abuse deprives the child of boundaries and any sense of entitlement, and this increases her or his vulnerability. For instance, an adult victim of abuse compared herself to an amoeba who did not know her boundaries and therefore had great difficulty setting any limits. Many victims learn to survive by subordinating their needs to those of the abusing adults. When privacy is nonexistent, it becomes difficult for the child to develop any sense of self. Absent a sense of self or entitlement, it is difficult to say no, and it is readily apparent why victims are vulnerable to reabuse.

Parents' denial of abuse may feed into the child's denial. Reality testing is affected, as when secrecy is rewarded but telling the truth is not, and the abusing parent is depicted as good and the child as bad. Secrecy reinforces the child's sense of isolation, precludes individuation, and cuts the child off from peers. The cost of secrecy and denial is high, requiring the use of denial, splitting, and dissociation. If the world does not know about the incest, then it does not exist and becomes split off. Summitt (1983, p. 180) notes that the secrecy surrounding the abuse "is both the source of fear and

the promise of safety." The child is lulled into believing that everything will be all right if she does not tell. Summitt believes that
unless the child shares the secret, she "is likely to spend a lifetime
in what comes to be a self imposed exile from intimacy, trust and
self validation" (p. 185).

Dissociation is a common way of dealing with abuse, especially
when the abuse occurs repeatedly and children learn to dissociate
in anticipation of the abuse (Terr 1991). Some may use counting
rituals—for example, counting the squares on the ceiling or flowers
on the wallpaper, or chanting certain phrases to induce as sort of
self-hypnosis. Dissociation serves as a survival tool in that it mentally
distances or removes the child from the trauma of abuse. This may
occur in a variety of ways: The child who depersonalizes convinces
herself or himself that "it is not happening to me." Alternatively,
she or he may use derealization to convince herself or himself that
it is not happening at all. At the extreme is dissociative identity
disorder, in which there is fragmentation of behavior, affect, sensation, and knowledge. The child may ascribe the victimization to an
alter personality or have no recall of the abuse.

Dissociation protects the child from knowledge of the abuse but
does so at a considerable cost. Because the event is not clearly remembered, the child fails to assimilate the full impact of the trauma
and learn from it. She or he is unable to assess danger signals and
consequently is unable to protect herself or himself from repeated
abuse. She or he may unconsciously seek to repeat the trauma as a
means of trying to master it. As Richard Rhodes (1990, p. 267)
notes, "Repetition is the mute language of the abused child." Rather
than work through the abuse, the child seeks to resolve the trauma
through repeating it. This may involve revictimization or identifying
with the aggressor and perpetrating abuse.

The abused child may handle sexual overstimulation and rage
by identifying with the perpetrator. Shengold (1989, p. 316) refers
to the "terrifying intensity of rageful wishes" experienced by adult
patients who have been sexually abused as children. He notes how
it invades all relationships and how these patients are crippled by
their attempts to defend against their rage. Their rage may be turned
upon self, others, or the therapist. If the sources of these feelings

are not recognized, they are likely to compound the victim's difficulty with trust. Abused children experience a loss of power and control. Identification with the perpetrator, either in play or in real life, becomes a way for them to view themselves as powerful rather than helpless and ineffectual. Premature sexualization is yet another factor contributing to a victim's becoming sexually aggressive.

Other defenses used to deal with sexual abuse include denial, repression, and suppression. Williams (1992) studied 100 women who had been seen in an emergency room as children or adolescents for sexual abuse. She found that 38% of the women on follow-up had no memories of the abuse or of having been seen at the hospital. Briere and Conte (1993) studied women in psychotherapy for sexual abuse and found that 30% to 40% of them had forgotten about their abuse at some point in their lives. These authors linked self-reported amnesia for abuse with more severe abuse in childhood. Herman and Schatzow (1987) arrived at similar findings.

A child who relies heavily on the defenses of dissociation, splitting, repression, and denial is likely to encounter learning problems in school, particularly around attention and memory. Surprisingly little has been written about this association even though it has often been observed by clinicians. PTSD is also likely to disrupt the child's ability to perform at school.

Sexual abuse may alter perceptions of self and information processing. Fine (1990) notes that faulty information processing may result from the use of any of the following: dichotomous thinking, selective abstraction, arbitrary inference, overgeneralization (e.g., the perpetrator was male, therefore all males are bad), time distortion, distortion in self-perception, excessive responsibility, circular thinking, and misassumption of causality. The child who assumes he was abused because he is bad and that he is bad because he was abused may have difficulty accepting praise because it is discordant with his self concept.

The question of whether child abuse victims differ from non-abused control subjects in their perceptions of locus of control was explored by Mannarino and Cohen (1996). Although no differences were found in this study, the authors did find that the abused group felt different from peers, blamed themselves for negative events, and had reduced interpersonal trust and lower perceived credibility.

Trauma shatters basic assumptions, beliefs, and expectations about oneself and the world (McCann and Pearlman 1990). Assumptions that are shattered include viewing oneself in a favorable light, personal invulnerability, and belief in a meaningful, orderly world. These are basic schemata that help individuals organize their life experiences and understand the world. A child who is deprived of these schemata is left with disorder, both internal and external. Her views of self and world are drastically altered and may get played out in expectations of a foreshortened future (Terr 1983).

One of the most insidious effects of child sexual abuse—one that is often difficult to measure in research studies—is violation of trust. This cuts across all child sexual abuse and is central to many of the ensuing emotional problems. Trust has been undermined by the perpetrator, who was usually someone in a position of authority who had responsibility for the child. Violation of trust makes it difficult for the child to trust people in the future and is likely to lead to conflicts around intimacy. It also renders therapy very difficult.

Long-Term Effects of Childhood Sexual Abuse

The early literature on long-term effects of child sexual abuse consists mostly of retrospective follow-up studies based on clinical populations of predominantly adult females. The problems inherent in these types of studies include lack of standardization, pooling of cases, absence of controls, retrospective bias, memory distortions, difficulty in determining the source of trauma, and lack of differentiation of the effects of abuse from the conditions that may have predisposed to it. Furthermore, many of the adults in these studies did not disclose abuse until later in life, and they received no treatment for the abuse at the time it occurred.

Findings from studies on the long-term effects of child sexual abuse have been summarized in several review articles (Beitchman et al. 1992; Green 1993; Schetky 1990). These studies, in spite of their shortcomings, do show some consensus regarding common sequelae of child sexual abuse, which include depression, anxiety, psychiatric hospitalization, substance abuse, self-abusive behavior, borderline personality disorder, somatization disorder, PTSD and dissociative disorders, revictimization, and poor parenting. In addition, eroticization in children, difficulty with trust and intimacy in later life, sexual dysfunction, and sexual aggression are noted. With such an extensive list, one might ask whether there are any disorders that are not related to sexual abuse? According to these studies, the long-lasting negative effects of child sexual abuse that were noted appeared to be correlated with abuse by father or stepfather, use of force, and lack of support by a close adult.

The past 10 years have seen the emergence of more sophisticated research on child sexual abuse utilizing standardized instruments, clinical and healthy control subjects, and prospective studies. The results of some of these studies are challenging our prior assumptions about the effects of child sexual abuse. Some newer outcome studies are reviewed below.

It should be noted that not all children become symptomatic following sexual abuse. Kendall-Tackett and colleagues (1993), in their review of the literature, found that between 21% and 36% of children were asymptomatic at the time of psychological evaluation. A word of caution in interpreting these findings is indicated, however, as some children may not become symptomatic until later on. Berliner (1991) suggests that the symptoms may be suppressed by the children or that they do not become manifest until subsequent developmental stages. Gomes-Schwartz and associates (1990) found that asymptomatic children were the ones most likely to show worsened functioning at 18 months follow-up, at which time 30% of them were symptomatic. Oates and colleagues (1994) suggest that there may be a sleeper effect wherein victims of child sexual abuse experience lower self-esteem over time.

Numerous authors have noted the discrepancy between parent ratings of abused children's symptoms and children's perception of themselves, with parents tending to see more psychopathology (Friedrich 1988; Mannarino et al. 1989). This raises questions as to whether children minimize their symptoms or parents read more into their children's behavior because of their anxiety about the sexual abuse. Alternatively, research tools may not be sensitive enough to detect the child's distress. These authors stress the importance of getting research data from multiple sources.

Friedrich (1988), in a study of 155 sexually abused children who were being seen for treatment or evaluation, concluded that the relationship between behavioral sequelae and abuse-specific variables was not very unitary or consistent. He compared 20 sexually abused boys with a sample of boys with conduct disorder and found very few differences between the two groups. The exceptions were that the boys with conduct disorder showed more aggressive behavior and the sexually abused boys exhibited more sexualized behavior. He then compared sexually abused children with control groups of healthy, nonabused children and psychiatric outpatients and again found that sexualization was the discriminating variable. Kolko and colleagues (1988) found more sexual behavior problems in sexually abused children when they were compared with physically abused or nonabused children.

Mannarino and colleagues (1991), using standardized instruments, compared sexually abused children with healthy and clinical control subjects. At initial assessment, ratings on the Sexual Problems subscale of the Child Behavior Checklist (CBCL) for the sexually abused children were significantly higher than those for the healthy subjects and higher than those for the clinical control subjects. The authors found no differences among subgroups of the sexually abused children in terms of type or extent of abuse. However, at 12-month follow-up, those children who had experienced sexual intercourse showed significantly more depression, anxiety, and self-esteem problems than those who had experienced only fondling. The former were also less socially competent and had more behavior problems. The authors found that group differences on the CBCL were maintained across the follow-up period, except that the clinical control subjects showed more sexual problems and less social competence at follow-up than at the time of the initial assessment. Social competence in the abused group was comparable to that in the control group despite the former's ongoing emotional and behavioral problems.

Tong and colleagues (1987) followed up sexually abused boys

and girls at an average of 2.6 years after abuse. Based on parent CBCL ratings and interviews with parents, the authors found that 76% of the children were less confident than before, 30% had fewer friends, and 20% were more aggressive. Schoolteachers noted behavior problems in 28% of the children and lower adaptive functioning on all dimensions compared with the control subjects. Furthermore, the abused children scored much lower than the control subjects on the Piers-Harris Self Concept Scale.

McLeer and colleagues (1988, 1992) found that 43% to 48% of clinically referred sexually abused children in their samples suffered from PTSD. These authors then compared prevalence of psychiatric disorders in a clinical sample of 92 sexually abused children and a sample of nonabused psychiatric outpatients (McLeer et al. 1994). PTSD was found to be the most prevalent diagnosis in each group. The prevalence of PTSD was 42% in the abused group versus 8% in the control group. The authors also noted significant comorbidity with DSM-III-R attention-deficit hyperactivity disorder (ADHD). Similar findings were reported by Glod and Teicher (1996). Famularo and colleagues (1992) found that 48% of sexually abused children in their sample were diagnosed with PTSD. In addition, many children who do not fulfill all of the criteria for the diagnosis of PTSD exhibit some symptoms of the disorder.

Several authors have reported increased rates of anxiety among sexually abused children (Gomes-Schwartz et al. 1990; Kolko et al. 1988). Kendall-Tackett and colleagues (1993) reviewed empirical studies on the impact of child sexual abuse that compared sexually abused children with nonclinical control subjects. They found that sexually abused children manifested more anxiety, sexualized behavior, depression, withdrawal, aggression, and internalizing and externalizing behavior. The biggest differences were found for acting-out behaviors such as sexualized behaviors and aggression.

The question of whether there is a link between eating disorders and child sexual abuse is controversial (Pope and Hudson 1992). Similarly, studies are conflicting as to whether a history of sexual abuse increases the likelihood of subsequent homosexual behavior, and most of these studies have dealt only with female victims (Beitchman et al. 1992).

Psychobiological Responses

It is well known that stress leads to increase in norepinephrine turn-over and may affect areas of the brain involved in regulation of emotions and memory. Heightened sympathetic arousal has been demonstrated in combat veterans with PTSD (Charney et al. 1993) as well as in animal studies. DeBellis et al. (1994b) demonstrated that sexually abused girls exhibit significantly greater total catechol-amine synthesis compared with control subjects. They noted that these findings are consistent with those in the adult literature on PTSD even though these girls did not show full-blown PTSD. Fifty-eight percent of the sexually abused girls demonstrated histories of severely depressed mood and suicidal behavior. They also demonstrated an increased incidence of hyperactivity, with the criteria for ADHD being met in 32% of them.

The hypothalamic-pituitary-adrenal axis is also involved in the regulation of stress. Blunted adrenocorticotropic hormone (ACTH) response to ovine corticotropin-releasing hormone (CRH) in sexually abused girls has been demonstrated by DeBellis et al. (1994a). These authors found that cortisol levels were consistently higher in sexually abused children and did not follow the normal diurnal curve. They attribute this finding to dysregulation of the hypotha-lamic-pituitary axis associated with hyporesponsiveness of the pituitary to exogenous CRH and normal overall cortisol secretion. The authors speculate that chronic or intermittent endogenous CRH hypersecretion occurred in these girls in response to the emotional and physical stress associated with sexual abuse. CRH hypersecre-tion may lead to downregulation of CRH reception in the anterior pituitary and possible hypertrophy or hypersensitivity of the adrenal cortices. The net effect would be adaptive changes in ACTH and cortisol secretion to reduce the amount of ACTH necessary to maintain normal cortisol secretions from hyperresponsive adrenals.

The hypopituitary-gonadal axis may also be involved in chronic physical or emotional stress. Laboratory studies with animals have linked stress with delayed puberty (Johnson et al. 1992). A few authors have suggested that sexual abuse may cause early onset of puberty in females (Herman-Geddes et al. 1988; Putnam and Trickett 1993).

It is well known that stress may cause immune suppression, presumably through the neuroendocrine and neurosecretory systems. To date, there has been only one study on this hypothesis involving children. DeBellis and colleagues (1996), in a small exploratory study of sexually abused girls and control subjects, found a significantly higher incidence of plasma antinuclear antibody (ANA) titers in the abused subjects compared with the control subjects. The authors speculate that the stress of severe sexual abuse may lead to suppression of T suppressor cells that actively suppress the auto-antibody-producing lymphocytes, thus increasing the incidence of positive ANA titers. They caution, however, that sexual abuse may be but one of many stressors in the homes of the abused girls.

More recent studies have explored the relationship between cortisol response to stress and alterations in memory. Bremner and colleagues (1993) described how the stress response shunts energy to the brain and muscles and activates attentional and memory systems. Although in the short run this response is beneficial and promotes survival, its long-term effects could be detrimental. Animal studies have demonstrated that the hippocampus is involved in new learning and memory. Bremner et al. reviewed clinical studies and noted that the increase in glucocorticoids that occurs in response to stress may cause neurotoxicity to the hippocampal neurons.

Outcome Variables: Developmental Framework

The impact of sexual abuse will vary according to the child's developmental stage. Surprisingly, very few studies have looked at the effects of sexual abuse across various age groups. Cole and Putnam (1992) discuss how sexual abuse can disrupt various developmental phases and emphasize that the impact may be cumulative in that the abuse takes on new meaning in subsequent stages of development and may need to be worked through again in therapy. They also urge that researchers look beyond mere assessment of self-esteem to the child's ability to understand and integrate multiple elements of self.

▶ Family Functioning

Children who receive maternal support following disclosure of sexual abuse fare better than those who do not (Everson et al. 1991a,

1991b; Gomes-Schwartz et al. 1990). Cohen and Mannarino (1998) and Deblinger and colleagues (1996) also emphasize the importance of parental support and of including parents in the treatment of sexually abused children. Bentovim and colleagues (1987) found that family consensus that abuse had occurred was an important factor in determining treatment outcome. Berliner (1993) noted increased pathology in children whose disclosures were met with disbelief or punishment. Support for the child's disclosure of abuse is most likely to be compromised when the perpetrator is a spouse or boyfriend of the mother (Gomes-Schwartz et al. 1990).

Oates and colleagues (1994) found that the major variable relating to improvement in sexually abused children was adequacy of family functioning. Peters (1988), studying a nonclinical sample of adult females who had experienced child sexual abuse, found that the risk of sexual abuse was related to certain family factors that in themselves may produce psychological problems in later life. Peters linked risk of sexual abuse with certain family characteristics that may be predictive of problems in later life. Specifically, lack of maternal warmth was noted to be a strong predictor of psychological difficulties in later life.

Friedrich (1988) noted that the family context of abuse had a strong relationship to the child's behavioral adaptation to sexual abuse. He found a relationship between family conflict and cohesion and whether or not a child developed internalizing or externalizing behaviors. He noted that a history of sexual abuse or psychiatric problems in the mother interacted with the child's response to sexual abuse and that the behavioral problems of the child were not solely attributable to the sexual abuse. Cohen and Mannarino (1996), in a controlled study, found that parental emotional distress related to the child's abuse predicted the child's posttreatment psychopathology regardless of type of treatment provided.

Conte and Schuerman (1987) found that nonabuse variables were associated with parents' scores on the CBCL and accounted for 22% of the variation in child behavior. These variables included a parent's negative outlook, number of stressful life events experienced by the child, parents' education, and number of children in the family. The authors also found a correlation between outcome and the victim's supportive relationship with an adult or sibling.

▶ Treatment

Few studies have looked at the impact of psychotherapy on outcome in child sexual abuse, and most of these have addressed only short-term therapy. In one study, the greatest amount of improvement was found among subjects who received treatment by the program run by the research team (Gomes-Schwarz et al. 1990). In contrast, Oates and colleagues (1994), in an 18-month follow-up of sexually abused children in New Zealand, found no correlation between therapy and outcome. Those children who entered therapy were likely to be more depressed than those who did not, and at 18 months follow-up only 41% were rated improved. In England, Bentovim and colleagues (1987) followed up 120 families and 180 victims of child sexual abuse. These families were noted for chaos, violence, and substance abuse. The authors pointed out that their treatment program was in its early stages and consisted of family treatment or group treatment for families and children over a 12- to 15-month period. No research tools were used either before or after treatment. Bentovim et al.'s clinical impression was that the "victim's circumstances" improved in 61% of cases, with the most noticeable change being a decrease in sexualized behaviors and emotional difficulties. A reabuse rate of 16% was found. Cohen and Mannarino (1997), in a study of treatment outcome among sexually abused preschoolers, found superior efficacy of cognitive-behavioral therapy over nondirective supportive therapy.

▶ Involvement in the Legal System

Child victims of sexual abuse may be involved in criminal, civil, and child protective proceedings. When a child testifies in court, there is potential benefit in allowing her or him to confront the abuser, feel believed, and see justice carried out. These proceedings are not without risk, as when the child is traumatized by seeing the perpetrator again, by the court proceedings, by the publicity surrounding them, or when the perpetrator is acquitted. Goodman and colleagues (1992) found that recovery was slower among children involved in court proceedings, particularly when the children had to testify many times. Everson and associates (1991a, 1991b), studying adolescents, reached similar conclusions. Runyan and colleagues (1988), on the other hand, found that recovery was related to how swiftly cases were resolved in court.

▶ Sex of Victim

Most studies to date have focused primarily on female victims of incest. Male victims may experience a double stigma in that not only have they been abused but the abuse is often homosexual. Another difference for male victims is that the abuse is more likely to be perpetrated by someone outside of the family. Some authors feel that male victims are held more responsible in that people see them as less vulnerable and assume they should have been able to prevent the abuse (Finkelhor 1984). Thus, a double standard may exist in regard to stigmatization. Kendall-Tackett and colleagues (1993) note that, despite the popular belief that boys are more likely than girls to exhibit externalizing symptoms, greater likelihood of externalizing behaviors in boys has not been substantiated.

▶ Female Perpetrators

Child sexual abuse perpetrated by females has been a neglected topic that many clinicians do not like to think about or ask patients about. Consequently, the prevalence of this problem has been underestimated. In addition, society allows more latitude to females in terms of what sort of touching is permitted in the name of hygienic care. Finkelhor (1984) estimates that females perpetuate about 5% of the abuse of girls and 20% of the abuse of boys. Sgroi and Sargent (1993) believe that abuse by a female is likely to be reported at a later age and is more likely to be met with disbelief. Abuse by females may occur in isolation or when the female is acting as a coperpetrator with her male partner.

No studies have compared the impact of abuse by females with that of abuse by males. Those describing the impact of sexual abuse by females on a female victim note problems around self differentiation and identity, with the victim feeling that she does not own her body (Sgroi and Sargent 1993). Further, adult victims may fear close relationships with women, may worry that they themselves might become perpetrators, and may choose to avoid parenting altogether (Sgroi and Sargent 1993).

▶ Relationship to Abuser and Duration of Abuse

In a New Zealand study, Merry and Andrews (1994) found no association between severity of abuse and relationship with the abuser to psychological outcome; nor did there seem to be any correlation of these variables with life events. In contrast, Oates and colleagues (1994) in Australia found that the number or type of events did not correlate significantly with the abused child's functioning but that the duration of the events did. They found that the long-term negative life events were associated with decline in self-esteem over time; children who experienced few such events sustained adequate functioning. The authors also failed to find any significant relationship between relationship of the abuser and child, type of abuse, duration, or use of coercion.

▶ Preabuse Variables

There has been notably little research on the issue of the effect of preabuse factors. Mannarino and colleagues (1994) found that sexually abused children had more prior developmental and psychiatric problems than did control subjects and suggested that sexual abuse exacerbated preexisting problems.

Conclusion

It is apparent that the effects of childhood sexual abuse involve a complex interplay of cognitive, emotional, biological, and social factors. One needs to consider each child's predisposing vulnerabilities, as well as family stability and support, in assessing treatment needs and predicting outcome. Studies on neurobiological dysregulation in abused children suggest that some symptoms associated with child sexual abuse may be biologically based. This has important implications for treatment. Clinicians need to consider multiple treatment modalities for sexually abused children, integrating cognitive, behavioral, and psychodynamic techniques when appropriate, as well as psychopharmacology in some cases.

We have more to learn about the impact of sexual abuse on

development, to what extent therapy affects outcome, and which treatment modalities are most effective. Additional research is needed to explore the comorbidity of sexual abuse with disorders such as attention-deficit/hyperactivity disorder and eating disorders. Other neglected areas of research include male victims of abuse and victimization by female perpetrators. It is encouraging to see the amount of well-designed research emerging on child sexual abuse, and we need to continue to work to see that these efforts receive adequate funding.

References

Beitchman J, Zucker K, Hood J, et al: A review of the long-term effects of child sexual abuse. Child Abuse Negl 16:101–119, 1992

Bentovim A, Boston P, Van Elbur A: Child sexual abuse—children and families referred to a treatment project and the effects of intervention. Br Med J 295:1453–1457, 1987

Berliner L: The effects of sexual abuse on children. Violence Update 1:1–10, 1991

Berliner L: Effects of sexual abuse on children. Paper presented at the annual meeting of the International Society for Traumatic Stress Studies, San Antonio, TX, October 1993

Bremner JD, Davis M, Southwick SM, et al: Neurobiology of posttraumatic stress disorder, in American Psychiatric Press Review of Psychiatry, Vol 12. Edited by Oldham JM, Riba MB, Tasman A. Washington, DC, American Psychiatric Association, 1993, pp 183–204

Briere J, Conte J: Self reported amnesia for abuse in adults molested as children. J Trauma Stress 6:32–31, 1993

Charney DS, Deutch A, Krystal J, et al: Psychobiological mechanisms of posttraumatic stress disorder. Arch Gen Psychiatry 50:294–305, 1993

Cohen J, Mannarino A: Factors that mediate the treatment outcome in sexually abused preschool children. J Am Acad Child Adolesc Psychiatry 35:1402–1410, 1996

Cohen J, Mannarino A: A treatment study for sexually abused preschool children: outcome during a one-year follow-up. J Am Acad Child Adolesc Psychiatry 36:1228–1235, 1997

Cohen J, Mannarino A: Factors that mediate treatment outcomes in sexually abused preschool children: 6- and 12-month follow-up. J Am Acad Child Adolesc Psychiatry 37:44–51, 1998

Cole P, Putnam F: Effect of incest on self and social functioning: a developmental perspective. J Consult Clin Psychol 60 (suppl 2):174–184, 1992

Conte J, Schuerman R: Factors associated with an increased impact of child sexual abuse. Child Abuse Negl 11:201–211, 1987

DeBellis M, Chrousos G, Dorn L, et al: Hypothalamic-pituitary-adrenal axis dysregulation in sexually abused girls. J Clin Endocrinol Metab 78 (suppl 2):249–255, 1994a

DeBellis M, Lefter L, Trickett P, et al: Urinary catecholamine excretion in sexually abused girls. J Am Acad Child Adolesc Psychiatry 33 (suppl 3): 320–327, 1994b

DeBellis M, Burke L, Trickett P, et al: Antinuclear antibodies and thyroid function in sexually abused girls. J Trauma Stress 9:369–378, 1996

Deblinger E, Lipman J, Steer R: Sexually abused children suffering post-traumatic stress symptoms: initial treatment outcomes. Child Maltreatment 1:310–321, 1996

Everson M, Hunter W, Runyan D, et al: Adolescent adjustment after incest: who fares poorly? Paper presented at the San Diego Conference on Responding to Child Maltreatment, San Diego, CA, 1991a

Everson M, Hunter W, Runyan D, et al: Maternal support following disclosure of incest. Am J Orthopsychiatry 59:197–227, 1991b

Famularo R, Kinscherff R, Fenton T: Psychiatric diagnoses of maltreated children: preliminary findings. J Am Acad Child Adolesc Psychiatry 31:863–867, 1992

Fine CG: The cognitive sequelae of incest, in Incest-Related Syndromes of Adult Psychopathology. Edited by Kluft RP. Washington, DC, American Psychiatric Press, 1990, pp 161–182

Finkelhor D: Child Sexual Abuse. New York, Free Press, 1984

Friedrich W: Behavior problems in sexually abused children: an adaptational perspective, in Lasting Effects of Child Sexual Abuse. Edited by Wyatt G, Powell G. Newbury Park, CA, Sage Publications, 1988, pp 171–191

Glod C, Teicher M: Relationship between early abuse, posttraumatic stress disorder, and activity levels in prepubertal children. J Am Acad Child Adolesc Psychiatry 35:1384–1393, 1996

Gomes-Schwartz B, Horowitz J, Cardarelli A: Child Sexual Abuse: The Initial Effects. Newbury Park, CA, Sage Publications, 1990

Goodman G, Taub E, Jones D, et al: Emotional effects of criminal court testimony on child sexual assault victims. Monogr Soc Res Child Dev 57 (suppl 2), 1992

Green A: Child sexual abuse: immediate and long-term effects and intervention. J Am Acad Child Adolesc Psychiatry 32 (suppl 5):890–902, 1993

Herman JL: Trauma and Recovery. New York, Basic Books, 1992

Herman JL, Schatzow E: Recovery and verification of memories of childhood sexual trauma. Psychoanalytic Psychology 4:490–494, 1987

Herman-Geddes M, Sandler A, Friedman N: Sexual precocity in girls: an association with sexual abuse? American Journal of Diseases of Children 142:431–433, 1988

Johnson E, Kamilaris T, Chrousos G, et al: Mechanisms of stress: a dynamic view of hormonal and behavioral homeostasis. Neurosci Biobehav Rev 16:115–130, 1992

Kendall-Tackett K, Williams L, Finkelhor D: Impact of sexual abuse on children: a review and synthesis of recent empirical studies. Psychol Bull 113 (suppl 1):164–180, 1993

Kolko D, Moser J, Weldy S: Behavioral/emotional indications of sexual abuse in child psychiatric inpatients: a controlled comparison with physical abuse. Child Abuse Negl 12:529–542, 1988

Mannarino A, Cohen J: Abuse-related attributions and perceptions, general attributions and locus of control in sexually abused girls. J Interpersonal Violence 11(12):162–180, 1996

Mannarino A, Cohen J, Gergor M: Emotional and behavioral difficulties in sexually abused girls. Journal of Interpersonal Violence 4 (suppl 2):437–451, 1989

Mannarino A, Cohen J, Smith J, et al: Six- and twelve-month follow-up of sexually abused girls. Journal of Interpersonal Violence 6 (suppl 4):494–511, 1991

Mannarino A, Cohen J, Berman S: The relationship between preabuse factors and psychological symptomatology in sexually abused girls. Child Abuse Negl 18:63–71, 1994

McCann L, Pearlman L: Psychological Trauma and the Adult Survivor: Theory, Therapy and Transformation. New York, Brunner/Mazel, 1990

McLeer S, Deblinger E, Atkins M, et al: Posttraumatic stress disorder in sexually abused children, II: a prospective study. J Am Acad Child Adolesc Psychiatry 27:650–654, 1988

McLeer S, Deblinger E, Orvaschel J: Sexually abused children at high risk for posttraumatic stress disorder. J Am Acad Child Adolesc Psychiatry 31:875–879, 1992

McLeer S, Callaghan M, Delmina H, et al: Psychiatric disorders in sexually abused children. J Am Acad Child Adolesc Psychiatry 33 (suppl 3):313–319, 1994

Merry S, Andrews L: Psychiatric status of sexually abused children 12 months after disclosure of abuse. J Am Acad Child Adolesc Psychiatry 33 (suppl 7):939–944, 1994

Oates K, O'Toole B, Lynch D, et al: Stability and change in outcome for sexually abused children. J Am Acad Child Adolesc Psychiatry 33 (suppl 7):945–953, 1994

Peters S: Child sexual abuse and later psychological problems, in Lasting Effects of Child Sexual Abuse. Edited by Wyatt G, Powell G. Newbury Park, CA, Sage Publications, 1988, pp 101–117

Pope HG Jr, Hudson J: Is childhood sexual abuse a risk factor in bulimia nervosa? Am J Psychiatry 149 (suppl 4):455–463, 1992

Putnam F, Trickett P: Child sexual abuse: a model of chronic trauma. Psychiatry 56:82–95, 1993

Rhodes R: A Hole in the World: An American Boyhood. New York, Simon & Schuster, 1990

Runyan D, Everson M, et al: Impact of legal intervention on sexually abused children. J Pediatr 1131:647–653, 1988

Schetky DH: A review of the literature on long-term effects on childhood sexual abuse, in Incest-Related Syndromes of Adult Psychopathology. Edited by Kluft RP. Washington, DC, American Psychiatric Press, 1990, pp –35–54

Sgroi S, Sargent N: Impact and treatment issues for victims of childhood sexual abuse by female perpetrators, in Female Sexual Abuse of Children. Edited by Elliot M. New York, Guilford Press, 1993

Shengold L: Child abuse and deprivations: soul murder. J Am Psychoanal Assoc 27:533–599, 1979

Shengold L: Soul Murder: The Effects of Childhood Abuse and Deprivation. New Haven, CT, Yale University Press, 1989

Summitt R: The sexual abuse syndrome. Child Abuse Negl 7:177–193, 1983

Terr L: Time sense following psychic trauma: a clinical study of ten adults and twenty children. Am J Orthopsychiatry 53:244–544, 1983

Terr L: Childhood traumas: an outline and overview. Am J Psychiatry 148 (suppl 1):10–12, 1991

Tong L, Oates K, McDowell M: Personality development following sexual abuse. Child Abuse Negl 11:371–383, 1987

Williams L: Adult memories of childhood abuse: preliminary findings from a longitudinal study. The Advisor (American Professional Society on the Abuse of Children), Summer 1992, pp 19–21

5

Transcultural Aspects of Sexual Victimization

Harriet P. Lefley, Ph.D.

Any consideration of sexual victimization, or the very concept of victimization itself, must take into account cultural views of appropriate and inappropriate sexual behavior. These views inform children's and adults' expectations of others and situations that involve betrayal of trust. The perception of a sexual act as abusive, violating, and self-diminishing, and the availability of resources to prevent its recurrence, are very much a function of societal attitudes toward sexuality and responses to breaches of normative patterns. Such patterns may also involve sexual rituals that vary widely in meaning from culture to culture.

In this chapter we face the very difficult task of examining culturally relative versus universally absolute ideas about morality and appropriateness in gender and adult–child relationships. Our purpose is neither to argue nor to equalize the merits of these bipolar viewpoints. Like all the contributors in this volume, this author is a member of Western culture and shares its dominant values. Rather, one aim of this chapter is to examine the importance of cultural context and social response in defining behaviors as sexually exploitative and in developing appropriate approaches to treating victims. In this connection, we first examine some relevant practices of distal cultures—those most sharply differentiated from our own—and then speak of more proximal cultures, namely, diverse ethnic groups within the United States.

Defining Culture

Culture is defined as the normative belief systems, attitudes, values, behavioral and religious practices, and overall worldview of a particular ethnic or national group, typically bound by common traditions and language, assessed at a particular point in its history. In contemporary social science, ethnic or national groups are loosely grouped together under the rubric of modern versus traditional or sometimes Western versus non-Western cultures. The former terms generally represent the industrialized world, the latter the developing countries. On a simplistic level, modern Western cultures are more often characterized as scientific, and traditional non-Western cultures as religious-magical, in their worldview. In almost all cultures, however, concepts of sexuality and appropriate sexual behavior are incorporated in the dominant religious tradition.

Our contemporary world is subject to mass migrations for both economic and political reasons, and ethnic groups from traditional cultures are likely to transport and transmit their views regarding human sexuality. Within industrialized societies, cultural attitudes toward sexuality also are affected by minority status, socioeconomic status, and interrelated sequelae of social deprivation. Sexual behavior may be affected by such variables as housing patterns and opportunities for assault, accessibility of potential victims, social discrimination and displaced rage, perceived criminality of specific types of sexual assault, and the degree to which censure of the larger society is contingent on the race or ethnicity of perpetrator and victim.

Cultural Norms and Views of Human Sexuality

Sexual victimization implies a subject–object relationship. Sexual assault involves the violation of both bodily and psychological boundaries against the will of a person seen as object. In an assessment of the salience and duration of negative psychological sequelae, the conceptualization of these boundaries may be all-important. Culture defines the extent to which a sexually aggressive act, whether bodily invasive or not, is perceived by significant others as an insult to the integrity of the assaulted individual.

Culture also determines the degree of censure applied to the perpetrator. Even when an act is negatively perceived, in many situations a particular cultural ambience may determine whether this assessment can even be acknowledged and acted upon by significant others and brought to the attention of legal authorities. In many contexts throughout the world, whether in war, slavery, or forced marriage, a member of an oppressed subculture may be sexually assaulted but understand that there is no possibility of punishing the perpetrator or preventing recurrence. The assault may be normalized or even sanctioned by the dominant power structure.

On a worldwide basis, various ethnic or national groups differ in their basic attitudes toward 1) the notion of a bounded, self-contained self with individual rights (Guisinger and Blatt 1994); 2) gender roles and appropriate prerogatives (Adler 1991); and 3) the rights of children and concepts of child abuse (Korbin 1981, 1987). A major factor is a culture's sex role differentiation and gender entitlement. To what degree is gender asymmetry—that is, male dominance and female subjugation—a factor in a culture's assessment of sexual assault? Although women in agrarian societies do heavy physical labor along with men, there is generally an inverse relationship between sex role differentiation and economic development. With industrialization and technological advances, societies offer greater opportunities for women of all classes to become more educated, assume productive roles in the labor market, demand equal rights, and reduce the distance between male and female prerogatives. Under these conditions there is greater acceptance of equal privilege both for sexual behavior and for the right of a woman or child to accept or reject sexual overtures.

The salience of fundamentalist religious beliefs is another aspect of gender asymmetry. In cultures that sanctify female subjugation on the basis of religious scripture or belief systems, sexual behavior is owned by the society rather than the individual participants. Women are typically categorized as chaste or unchaste based on their sexual history, even when they have been helpless to resist rape. Yet the culture may condone nonconsensual sexual assault on chaste women through forced marriage or punish unchaste women for consensual sexual activity. In either case the man is held blameless; it is the woman's status that establishes the appropriateness of the man's behavior (Adler 1991).

Commodification of women and children is an extremely important variable. In some cultures, women and children are perceived as property of their husbands or parents. Marriageable girls are owned by their fathers and are salable to others in order to improve the fortunes of the family. Children of either sex may be sold into prostitution. Ownership of women and children as sexual property has a long historical tradition in Western as well as non-Western cultures. This has been manifested in practices ranging from droit du seigneur, the codified right of a feudal lord to have sexual relations with a vassal's bride on her wedding night, to involuntary impregnation of female slaves.

Loh (1981) suggested that even in the United States, until very recently our legal definitions of rape have been based on common-law statutes that embody Victorian values of women as property. Rape has been viewed in terms of reducing the marketability of this property rather than as an assault on the bodily and psychological integrity of women. He states that rape legislation reform as late as the 1970s "reflects a shift . . . from protecting a tangible property interest to one of safeguarding an intangible, personal right" (p. 32).

Cultural Constructions of Child Sexual Abuse, Incest, and Rape

Child Sexual Abuse

Korbin (1987) states that "from a cross-cultural perspective, child sexual abuse can be defined as proscribed *sexual conduct* between an adult and a *sexually immature* child for purposes of the adult's *sexual pleasure* or for economic gain through child prostitution or pornography" (p. 248). The words are underlined in the original text to convey the idea that the concepts are culture-bound. Korbin points out that a man or woman's grasping the testicles of an adult male would be construed as sexual conduct in the United States, but would be considered a form of nonsexual greeting in Highland New Guinea. Kissing children's genitals would be considered sexual abuse in the United States but a manifestation of pride in certain areas of Turkey.

Sexual maturity is defined differently according to a society's values and needs, and sexual pleasure may take various cultural forms. Thus, the following criteria outlined by Korbin (1987, pp. 249–250) would yield a more functional cross-cultural definition:

1) *Violation of family roles/statuses.* Child sexual abuse is best conceptualized as the disruption of expected roles, relationships, and behaviors. . . . The precise sexual act is likely to be less important than the nature of the relationship that was violated. . . .

2) *Coercion.* A measure for assessing sexual abuse is the degree to which force, threat, or deceit must be brought to bear in order to obtain a child's compliance. . . . In most societies children are taught to obey adults, whether or not they wish to comply.

3) *Consent.* Sexual abuse may also be determined by the extent to which a child is capable, by virtue of age, power differentials, and the nature of the relationship[,] to freely consent. . . . A lack of physical or verbal resistance by a child does not necessarily imply consent.

4) *Secrecy.* Proscribed sexual conduct with children is likely to occur in extreme secrecy. If children are masturbated casually with other adults present, this must be considered differently than fondling of children that takes place secretly, with warnings to the child not to reveal what has transpired.

5) *Age discrepancy.* If there is an age discrepancy such that the child and the adult could not be considered appropriate marriage and/or sexual partners, the sexual conduct can more appropriately be categorized as abusive. Cultural practices such as child betrothal and marriage, however, complicate the issue.

In an earlier volume, Korbin (1981) described in great detail a range of cross-cultural child-rearing practices that would be considered highly abusive in modern cultures and abhorrent to Western sensibilities. According to LeVine and LeVine (1981), these practices have special indigenous meanings and reflect parental beliefs that they are acting in the best interests of their children. For the most part they are performed to help rather than harm children within the worldview of the culture. These practices range from elongating infants' skulls through bark bindings to cutting off small girls' finger joints during mourning ceremonies. Initiation ceremonies may require circumcision without anesthesia, clitoridectomies, or ritual mutilation. Langness (1981) cites a New Guinea practice of ritual defloration accompanying first menstruation. For betrothed girls, sexual intercourse first takes place with a male assigned this task by the bridegroom's father, then by the bridegroom's father, and only many months later by the bridegroom himself.

Sexual conduct with children may occur during religious or ceremonial events. In some parts of New Guinea, ritualized homosexuality is a component of male initiation rites. This is based on the assumption that boys acquire masculinity through the intake of semen during the prolonged practice of fellatio with older, sexually mature males. The intake of semen is symbolically equated with mother's milk as essential for development.

Sexualized behaviors with children may also be a common aspect of daily living. Korbin (1987) maintains that in several different societies it is normative for adults to nuzzle, blow on, sniff, and praise their children's genital organs since this behavior is associated with the child's eventual fertility. Children are sometimes encouraged to participate in games that pair sexuality with aggression. "Among the Bena Bena of New Guinea," Langness (1981) notes, "young boys are sometimes given sticks and encouraged to chase and beat girls, the adults urging them to 'stick it up her vagina' or 'go and hit her hard'" (p. 16).

Sexual aggression against females is culturally condoned in a variety of settings. In Turkey, Olson (1981) described child brides and bride kidnapping against the girl's wishes; a reputedly high incidence of wife beating; and abuse by in-laws. A common practice during sexual consummation of a marriage is for kin and wedding guests to wait outside in order to witness the bloodied sheet that proves the bride's virginity. Lack of such proof may lead to rejection and ostracism of the bride by husband and family. Seduction or rape can lead a child into prostitution, often the only recourse for a violated and abandoned young girl. This pattern is reportedly found throughout the Middle East, North Africa, and the Indian subcontinent. The selling of young girls by impoverished families has provided a sex market for Western tourists in some of the major cities of Southeast Asia.

Incest

The taboo against sexual intercourse or marriage between parents and children or siblings is presumed to be universal with respect to the nuclear family (Ember and Ember 1992). In many cultures these restrictions also apply to members of the extended kinship or clan network. Conversely, there may also be culturally exempted categories. In Bali, for example, twins were exempted from restrictions on brother–sister incest because they were presumed to have been previously intimate in the womb (Korbin 1987). The Incan, Hawaiian, and ancient Egyptian royal families permitted and even required incestuous marriages in order to perpetuate dynasties, but the incest prohibition has generally been strictly applied to commoners in all societies.

Numerous theories—both functionalist (society-maintaining) and psychoanalytic (defense against forbidden unconscious sexual desires)—have been advanced to explain this universality. These explanatory models are framed in terms of the social utility of the incest taboo to adult members of society, rather than the harm done to victims when the taboo is breached. La Fontaine (1987) has pointed out that anthropology has largely concerned itself with explaining the incest taboo but has had little to say about its violation. It is primarily in the context of Western cultures that social scientists have discussed pedophilic incest, as well as forced incest between stronger and weaker siblings, as an issue of child abuse.

LeVine and LeVine (1981) have reported in tropical Africa cases of rape of prepubescent girls by adult men who are closely related and are considered classificatory fathers of their victims. These authors have also come across cases of actual father–daughter incest and the seduction of pubescent girls by schoolteachers. The latter is a source of recurrent scandals in Nigeria and Kenya, and the teachers lose their jobs. Intrafamilial incest, however, is treated as a religious offense rather than a civil crime.

Finkelhor (1984) has estimated that within the United States, 1 in 20 females will be subjected to sexual contact ranging from fondling to full intercourse with a father or stepfather before the age of 18 years. There is an ironic relationship between the pace of industrial development and the incidence of socially recognized child abuse. Modernization is likely to be accompanied by more legal constraints against child abuse and sexual assaults against women and children. However, anthropologists report an actual increase in both child battering and sexual molestation under conditions of modernization and conspicuous social change (LeVine and LeVine 1981). With the stresses of rapid cultural transition, frustrations are displaced onto weaker victims and traditional norms and values lose their power to restrain formerly forbidden impulses.

Rape

From a random sample of 35 societies taken from the anthropological Human Relations Area Files, Rozee-Koker (1987) derived cross-cultural codes on seven types of female rape. Her sample included both matrilineal and patrilineal cultures. The codes were based on a conceptualization that takes into account "both the societal prescriptions for human genital contact and the individual woman's right and opportunity to choice in the matter" (p. 105). The essential feature of her model was normative (societally condoned) versus nonnormative (uncondoned) rape. Societal approval was considered present when 1) there is no punishment of the male or the female only is punished; 2) the rape itself is condoned as a punishment of the female, or 3) the rape is embedded in a cultural ritual such as an initiation ceremony.

Types of normative or socially condoned rape found in Rozee-Koker's sample of cultures included the following:

1. *Marital rape*. A woman has no rights or choice in consummating the marriage and/or in subsequent husband–wife genital contact.
2. *Exchange rape*. Males use female genital contact as a bargaining tool in woman-exchange, woman-sharing, women as stakes in gaming, and so forth.
3. *Punitive rape*. The woman is punished for going against male authority or for breaking social rules.
4. *Theft rape*. Women are involuntarily abducted to be used as sexual or reproductive objects, for prostitution, as spoils of war, and so forth.
5. *Ceremonial rape*. Types of ceremonial rape include defloration rituals, manhood rituals that require female submission, or other ceremonial practices involving females' participation in sexual intercourse, whether or not they are willing to participate.
6. *Status rape*. This form of rape is considered present when unchosen genital contact occurs as a result of differences in status, such as master and slave, chief and clanswoman, nobleman and commoner, or priest and parishioner.

Socially condoned, normative rape was found in all but one of the societies, whereas nonnormative or uncondoned rape was found in 63% of the societies. In 60% of the societies, both normative and nonnormative rape were found in the same culture. Rozee-Koker feels that these findings highlight the social complexity of the concept of rape. She notes that in most societies the simple definition of nonconsensual sexual relations simply does not obtain. There appears to be regulation, rather than prohibition, of forced genital contact with an unwilling female.

Definition of Sexual Assault and Attribution of Culpability in Modern Societies

In this section, we turn to cultural differences that inform the definition and handling of sexual assault in the Western world, with special reference to the United States. In many respects, it is easier to attribute harshly proprietary attitudes toward child and female sexuality to cultures perceived as less enlightened than our own. Most Western cultures have sanctions against adult genital contact with children, who presumptively lack the capacity for informed consent. Adult women, however, are presumed to have choice, and cultural definitions of rape are contingent precisely on the woman's implied consent. Bourque (1989) cited six surveys involving community assessments of simulated sexual encounters as rape or nonrape. All involved coercion, typically with a weapon, but the circumstances and the behavior and/or appearance of the victim were varied. The findings demonstrated that evaluations of the victim–perpetrator relationship and the social context of the encounter were as important as the element of force in defining rape.

Rape myths involve situations in which victims of coerced sex are viewed as seductive and therefore culpable. A four-nation study found that cultural acceptance of rape myths was significantly correlated with restrictive beliefs about women's social roles and rights (Costin and Schwartz 1987). In numerous studies, males are more likely than females to assess women's dress or behavior as a contributory factor in sexual assault (Bourque 1989). However, culture is sometimes more important than gender in assigning moral and causal responsibility (Kanekar and Vaz 1988). Thus, a rapist on trial may be rated more guilty when the victim is from the rater's own cultural group than from a cultural outgroup (Bagby and Rector 1992). Conversely, a victim from an outgroup may be perceived as having more contributory responsibility. Among White-American university students, for example, rape culpability attributions were greatest against Black rape victims and against White victims who had dated Black defendants (Willis 1992).

Victims may be injured not only by the often terrifying experience of rape itself but also, and possibly even more so, by a type of public response that Williams and Holmes (1981) termed the "Second Assault." Implicit in this public response are cultural attitudes toward rape that lead to denial or minimization of the experience, withholding of sympathy, and even condemnation of the victim. These cultural attitudes typically are internalized by the victims and presumably shape their psychological response to sexual assault.

Ethnic and Cultural Differences in Victims' Responses to Rape

The relationship between cultural attitudes toward rape and victims' responses was assessed in two interrelated studies by Williams and Holmes (1981, 1982) in San Antonio, Texas. The first study involved triethnic samples of African-American, Anglo, and Mexican-American female rape victims ($N = 61$). The second study surveyed public attitudes toward rape among 336 African-American, 335 Anglo, and 340 Mexican-American respondents in the same city. Victims' responses to rape were measured in terms of crisis response, feelings about men, health concerns, and general functioning. Public attitudes were tapped in a series of nine vignettes of forced sex that included "two stereotypic street rapes, two bar pickups, two hitchhikers, a date rape, a husband-wife assault, and the rape of a prostitute" (Williams and Holmes 1982, p. 157).

Mexican-American public attitudes reflected significantly more victim-blaming and less willingness to define situations as rape than did those of the other two groups, and Mexican-American victims were more adversely affected by the rape in terms of crisis response, negative feelings about men, and general functioning. In contrast, African-American victims evidenced the least severe degree of crisis, least impairment of functioning, and fewest health concerns, although they also reported negative feelings toward men. Anglo victims were least negatively affected in their attitudes toward men, but their responses were midway on the other measures. In the second, triethnic public attitudes study, however, Anglo respondents were least victim-blaming and most likely to assess situations as rape, while the African-American respondents were midway between the other two groups in terms of these measures. In the Williams and Holmes's studies, accordingly, the concordance between public attitudes and personal psychological response appeared to be consistent only for the Mexican-American respondents.

The questions posed in this research were partially replicated in a later study in Miami, Florida (Lefley et al. 1993). The sample comprised 101 African-American, Hispanic-American, and White-American female rape victims and 89 nonvictim control subjects aged 18 to 50 years (mean = 32 years). The victims were selected from 881 consecutive admissions to the rape treatment center of a large county hospital. The nonvictim control subjects, randomly selected from the same neighborhoods as the victims, were matched for ethnicity, marital status, age, and socioeconomic status (SES). In both groups, women with predisposing factors that might affect their psychological response, such as a history of mental illness, cognitive impairments, or a prior experience of rape or incest, were not included in the study.

All subjects responded to 1) nine rape scenarios involving forced sex with the assailant holding a weapon and 2) a 10-item questionnaire based on the instruments developed by Williams and Holmes (1981, 1982). In lieu of a public survey, the study assessed the subjects' own perceptions of how most men and most women in their cultural group would respond. The design for both measures was a group (victim/nonvictim) by ethnicity, by reference group (self, most men, most women) analysis. All respondents were tested with the Revised Symptom Checklist–90 (Derogatis 1977), and the rape victims were also administered the Impact of Events Scale (Horowitz et al. 1979). The latter yields factor scores on two maladaptive coping styles: intrusion ("unbidden thoughts and images") and avoidance ("denial of the meaning and consequences of an event, blunted sensations, and awareness of emotional numbness").

The authors found a significant main effect for the reference group and a significant ethnicity–by–reference group interaction. Within each ethnic group there was remarkable concordance of victims and nonvictims in their attributions of public beliefs about rape in their communities. All subjects found men to be more punitive than others toward victims, but African-American women were most likely to perceive men in their community as victim-blaming. Overall, however, Hispanics were most likely, and Whites least likely, to attribute victim-blaming to most men and most women in their ethnic communities and to include themselves in these sentiments.

There were highly significant differences between victims and nonvictims on scores from a battery of psychological instruments. Throughout, there were almost no ethnic differences in the mean scores of nonvictims. In contrast, the scores of victims on measures of psychological distress were found to be highest among Hispanics and lowest among Whites, with those of African Americans falling midway between the scores of the other two groups. On the SCL-90-R, Hispanic victims had higher mean Global Severity and significantly higher scores on the Obsessive-Compulsive scale ($P < .04$) compared with the other two groups of victims. On the Impact of Events Scale, Hispanic victims were most likely, African-American victims mediately likely, and White victims least likely to report both thought intrusion and avoidance as coping mechanisms. Hispanic victims were significantly more likely than the others to utilize avoidance as a response to anxiety-provoking situations ($P < .005$) (Lefley et al. 1993).

The findings in this study seemed to confirm that victims' psychological response to rape may reflect their internalization of cultural attributions regarding women's culpability in situations involving coercive sex. Similar findings in two very different samples of Spanish-speaking nationality groups—Mexican women in Texas and primarily Cuban women in Miami—suggest the persistence of pan-Hispanic cultural forms governing the behavior of men and women. Psychoculturally, we may speculate that cognitive dissonance is set up when *machismo*, the cult of virility, is counterposed to *marianismo*, the ennoblement of female chastity. Thus, people may find it natural for men to want to seduce women but, on the other hand, threatening to think of chaste women as being violated against their will. This dynamic may well underlie attitudes toward rape in many cultures that are highly sex-differentiated. Internalized cultural attitudes are manifested not only in victims' psychological reactions. They also may mediate the willingness of victims and their families to report sexual assault and to use the remedial resources offered by the larger society.

Cultural Differences in Risk Factors, Reporting, and Service Utilization

In the Lefley et al. study (1993), described in the previous section, some rape victims were excluded from the study because of characteristics that might have confounded interpretation of their psychological responses. These characteristics were also empirical risk factors for rape. Because they composed 49% of the potential subject pool, these victims were studied separately to determine if there were possible differences in risk factors among ethnic groups (Scott et al. 1993).

The study sample comprised 432 women, aged 18 to 50, who had been screened out of the 881 consecutive admissions to the rape treatment center. The group had failed to meet the following exclusionary criteria that were also risk factors: 1) history of previous rape and/or incest, 2) history of psychiatric hospitalization, and 3) mental retardation, current substance abuse, or other variables affecting cognitive capacity and alertness. Subjects with no local address were screened out because they were not accessible for follow-up interviews. Risk factors especially relevant in this group of victims (those with no fixed local address) subsumed 4) tourist or visitor status (site unfamiliarity) and 5) homelessness or temporary shelter (exposure and vulnerability).

Highly significant cultural differences were found in the following characteristics in proportion to the representation of the three ethnic groups. African-American women ($n = 181$) had a greater history of previous rape and/or incest ($P < .0001$). Hispanic women ($n = 83$) had a greater history of prior psychiatric hospitalization ($P < .004$). Tourists or visitors were more likely to be White ($n = 168$) ($P < .004$). Only 13 of the 432 screened-out victims were homeless street persons or in transient shelters, and the majority (77%) of these were White.

Socioeconomic differences may be salient factors in the differential history of prior rape among African-American women. That is, a greater number of victims may live in poorly protected crime-ridden neighborhoods. Research indicates that Hispanic women are least likely of all ethnic groups to utilize inpatient mental health services (Russo et al. 1987). Our highly disparate finding may indicate that only the most disabled Hispanic female rape victims are likely to present at the county hospital (those with prior experience with the system), whereas the Hispanic victim with more means is likely to avoid the public sector and go to a private physician.

Selective utilization of services may also affect statistics on homeless rape victims. Among the original 881 victims screened for the research project, just over 1% of the women reporting to the rape treatment center were living on the streets or in shelters. This seemed like a gross underestimate of a category of women who actually may have been raped during the study period. One speculation is that many homeless women, especially those with children, will not report rape because they fear that exposure to the police, health care, or social welfare systems may worsen rather than improve their lives.

The findings of more previous rape or incest among African-American women are contrary to those of Wyatt (1985). In a multistage, stratified probability sample of 284 African-American and White-American women in Los Angeles County, she found that 62% reported at least one incident of sexual abuse prior to age 18 years. However, abuse was reported by 57% of the African-American women, in contrast to 67% of the White-American women. The differences in the findings from the Wyatt (1985) and Scott et al. (1993) studies are not necessarily inconsistent. They may indicate that 1) there is less child sexual abuse in the African-American community, but 2) current black female rape victims are more likely to be repeat victims. Another interpretation is also likely, however. The findings from Scott et al.'s study may reflect more openness and less reluctance to disclose their past experiences by women who have already been identified as rape victims. This interpretation is reinforced by the large number of Hispanic women willing to disclose their psychiatric histories in the same study.

Despite this openness on the part of victims who have previously been admitted for treatment, the initial decision to reveal one's rape appears to be a function of the perceived benefits of obtaining treatment. This decision is related to the anticipated consequences of the revelation both within one's own culture and within the larger society. In a later study by Wyatt (1992), the findings indicated that African-American women were less willing than White women to disclose incidents involving rape. If the rapist is White, the victims may fear devaluation of their pain and also doubt evenhanded pursuit of the rapist by the police. If the rapist is Black, the victims may become protective of the image of black men, reluctant to contribute further to the racial myths and sexual stereotypes of the larger society.

The finding in the study by Scott et al. (1993) that a minuscule number of homeless women present for rape treatment suggests both a suppressed response in a life with multiple and often horrendous stressors and the possibility that interactions with "the system" may be feared even more than the sequelae of rape. Since women who live and sleep in the open are extremely vulnerable, the data imply vast underreporting of the actual prevalence of sexual assault in this population.

Long (1986) points out that cultural values and beliefs, particularly loyalty to one's group, have a marked impact on the reporting of abuse to authorities and the assessment and treatment of victims. She notes that in small rural towns and on American Indian reservations it is often impossible to prevent community awareness of victims, perpetrators, and informants. "Sanctions within a tribal clan or other subgroup are often more severe in relation to the informant than in relation to the abuser. . . . There may be negative consequences for the victim once outside intervention occurs. These consequences can include desertion, more severe abuse, and social isolation or stigmatization" (p. 133). In Long's analysis, the subculture and loyalties of healthcare professionals were given equal weight with those of other subcultural groups. One case study involved a psychiatrist who refused to acknowledge symptoms of sexual abuse in the clinically depressed daughter of a prominent surgeon. The psychiatrist reluctantly agreed to transfer the case only after the patient had clearly disclosed paternal sexual abuse to an inpatient nurse.

Patterns found in the National Study of the Incidence and Severity of Child Abuse and Neglect are even more salient with respect to bias in reporting. Of 77,000 recognized cases of child abuse in a 1-year period, hospitals tended to report to child protection agencies children who were African American, were younger, lived in lower-income urban areas, and had more serious injuries. Hospitals failed to report to child protection agencies almost half the cases in which the individual's experience met the study's definition of abuse. Discriminant analysis revealed that a disproportionate number of unreported abuse cases were from White families of higher income (Hampton and Newberger 1985).

Ethnic Differences in Child Sexual Abuse and Juvenile Offending

Child Sexual Abuse

Okamura and colleagues (1995) point out that reporting of child sexual abuse is very much a function of cultural factors of shame and denial. Thus, the basic data set utilized for ethnic comparison may in itself reflect not veridical differences in frequencies, but cultural differences in the willingness of both families and children to disclose information to authorities. As suggested previously, assessment and subsequent reporting of sexual abuse may also be affected by racial/ethnic prejudgments of the initial referral source.

Nevertheless, a substantial number of cases of physical and sexual abuse do reach the attention of authorities, and it must be assumed that existing data sets at least represent the distribution of the most severe cases. A study analyzed 4,132 cases of child physical abuse and sexual abuse reported in Los Angeles County with respect to ethnic differences (Lindholm and Willey 1986). This research produced interesting findings with regard to gender and ethnicity. Overall, in Anglo and Hispanic families fathers were more likely to inflict physical abuse, whereas in African-American families mothers more often inflicted such abuse. The trend of physical abuse by females was directly related to single-parent families in each ethnic group, with the higher rate among African-American families apparently attributable to the higher number of female-headed households.

Across racial/ethnic groups, however, suspected perpetrators of sexual abuse were in most cases male (95% were male, 5% were female). Among victims of physical abuse, males (88.3%) received more abuse than did females (64.7%). Among victims of sexual abuse, the ratio of females to males was almost 5:1. With respect to ethnicity, African-American children were more likely to have been physically abused, but less likely to have been sexually abused, than were Anglo or Hispanic children. The proportion of physical abuse to sexual abuse for African-American children was 81.3% versus 16.6%; for Hispanic children 73% versus 28.2%; and for Anglo children 73% versus 26.7%. The last two groups had remarkably similar proportions of physical to sexual abuse.

Overall, child sexual abuse occurred in 24.5% of the cases studied. There was a highly significant relationship between ethnicity and type of sexual abuse ($P < .0001$). Fondling occurred half as often among African Americans (4.9%) as among Hispanics (11.7%) and Anglos (11.2%). However, fewer Anglo females had to participate in sexual intercourse than Hispanic or African-American females. These patterns were similar to those reported by Rao and colleagues (1992) for an equally large sample of reported cases. They found that Asians and Whites were least likely to experience genital or anal intercourse (36% for each), while Hispanics (50%) and Blacks (58%) were most likely to have been victims of vaginal or anal intercourse.

In the Lindholm and Willey (1986) study, oral copulation was rare but was inflicted more often on Anglo children. Sodomy was also rare, but Hispanic boys were more likely to have been sodomized than Anglo boys, and African-American boys were not sodomized at all. Anglo children and females were more likely to have endured a combination of sexual abuse, including genitals, hands, mouth, and penetration by objects.

Ima and Hohm (1991) reported that physical abuse was much more common and sexual abuse much less common among Asians when compared with the general United States population.

A 2-year study of 2,007 victims of child sexual abuse presenting at a California child and adolescent sexual abuse treatment center evaluated cases involving Black (37.6%), White (25.9%), Hispanic (21.9%), Asian (6.6%), and racially mixed/other (7.2%) victims (Rao et al. 1992). Highly significant differences were found in the characteristics of the victim, the family, the assailant, and the abusive incidents. The mean age of the victims on presentation differed across ethnic groups. In mean years, Asian (11.5) and Hispanic (10.5) victims were significantly older than White (9.0) and Black

(8.7) victims. Asian and Hispanic victims and their families were also more likely to be immigrants to the United States and to have more intact families. The proportion of families in which the parents were living together differed across ethnic groups: Asians 54.0; Hispanics 27.0; Whites 23.9; and Blacks 12.7 ($P < .0001$ across all groups). Asian victims were significantly more likely than the others to be living in a shelter at the time of evaluation. These children had been sent to shelters by authorities to protect the victim after discovery of intrafamilial sexual abuse. The families were equivalent in SES. Asian, White, and Hispanic victims were more likely to have their mothers as primary caretakers, whereas Black victims were more likely to be cared for by another relative. Asian primary caretakers were only half as likely as primary caretakers in the other ethnic groups to report the abuse to authorities; 60% to 67% of those who brought the abuse to the attention of authorities in other ethnic groups were primary caretakers. Asian children were least likely to first disclose the abuse to their mothers (24.7%), compared with Black children (60%) and Hispanic children (52%).

In the Los Angeles study of Lindholm and Willey (1986), Hispanics had the highest rate of reported child sexual abuse. The findings are inconsistent with recalled sexual abuse in the Los Angeles Epidemiologic Catchment Area (ECA) Project survey. In this community survey, the prevalence rate of child sexual victimization was higher for non-Hispanic whites (8.7%) than for Hispanics (3.0%) (Siegel et al. 1987). Lindholm and Willey's lower rate of reported sexual abuse among Black children is congruent with Wyatt's (1985) finding in a probability sample of the general population, in which African-American women reported somewhat lower percentages of child sexual abuse than did White-American women. However, the lower rate is inconsistent with the significantly higher history of prior rape or incest reported by African-American women who are repeat rape victims (Scott et al. 1993) and must be evaluated within the context of Wyatt's (1992) contention that African-American women are less likely to disclose sexual assault to authorities.

Putative underreporting is related to the potential importance of disclosure to vulnerable lower-SES Black families. Abney and Priest (1995) suggest that in this social context, disclosure of sexual abuse by the victim brings not only shame but also fear of being believed, fear of being removed from the caretaker's home, and a belief that disclosure may lead to the dissolution of the family. This may be true of other minority groups as well.

Juvenile Sexual Offending

Barbaree and colleagues (1993) point out that among all of the offenses that were committed by adolescents and reported in the criminal justice statistics, 74% of the offenders were White. However, for sexual offenses the proportion drops to 64%, and for forcible rape, to 42% (Brown et al. 1984). Koss and Harvey (1991) state that "the typical image of a rapist, derived primarily from crime statistics, is that of a young, black, urban male, often of lower class status. However, other information suggests that the image is incorrect" (p. 38). They then go on to cite several studies that found no significant differences in the incidence and prevalence of rape as a function of race, social class, or place of residence. Again, this highlights the difficulties in assessing the true picture—that is, whether the racial/ethnic differences in the prevalence of sexual assault reflected in the crime statistics represent actual differences or are an artifact of biased treatment by the police and criminal justice system. Racial discrimination in the frequency and severity of charges for rape has been well documented (Bradmiller and Walters 1985).

In their cross-cultural study of more than 2,000 cases of child sexual abuse victims (aged 9 to 11.5 years), Rao and colleagues (1992) found significant differences among Black, White, Hispanic, Asian, and other victims but found no significant racial/ethnic differences in the 15% to 25% of abusers who were under 18 years of age.

The picture of the typical rape victim is similarly unclear. A national probability sample of all U.S. households found that the typical profile of the rape victim was a young, unmarried black woman of lower SES living in an urban area. Among female adolescents, however, the risk of forcible rape was higher for White teenagers than for Black teenagers among 13- to 15-year-olds (Ageton 1983).

In contrast, the more current ECA survey of 3,000 adult community residents in the Los Angeles area indicated that the highest rates of rape were reported by young non-Hispanic White women with some college education. In the most recent assault, three-fourths of the victims knew their assailant, and over half sustained physical injury (Siegel et al. 1987). In the ECA survey, Hispanics reported significantly lower rates of lifetime sexual abuse than did non-Hispanics, and men reported significantly lower rates of lifetime sexual abuse than did women. In cases of repeat victimization, however, after individuals had been victimized once, neither ethnicity nor gender was related to their probability of being sexually assaulted again (Sorenson and Siegel 1992).

Another variable relates to the degree of injury sustained during the rape. In a study of 440 cases of reported rape, White victims sustained both genital and nongenital injury almost twice as often as did Black victims. Survivors attacked by a single assailant were injured as often as survivors of gang rape (Cartwright 1987). This pattern suggested that hostility and bodily harm were more likely to be directed toward the White victims.

We have noted earlier in this section the apparent overrepresentation of African-American juvenile sex offenders in the statistics for forcible rape (Brown et al. 1984). Davis and Leitenberg (1987) suggested that this overrepresentation may be attributable to the predominant female head-of-household pattern in lower-SES African-American families, an explanation contested by Knight and Prentky (1993) as being discordant with other data. The large data set explored by Lindholm and Willey (1986) showed a correlation between maternal-headed families among African Americans and more physical abuse but less sexual abuse among African-American children when compared with Anglo and Hispanic children. Moreover, being raised in a maternal-headed low-SES home is not necessarily correlated with antisocial sexual behavior. A study of 305 adolescent sex offenders in which all social classes were represented found that 57% of the offenders were living in a two-parent household, 23% in a single-parent household, and 20% in other settings (Fehrenbach et al. 1986).

Ethnic Diversity, Minority Status, and Treatment Implications

Wyatt (1990) has developed what she terms the *Four Traumagenic Dynamics* model, in which the effects of sexual abuse on children from racial/ethnic minorities are compounded by their status and learned experiences within the majority culture. Traumatic sexualization—that is, the shaping of a child's sexuality in developmentally inappropriate and interpersonally dysfunctional ways (Finkelhor 1984)—occurs through numerous messages from society that people of color are as children sexually precocious and as adults hypersexual and have arcane erotic skills. Betrayal also emanates from the larger society as minority children learn the impact of various forms of racial discrimination. They are betrayed additionally by their parents' inability to protect them and ward off harm. Stigmatization shatters children's assumptions of a secure world, tarnishes self-image, and diminishes self-esteem. Powerlessness results when children perceive that the adults in minority groups lack a sense of control of their lives in such areas as employment or housing and are portrayed in the media as members of an underclass or as criminals. Other forms of victimization of minority children come from witnessing violence, death, and other terrorizing events. The cumulative impact of these various forms of victimization may exacerbate the effects of sexual victimization, and this may lead to posttraumatic stress disorder reactions that may be difficult for clinicians to evaluate and treat.

Wyatt recommends that clinicians assess the variety of victimization experiences that children have encountered and conceptualize how these experiences may be manifested in social, emotional, cognitive, and sexual functioning. She suggests that treatment programs include a variety of therapeutic techniques, including drawing, role playing, reading, family history taking, keeping diaries, and play therapy, as well as consultation with therapists from the victim's own cultural background.

African Americans

Although Wyatt's (1990) model applied to all ethnic minority groups, it has particular applicability to African Americans. Compared with other minorities, African Americans have had the greatest exposure to legally sanctioned oppression from the majority culture, in the form of slavery and of de jure as well as de facto segregation. The institution of slavery, with its practices of culturally endorsed rape, enforced miscegenation, arbitrary separation of parents and children, and deliberate deculturation policies, had a profound impact on black family life and generated both adaptive and maladaptive reactions.

According to Ho (1992), certain strengths were born of this heritage among many African-American families. These include strong kinship bonds; strong work, education, and achievement orientation; strong commitment to religious values and church participation; a humanistic orientation; and endurance of suffering. The humanistic orientation is described as an authentic, natural type of interpersonal connectedness "without the Puritan influences such as task-center[ed]ness and materialistic achievement that are characteristic of White middle-class American values. In adjusting to the victim system and adversity, Black Americans have developed great tolerance for conflict, stress, ambiguity, and ambivalence . . ." (Ho 1992, p. 78).

The higher tolerance thresholds that have enabled African Americans to endure suffering may also be inimical to their seeking help from mental health professionals. In Ho's schema, these characteristics derive from a strong religious orientation "which views emotional difficulties as 'the wages of sin' and interpersonal conflicts as not following 'the Lord's teachings.' To seek help from a therapist rather than through prayer may signify an absence of trust in God" (Ho 1992, p. 79).

Despite the continuing growth of the African American middle class, the sequelae of segregation and discrimination continue to include lower SES among African Americans as a group, a proliferation of single-parent households with multiple children in poverty, and numerous psychological problems among African American youth. According to Gould and Canino (1981), poor urban Black children showed higher rates of psychopathology and psychiatric impairment than all other ethnic groups. These problems ranged from low self-esteem (partially manifested in the skin-color discrimination that exists among Blacks themselves) to clinical depression. Black juvenile delinquents were found to have higher rates of depression and other psychological and neurological symptoms than do comparable White juvenile delinquents (Dembo 1988). Black inner-city youth were found to have school dropout rates ranging from 40% to 60%, primarily among males, with a high rate of functional illiteracy (Reed 1988).

Ho (1992) notes inordinately high birth rates (as high as nearly 90%) among unmarried Black women between the ages of 15 and 19 years. He points out that for many low-income Black teenagers, early parenthood may be viewed as a rite of passage and source of pleasure; however, having a child at an early age also interferes with opportunities for a productive and satisfying life. Female-headed households in poverty also provide a fertile ground for sexual abuse. If the woman is working, she has few options for selectivity of caregivers and often must leave her children with older siblings or untrained teenagers for many hours. Also, Abney and Priest (1995) note that "African American children may be exposed to adult males who are not their biological fathers for an extended period of time based on parental dating or live-in arrangements. This extended exposure to males who are not their biological fathers may place children at an increased rate of sexual victimization" (pp. 16–17).

Although the data suggest relatively lower rates of sexual abuse of African-American children, the reported abuse seems to be more severe. In a comparative study of female victims of incest, Russell and colleagues (1988) found that African-American victims were more severely abused than White victims in the sex acts performed. Their abuse was more often accompanied by force. They were older than White victims at the time of their first abusive experience, but the perpetrators were younger, indicating more adolescent offenders. The incest was more likely to occur with nonblood relatives than it was among White victims, although there were equal rates of abuse by fathers in the two groups. African-American women reported more long-term effects and more negative life experiences and were more upset by their experience than were White-American women, presumably because of the greater degree of dehumanization and violence accompanying the incest.

Abney and Priest (1995) suggest that for poor African-American families there is a cost-benefit ratio that must be taken into account in reporting sexual abuse to authorities. Included are the relative importance of the offender as a financial resource to the family and the possible effects of his loss on family stability. There is also the potential for long-term incarceration. As Abney and Priest (1995) note, "Some African American victims of sexual abuse may decide to suffer in silence to protect the African American male perpetrator, who is likely to receive more severe legal penalties for his behavior than a white male" (p. 16). With these pressures, child victims may be faced with a massive double bind that militates against disclosure to adults. If the family is defensive and refuses to believe that the abuse took place, the child will be accused of lying, punished, and further ostracized. If the child is believed, the disclosure may lead to separation and breakup of the family.

Abney and Priest (1995) emphasize the importance of establishing a safe therapeutic environment in which victims can discuss their feelings and concerns. They note that it is not unusual for African-American survivors of childhood sexual abuse to blame themselves for the victimization and to feel a need to shield the offender. Like Wyatt (1990), they believe that multiple layers of societal victimization may have contributed to this self-blame. In their experience, it is important to address in therapy the clients' cognitions regarding protection of sex offenders in the African-American community and to establish the appropriate target of accountability. As described by Abney and Priest (1995), "Specifically, the clients were encouraged to examine their beliefs that disclosing their childhood sexual victimization would in some way betray African Americans. Clearly there was a need to hold the offender accountable and for the client to be accountable to themselves and other potential victims" (p. 28).

These dynamics clearly apply in working with African-American child victims and their families. The tendency to protect offenders may be even more salient among adult household members who have not observed the abuse and who may minimize its impact on the child. In addition to the impact on victims being emphasized, cognitive strategies may be used in reframing assumptions that the offender will be prosecuted because of race rather than for criminal sexual abuse. It may be pointed out that protecting an African-American sex offender from "betrayal" means betrayal of an African-American child.

Asian Americans

Ima and Hohm (1991) reviewed 158 cases of child maltreatment among Asian-American and Pacific Islander clients that were reported to and handled by the Union of Pan Asian Communities in San Diego, California. They found that physical abuse was much more common and sexual abuse much less common in the Asian-American group compared with the general U.S. population. Continuity of social support systems and families' ability to cope with cultural conflicts were important factors in preventing and dealing with child abuse.

Ho and Kwok (1991) suggest that the Chinese pattern of child rearing from initial permissiveness to unquestioned obedience may facilitate using children as sexual objects. Yet any acknowledgment may bring such disgrace to the family that the likelihood of reporting sexual abuse to authorities or even to other family members remains minimal. This may explain why, in the study of child sexual abuse cases by Rao and colleagues (1992), more than 60% of Asian-American child victims never spontaneously disclosed the abuse and fewer than 25% disclosed the abuse to their mothers. It may also explain why primary caretakers in Asian families were 50% less likely than Black, Hispanic, and Anglo primary caretakers to report child sexual abuse to authorities.

Even past sexual victimization may bring disgrace. Writing about counseling Asian immigrants, Tsui (1985) points out that

> [w]ith sexual assault victims, the treatment issues are greatly complicated by the role of the family. A person's self-worth is often closely connected with upholding the family name and honor. Any person's disgrace or humiliation is perceived as bringing shame to the family, and this in turn is seen as a cultural infraction and personal failure. (p. 359)

Tsui goes on to say that this obtains even when family members are no longer in the picture or are deceased. Thus, Indo-Chinese refugees who had suffered rape or assault in their escape from Southeast Asia may still feel responsible for having brought shame to the deceased members of their family.

The particular emphasis on family disgrace may explain the unique demographic profile of Asian-American victims of child sexual abuse. In their cross-cultural study, Rao and colleagues (1992) reported clinically relevant differences between Asians and Black, Hispanic, and White victims and their families. Asian victims suffered less physically invasive abuse, were more likely to come from intact families, and were likely to be abused by a male relative living in the household. Asian victims had distinctive responses from the others. There was little sexual acting-out. This was attributed to cultural pressures against sexual behaviors and also a possible reporting bias due to cultural taboos against families or victims discussing sexual behaviors with outsiders. Asian victims were less likely to express anger and hostility but most likely to express suicidal impulses—a pattern also concordant with cultural norms against expressing hostility and with internalization of severe conflict.

Asian-American families were unique in their response to the abused child. They were least likely among the other ethnic groups to report the abuse, to refer the victim to authorities, or to be involved in the evaluation and treatment process. Overall, they were least likely to believe the abuse had occurred and were least supportive of the victim. This pattern of response may have been the result of, on the one hand, fear of blame and rejection by their community and, on the other hand, fear of the authorities, particularly because of the unique legal vulnerabilities of immigrant status.

Okamura and colleagues (1995) provide a series of guidelines in the treatment of Asian-American child victims, which involve 1) interviewing the child with a trusted adult; 2) avoiding repeated interviews; 3) recognizing the child's ambivalence, while providing a specific explanation of what will happen in the process of disclosure; and 4) when separation is necessary, matching the ethnicity of the child and the foster families and continuing contact with accepting family members. They note that treatment objectives include educating the entire family about abuse; their roles and responsibilities for supporting the victim; ways to avoid scapegoating the victim; and a commitment to the process of healing. For the child, there must be permission to express fears, anger, grief, and hopes for recovery.

Hispanic Americans

Like Asian Americans, Hispanic Americans tend to be underrepresented in case registers of child sexual abuse (Lindholm and Willey 1986; Siegel et al. 1987) as well as in reported sexual assault of women (Sorenson and Siegel 1992; Sorenson et al. 1987). Since many Hispanic Americans are immigrants, they also tend to be from more traditional cultures and to suffer the disclosure fears of groups already weakened by translocation, potentially vulnerable immigration status, and, in many cases, negative encounters with authorities.

Even among Hispanics who have had no problems with legal entry, prior experiences of colonialization may affect their self-image and cultural value system. With respect to Puerto Ricans, for example, Comas-Diaz (1995) states, "The sociopolitical context and the psychology of colonization provide a frame of reference for the internalization of oppression and victimization through sexual abuse" (p. 31). Comas-Diaz applies a sociodynamic explanatory model of sexual abuse in which the abuse is viewed not as an individual psychological aberration inflicted on a helpless victim, but as a product of powerlessness of men and enslavement of women and children.

As noted earlier, Scott and colleagues (1993) found that an unusually high number of Hispanic women reporting for rape treatment at a county hospital had a history of psychiatric hospitalization. This finding was highly at variance with the significant underrepresentation of Hispanic women in inpatient psychiatric facilities (Russo et al. 1987) and with the risk factors reported by victims from other ethnic groups. It was suggested that Hispanic women willing to appear at a county rape treatment center were likely to be those already identified with public-sector services. In the largely middle-class, predominantly Cuban population of Miami, we speculated that perhaps the majority of nonpsychiatric Hispanic rape victims were using private physicians and maintaining secrecy, so the information never appeared in any case register.

It is of course possible that the disproportionately low numbers of Hispanic child and adult victims may be the result of, at least partially, more intact and extended families, with less privacy and greater oversight of children, and a more homebound role for women. However, the disclosure issues previously discussed may have a major impact on reporting and comparative statistics. Fear of disclosure and underreporting are particularly salient in a cultural milieu with strong views about male and female sexuality and equally strong views about relations with authority.

Comas-Diaz (1995) has noted the relevance of *respeto* (respect), particularly respect for older people and authority figures, to the problem of sexual assault in Puerto Rican culture. "Respeto may play a central role in the sexual abuse of Puerto Rican children. A child may become the victim of sexual abuse by someone deserving respect. Similarly, a sexually abused child may fear breaking the silence due to respect for the abuser and fear of the consequences of breaking a cultural taboo" (p. 39).

Another issue in Puerto Rican culture involves sexual abuse of males in relation to homophobia. The popular belief that male survivors of sexual abuse become homosexuals militates strongly against disclosure by child victims. Paradoxically, the offender may be forgiven and the victim scorned. Comas-Diaz (1995) notes that

> [m]ales are considered to have a deep urgent need to satisfy their sexual appetites. Men who act frequently on these needs with a variety of partners are called *bugarrones*. If there are no females available (partly because marianista women are not allowed to have premarital sex), then another male can serve as a sexual partner. Because the *bugarron* is the aggressor, he is not considered a homosexual, as opposed to the male in the receptive role, who is considered homosexual . . . A pedophile could take advantage of the existence of the role of the bugarron as a potential justification for his abusive behavior with children. (p. 43)

Women rape victims are sometimes likely to be more scorned than their macho abusers, on the premise that the men could not control themselves but the women should have been able to avoid their defilement. The studies reported by Williams and Holmes (1981, 1982) and by Lefley and colleagues (1993) indicated that Hispanic rape victims suffered greater psychological distress than their African-American or White-American counterparts and also were more likely to blame themselves. Their distress correlated with more victim-blaming and greater subscription to rape myths in the assessed or ascribed attitudes of the Hispanic community. Separate research projects indicated that Hispanic female victims in two different sites and of very different national backgrounds were more likely than Black or White female victims to feel despoiled and somewhat to blame for having experienced sexual assault.

As in Asian cultures, the violation extends to the victim's significant others. In Hispanic cultures, *familismo* means that the individual is an integral part of the group, so anything that stigmatizes the victim inevitably stigmatizes the family as well. *Machismo* connotes virility, but it also means that "the man is the provider and is responsible for the welfare, honor, dignity, and protection of the family" (Comas-Diaz 1995, p. 40). This means that any violation of a woman or a child violates the men who have been unable to protect them.

In the treatment of female rape victims from traditional cultures, the family support system should be engaged as soon as possible. Male family members may be heavily invested in outrage and vengeance toward the offender, so it is important that therapists acknowledge that rape harms an entire family but that there are clear boundaries between primary and secondary victimhood. The message must be conveyed that the family's primary efforts should focus on returning the victim to psychological well-being rather than avenging family honor. Counselors should make special efforts to treat the victim with pronounced respect as well as sympathizing with her ordeal. If possible, other authority figures should be enlisted to model respect and reinforce the victim's value as a person, defining her as an individual who has been violated but not sullied.

Among the Hispanic victims in the study reported by Lefley et al. (1993), the tendency toward avoidance as a coping strategy, the tension between avoidance and intrusive thoughts, and the use of obsessive-compulsive mechanisms suggested ongoing investments of energy in trying to block the traumatic event. Because avoidance is such a powerful defense among these victims, and the level of distress is so high, counselors should be alert to appropriate pacing of interventions and initially limit them to empathy and support. Ultimately, victims can be led toward open discussions of the assault and toward an understanding of their own altered cognitive schemas, a typical legacy of rape (Koss and Harvey 1991). These schemas, which may range from self-punitive assumptions that the victim could have prevented the rape to an undue fear of recurrent pervasive dangers, should be confronted so that negative self concept and phobic reactions can be counteracted.

Conclusion

This chapter began with references to some normative practices in distal tribal cultures that would very likely be considered sexually abusive by all groups living in Western cultures, including those representing diverse ethnic backgrounds. However, research suggests differences among some racial/ethnic groups in the United States with respect to the definition of rape of adult women. Even when sex is coerced with a weapon, rape definitions appear to some extent at least to be contingent on behavior, situation, and status of the participants. In these situations, members of minority groups appear to be least likely, and White Americans most likely, to define any type of coerced sex as rape. Beliefs about sexual encounters, however, may reflect sociological realities as well as ethnological perceptions. With a long history of discrimination and police bias, combined with cultural myths about hypersexuality and sexual prowess of Black and Hispanic males, members of minority groups may have less inclination to interpret as rape the types of sexual encounters that can lead to criminal prosecution. Nevertheless, it is apparent that Hispanic and African-American women who are raped pay a heavy price for the perceived diminishment of their experience in their own culture.

Although similar research is lacking on definitions of child sexual abuse, in anecdotal and clinical materials there appears to be unanimity among ethnic minority cultures on the unacceptability of adult sex with children (Fontes 1995b). In fact, some writers have contended that children from minority groups are constantly exposed to rapelike experiences of institutional racism in terms of attributed hypersexuality, betrayal of trust, and stigmatization (Wyatt 1990) and/or a cultural ambience of powerlessness of men and subjugation of women and children (Comas-Diaz 1995). In this conceptual model, sexual abuse must be clinically treated within the sociocultural context of multiple forms of victimization and internalized helplessness.

The analyses offered by Comas-Diaz (1995) and Wyatt (1990) frame sexual abuse within the context of social oppression of Hispanics and African Americans, as well as other minority groups. This perspective may involve a number of psychodynamic issues that would benefit from exploration both in research and in therapy. For ethnic minority groups, these include the following assumptions:

1. Sexual assault is an additional burden and compounds the agony of victims who have been violated in many other ways by the society in which they live.
2. Sexual abuse may reflect displacement of the rage of powerless men against women and children.
3. Victims are likely to have low self-esteem and believe they deserve what happens to them.
4. Fear of disclosure may be both personally and socially protective.

Disclosure is threatening to vulnerable family systems, and maintaining silence will keep the child victim from being punished or separated from the family. Because of cultural myths about the sexuality of people of color, adult female rape victims will tend to protect the image of males in their society. They will also be reluctant to expose their own weakness and/or violation.

In terms of acknowledgment and definition of child sexual abuse, it appears that the more traditional the ethnic group, the more shameful the behavior and the greater the disgrace to the victim and family. If the abuse takes place within the household, the disgrace is so great that there may be an immediate effort to deny the act and thereby protect the perpetrator. Paraphilias are a source of family shame in any culture but are likely to be exceptionally threatening to the stability of traditional or group-oriented family systems. To a far greater extent than groups from mainstream American culture, ethnic minority groups continue to maintain sociocentric rather than individualistic value systems. These values are both traditional and adaptive for groups that tend to band together for mutual self-protection. In sociocentric cultures, however, the disgrace of the abuser and the disgrace of the abused both bring shame to everyone in the family. Open acknowledgment may also result in culturally insensitive and grossly destabilizing interventions from the welfare and criminal justice systems.

Various authors have offered guidelines for working with victims from specific ethnic groups (Fontes 1995b). Fontes (1995a) cautions that specific treatment recommendations based on the client's culture should be seen not as rigid prescriptions, but more as suggestions for consideration. It is important, however, that clinicians be aware of widely prevalent fears of minority and immigrant groups that agencies will take their children away and may use children's accusations to destroy families. For this reason, it is doubly important that the family feel welcomed and respected by the clinician in any type of intervention. The essence of cultural competence is to make the family feel validated, supported, and understood rather than to know bits of information about the culture that may or may not be relevant to treatment.

In a sociocentric culture, the family is the victim's lifetime support system, and acceptance by significant others is essential. Therefore, suggestions for working effectively with family members should be given equal weight to treating the victim. Some general suggestions are given below, with the caveat that each group is different not only culturally but in terms of its experiences with the health, welfare, criminal justice, and immigration systems. African-American families, for example, may have more reason to fear foster-home placement for an abused child. American Indian families are sociocentric but are less likely than traditional immigrants to feel that the actions of one member reflect badly on the others. Hispanic-American and Asian-American families are more likely to be immigrants or refugees and to feel threatened by the criminal

status of an offender-family member. Depending on their prior experiences, some may feel singled out for unjust accusations. Moreover, most members of ethnic minorities are poor. Facing threats of
deportation or imprisonment of a breadwinner, some families may
exert exceptional pressures on the victim to recant. In these situations, the clinician must be able to distinguish between desperation
and denial and to convey an attitude that is both understanding and
supportive as well as authoritative.

In working with families of traditional cultures, the therapist
should emphasize his or her role as a respected expert. The expert
must be able to explain the victim's fears of disclosing abuse, his or
her reactions and subsequent behaviors, and the need for the family
to avoid scapegoating and provide loving support. The family may
expect explanations for the offender's behavior, particularly if he
or she is a relative or friend. In this case, the expert may have to
"normalize the abnormal" with reassurances that these events occur
in other families as well, across cultures and social classes. The expert's explanation of a paraphilia as a recognized disorder, and the
message that the family is to be sympathized with rather than dis-
graced, are important therapeutic mechanisms for changing attitudes and attributions.

References

Abney VD, Priest R: African Americans and sexual child abuse, in Sexual
    Abuse in Nine North American Cultures. Edited by Fontes LA. Thou-
    sand Oaks, CA, Sage Publications, 1995, pp 11–30
Adler LL (ed): Women in Cross-Cultural Perspective. New York, Praeger,
    1991
Ageton SS: Sexual Assault Among Adolescents. Lexington, MA, Lexington
    Books/DC Heath, 1983
Bagby RM, Rector, NA: Prejudice in a simulated legal context: a further
    application of social identity theory. European Journal of Social Psychol-
    ogy 22:397–406, 1992
Barbaree HE, Hudson SM, Seto MC: Sexual assault in society: the role of
    the juvenile offender, in The Juvenile Sex Offender. Edited by Barbaree
    HE, Marshall WL, Hudson SM. New York, Guilford, 1993, pp 1–24
Bourque LB: Defining Rape. Durham, NC, Duke University Press, 1989

Bradmiller LL, Walters WS: Seriousness of sexual assault charges: influencing factors. Criminal Justice and Behavior 12:463–484, 1985

Brown EJ, Flanagan TJ, McLeod M (eds): Sourcebook of Criminal Justice Statistics–1983. Washington, DC, U.S. Department of Justice, Bureau of Justice Statistics, 1984

Cartwright PS: Factors that correlate with injury sustained by survivors of sexual assault. J Obstet Gynecol 70:44–46, 1987

Comas-Diaz L: Puerto Ricans and sexual child abuse, in Sexual Abuse in Nine North American Cultures. Edited by Fontes LA. Thousand Oaks, CA, Sage Publications, 1995, pp 31–66

Costin F, Schwartz N: Beliefs about rape and women's social roles: a four-nation study. Journal of Interpersonal Violence 2:45–56, 1987

Davis GE, Leitenberg H: Adolescent sexual offenders. Psychol Bull 101:417–427, 1987

Dembo R: Delinquency among black male youth, in Young, Black, and Male in America: An Endangered Species. Edited by Gibbs J. Dover, MA, Auburn House, 1988, pp 174–189

Derogatis LR: SCL-90-R: Administration, Scoring and Procedures Manual II, 2nd Edition. Towson, MD, Clinical Psychometric Research, 1977

Ember CR, Ember M: Cultural Anthropology, 7th Edition. Englewood Cliffs, NJ, Prentice-Hall, 1992

Fehrenbach PA, Smith W, Monastersky C, et al: Adolescent sexual offenders: offender and offense characteristics. Am J Orthopsychiatry 56:225–233, 1986

Finkelhor D: Child Sexual Abuse. New York, Free Press, 1984

Fontes LA: Culturally informed interventions for sexual child abuse, in Sexual Abuse in Nine North American Cultures. Edited by Fontes LA. Thousand Oaks, CA, Sage Publications, 1995a, pp 259–266

Fontes LA (ed): Sexual Abuse in Nine North American Cultures. Thousand Oaks, CA, Sage Publications, 1995b

Gould M, Canino I: Estimating the prevalence of childhood psychopathology. J Am Acad Child Adolesc Psychiatry 20:462–476, 1981

Guisinger S, Blatt SJ: Individuality and relatedness: evolution of a fundamental dialectic. Am Psychol 49:104–111, 1994

Hampton RL, Newberger EH: Child abuse incidence and reporting by hospitals: significance of severity, class, and race. Am J Public Health 75:56–60, 1985

Ho MK: Minority Children and Adolescents in Therapy. Newbury Park, CA, Sage Publications, 1992

Ho TP, Kwok WM: Child sexual abuse in Hong Kong. Child Abuse Negl 15:597–600, 1991

Horowitz M, Wilner N, Alvarez W: Impact of Events Scale: a measure of subjective stress. Psychosom Med 41:209–218, 1979

Ima K, Hohm CF: Child maltreatment among Asian and Pacific Islander refugees and immigrants: the San Diego case. Journal of Interpersonal Violence 6:267–285, 1991

Kanekar S, Vaz L: Attribution of causal and moral responsibility to a victim of rape. Applied Psychology 37:35–49, 1988

Knight RA, Prentky RA: Exploring characteristics for classifying juvenile sex offenders, in The Juvenile Sex Offender. Edited by Barbaree HE, Marshall WL, Hudson SM. New York, Guilford, 1993, pp 45–83

Korbin JE (ed): Child Abuse and Neglect: Cross-Cultural Perspectives. Berkeley, CA, University of California Press, 1981

Korbin JE: Child sexual abuse: implications from the cross-cultural record, in Child Survival: Anthropological Perspectives on the Treatment and Maltreatment of Children. Edited by Scheper-Hughes N. Dordrecht, The Netherlands, D Reidel, 1987, pp 247–265

Koss MP, Harvey MR: The Rape Victim. Newbury Park, CA, Sage Publications, 1991

La Fontaine JS: Preliminary remarks on a study of incest in England, in Child Survival: Anthropological Perspectives on the Treatment and Maltreatment of Children. Edited by Scheper-Hughes N. Dordrecht, The Netherlands, D Reidel, 1987, pp 267–290

Langness LL: Child abuse and cultural values: the case of New Guinea, in Child Abuse and Neglect: Cross-Cultural Perspectives. Edited by Korbin JE. Berkeley, CA, University of California Press, 1981, pp 13–34

Lefley HP, Scott CS, Llabre M, et al: Cultural beliefs about rape and victims' response in three ethnic groups. Am J Orthopsychiatry 63:623–632, 1993

LeVine S, LeVine R: Child abuse and neglect in sub-Saharan Africa, in Child Abuse and Neglect: Cross-Cultural Perspectives. Edited by Korbin JE. Berkeley, CA, University of California Press, 1981, pp 35–55

Lindholm KJ, Willey R: Ethnic differences in child abuse and sexual abuse. Hispanic Journal of Behavioral Sciences 8:111–125, 1986

Loh WD: What has reform of rape legislation wrought? Journal of Social Issues 37 (suppl 4):28–52, 1981

Long KA: Cultural considerations in the assessment and treatment of intrafamilial abuse. Am J Orthopsychiatry 56:131–136, 1986

Okamura A, Heras P, Wong-Kerberg L: Asian, Pacific Island, and Filipino Americans and child sexual abuse, in Sexual Abuse in Nine North American Cultures. Edited by Fontes LA. Thousand Oaks, CA, Sage Publications, 1995, pp 67–96

Olson EA: Socioeconomic and psychocultural contexts of child abuse and neglect in Turkey, in Child Abuse and Neglect: Cross-Cultural Perspectives. Edited by Korbin JE. Berkeley, CA, University of California Press, 1981, pp 96–119

Rao K, DiClemente RJ, Ponton LE: Child sexual abuse of Asians compared with other populations. J Am Acad Child Adolesc Psychiatry 31:880–886, 1992

Reed R: Education and achievement of young black males, in Young, Black, and Male in America: An Endangered Species. Edited by Gibbs J. Dover, MA, Auburn House, 1988, pp 65–78

Rozee-Koker PD: Cross-cultural codes on seven types of rape. Behavior Science Research 21:101–117, 1987

Russell DEH, Schurman RA, Trocki K: The long-term effects of incestuous abuse: a comparison of Afro-American and White-American victims, in Lasting Effects of Child Sexual Abuse. Edited by Wyatt GE, Powell GJ. Newbury Park, CA, Sage Publications, 1988, pp 119–134

Russo NF, Amaro H, Winter M: The use of inpatient mental health services by Hispanic women. Psychology of Women Quarterly 11:427–441, 1987

Scott CS, Lefley HP, Hicks D: Potential risk factors for rape in three ethnic groups. Community Ment Health J 29:133–141, 1993

Siegel JM, Sorenson SB, Golding JM, et al: The prevalence of childhood sexual assault: the Los Angeles Epidemiologic Catchment Area Project. Am J Epidemiol 126:1141–1153, 1987

Sorenson SB, Siegel JM: Gender, ethnicity, and sexual assault. Journal of Social Issues 48:93–104, 1992

Sorenson SB, Stein JA, Siegel JM, et al: The prevalence of adult sexual assault: the Los Angeles Epidemiologic Catchment Area Project. Am J Epidemiol 126:1154–1164, 1987

Tsui AM: Psychotherapeutic considerations in sexual counseling for Asian immigrants. Psychotherapy 22 (suppl 2):357–362, 1985

Williams JE, Holmes KA: The Second Assault: Rape and Public Attitudes. Wesport, CT, Greenwood Press, 1981

Williams JE, Holmes KA: In judgment of victims: the social context of rape. Journal of Sociology and Social Welfare 9:154–169, 1982

Willis CE: The effect of sex role stereotype, victim and defendant race, and prior relationship in rape culpability attributions. Sex Roles 26:213–226, 1992

Wyatt GE: The sexual abuse of Afro-American and white-American women in childhood. Child Abuse Negl 9 (suppl 4):507–519, 1985

Wyatt GE: Sexual abuse of ethnic minority children: identifying dimensions of victimization. Professional Psychology: Research and Practice 21:338–343, 1990

Wyatt GE: The sociocultural context of African American and white American women's rape. Journal of Social Issues 48:77–91, 1992

Phenomenology and Assessment of Sexually Aggressive Behavior and Treatment Considerations

6

Male Adolescent
Sex Offenders

Jon A. Shaw, M.D.

Acts of sexual aggression have become increasingly commonplace in our society. The increase in youth violence, homicides, and sexual aggression has been well documented (Elliott 1994a, 1994b, 1994c; Office of Juvenile Justice and Delinquency Prevention 1994). For example, arrests of juveniles for forcible rape increased 20% between 1983 and 1992 (Office of Juvenile Justice and Delinquency Prevention 1994). Sexual assault and sexual exploitation of children is widespread. A survey of high school students revealed that one out of five had been involved in committing acts of forced sex and that 60% of the boys found it acceptable in one or more situations to force sex on a girl (Davis et al. 1993).

Studies of adult sex offenders have consistently demonstrated that the majority admit the onset of some form of sexual offending behavior before 18 years of age (Abel et al. 1985; Longo and Groth

1983). The age at which the peak number of sexual assaults are committed by males is 17 years (Elliott 1994c). Twenty percent of all rapes and 30% to 50% of all child molestations are committed by juveniles under 18 years of age (Deisher et al. 1982). Ageton (1983) concluded from a probability sample of male adolescents aged 13 to 19 years that the rate of sexual assault per 100,000 male adolescents ranged from 5,000 to 16,000.

A *sexual offender* is an individual who has committed an act of sexual aggression that has "breached societal norms and moral codes, violated federal, state, municipal law, statute or ordinance and which usually but not necessarily results in physical or psychological harm to the victim" (National Task Force on Juvenile Sex Offending 1993, p. 10). Generally, the term *sex offender* refers to an individual who 1) has been convicted of committing a sex crime in violation of the state or federal laws, 2) has been awarded deferred adjudication for a sex crime under state or federal laws, 3) admits to having violated state and federal laws with regard to sexual misconduct, or 4) evidences a paraphiliac disorder as defined by DSM-IV (American Psychiatric Association 1994).

This chapter addresses the profile of the male adolescent sex offender, types of sexual offenses, psychiatric comorbidity, coexisting academic and school problems, social and family environment, the role of sexual victimization in the history of the sex offender, and treatment considerations.

Profile of the
Male Adolescent Sex Offender

Studies of adolescent sex offenders indicate that the majority of these individuals commit their first sexual offense before 15 years of age, and not infrequently before 12 years of age (Araji 1997; Awad et al. 1984; Longo 1982; Shaw et al. 1993). Early studies were concerned with trying to define a child molester syndrome or profile. Schoor and colleagues (1966) described the juvenile sex offender as generally being a loner. He was found to be sexually naive and immature and to prefer to play with younger children. Abel and colleagues (1985) characterized the sex offender as manifesting impaired social skills, lack of assertiveness, deviant sexual fantasies, and inappropriate sexual belief. Knight and Prentky (1993) suggest that it may be useful to classify adolescent sex offenders along two dimensions: 1) adolescent sex offenders who continue to offend into adult life versus those who desist; and 2) adolescent sex offenders who are rapists versus those who are child molesters. Efforts to categorize subsets of adolescent sex offenders have the value of delineating risk and protective factors that may shape course and outcome. The complex, multidetermined nature of adolescent sexual offending behavior, however, has made it difficult to set up a predictable taxonomic system. At present, there is considerable evidence that no one profile or typology is characteristic of the adolescent sex offender (Becker and Hunter 1993; Levin and Stava 1987).

Adolescent sex offenders are a heterogenous population. Although the overwhelming majority are male, they are represented in every socioeconomic status (SES) and every racial, ethnic, religious, and cultural group (Ryan et al. 1996). However, a number of factors have been found with uncommon regularity in the history of the adolescent sex offenders. These factors, as outlined by Becker and Hunter (1993), include

- Impaired social and interpersonal skills
- Delinquent behavior
- Impulsivity
- Academic difficulties
- Family instability
- Family violence
- Abuse and neglect
- Psychopathology

Sexually aggressive youth are more likely than youth in the general population to endorse traditional sex role stereotypes, themes of male dominance, rape-supportive myths, and interpersonal violence as a way of resolving conflict (Epps et al. 1994; White and Koss 1993).

Although a number of theories have been proposed as to why individuals become sex offenders, there is little empirical evidence to support any one of them. What is clear is that there is no single causal factor but rather a multiplicity of casual determinants and pathways to sexually aggressive behavior (Becker 1994). There are essentially four kinds of sexual offending behavioral patterns (Becker 1988), with most adolescent sex offenders combining various features of each:

1. Truly paraphiliac behavior with a well-established deviant sexual arousal pattern
2. Sexual offending behavior that is but one facet of the opportunistic exploitation of others
3. Sexual offending behavior that is related to a psychiatric or neurobiological substrate disorder such that the offender is unable to regulate and modulate his impulses
4. Impairment of social and interpersonal skills resulting in the offender's turning to younger children for sexual gratification unavailable from his peer groups

Types of Sexual Offenses and Victim Profiles

Sexual offending behavior ranges from noncontact sexual behavior such as obscene phone calls, exhibitionism, voyeurism, and lewd photographs to varying degrees of child molestation involving direct sexual contact such as frottage, fondling, digital penetration, fellatio, sodomy, and various other aggressive sexual acts. There is considerable diversity and range of severity of sexual offending behavior. In some instances the sexual offending behavior may be related to social and emotional immaturity, curiosity, and experimentation. In others the sexually aggressive acts are but one facet of a pattern of aggressive-violent acts against others or a manifestation of severe emotional, behavioral, and developmental psychopathology.

The spectrum of sexual offending behavior reported in the literature varies from one sample to another. Understandably, there are differences in behavior among those sex offenders incarcerated, those placed in residential centers, and those seen in outpatient clinics. In a descriptive study of male adolescents accused of committing sexual crimes and evaluated at the University of Washington Adolescent Clinic, it was noted that the most common offenses were "indecent liberties" or sexual touching (59%), rape (23%), exhibitionism (11%), and other noncontact sexual offenses (7%) (Fehrenbach et al. 1986). Wasserman and Kappel (1985), reporting on the sexually abusive behaviors of a group of adolescent sex offenders under 19 years of age, found that the spectrum of sexually aggressive acts included some form of penetration (59%), intercourse (31%), oral-genital contact (12%), genital fondling (16%), and noncontact sexual offenses (12%). Shaw and colleagues (1993) studied adolescent sex offenders in a residential treatment program and found a high proportion of violent and invasive sexual acts; 56% had committed vaginal rape, and 44% had perpetrated acts of anal sodomy, and the average offender had committed over nine sexual crimes and had victimized four to five persons. Abel and colleagues (1986) noted that the average juvenile sex offender under 18 years of age had committed eight sexual offenses and victimized an average of 6.7 persons. A review of a national sample of 1,600 sexually abusive youths from inpatient and outpatient samples, aged 5 to 21 years, reported that 68% of the sexual offenses involved penetrating and/or oral-genital behavior and that the offender had victimized an average of 7.7 persons (Ryan et al. 1996).

Most studies suggest that the victims of these young sex offenders are younger children. Abel and Osborn (1992) observed that 55% of the victims of adult sex offenders were 13 years of age or younger. Fehrenbach and colleagues (1986), in their study of adolescent sex offenders, noted that 62% of the victims were under 12 years of age and 44% were 6 years of age or younger. The great majority of victims are under 10 years of age (Ryan et al. 1996). Shaw and colleagues (1993), in their study of adolescent sex offenders, reported that the average age of the first victim was 6 years and the average age of the offender when committing the first sexual offense was 10 years.

The victims of male sex offenders are usually female. The proportion of female victims among those victimized by adolescent sex offenders ranges from 55% to 95% (Davis and Leitenberg 1987; Fehrenbach et al. 1986; Longo 1982; Schoor et al. 1966). Male victims of juvenile sex offenders tend to be younger than their female counterparts (Schoor et al. 1966). Hunter and Becker (see Chapter 8, this volume) note that assaults by juvenile sex offenders account disproportionately for the majority of assaults against boys. From 65% to 70% of male child molestations are carried out by juvenile sex offenders.

It has been generally recognized that although adolescents usually use coercion in the process of committing sexual offenses, they are less likely to harm their victims when compared with adult sex offenders. The coercion is usually expressed as bribery, intimidation, threats of harm or violent injury, physical force, and, rarely, use of a weapon (Fehrenbach et al. 1986; Knight and Prentky 1993; Ryan et al. 1996). Nevertheless, it is well known that victims report higher levels of coercion and force than are self-reported by offenders (Davis and Leitenberg 1987). Fehrenbach and colleagues (1986) found that 22% of the offenders in their sample continued their sexually aggressive acts even when the victims expressed "hurt or fear."

Psychiatric Comorbidity

Adolescent sexual offending behavior is often associated with a matrix of behavioral, emotional, and developmental problems (Awad et al. 1984). It is only in the last two decades that investigators have begun to examine adolescent sex offenders in an effort to explicate the spectrum of psychopathology (Becker 1988; Kavoussi et al. 1988; Lewis et al. 1979; Shaw et al. 1993, 1996). The findings are understandably affected by factors such as the assessment/evaluative approaches, diagnostic instruments, sample selection (e.g., inpatient vs. outpatient), and severity of offending behavior.

Lewis and colleagues (1979) studied 17 violent sex offenders and found a high prevalence of psychological comorbidity (ranging from 46.7% to 75%). The most common findings were symptoms of depression, auditory hallucinations, paranoid symptoms, and illogical thought processes. They found little difference between violent sex offenders and nonsexually violent delinquents on these measures. The sexually assaultive youth were described as having been violently antisocial since early childhood, and "violence in general rather than sexual aggression characterized their childhood" (p. 1195). Tartar and colleagues (1983) compared violent and non-violent delinquents and sex offenders across a broad range of intellectual, neuropsychological, and psychoeducational variables and found no differences between the groups. Awad and colleagues (1984) compared 24 adolescent sex offenders with a matched group of non–sexual-offending delinquents and found that the two groups were more alike than different. They were comparable in terms of variables such as the prevalence of psychiatric disturbance, violence, and sexual deviancy among parents, disrupted child–parent relationships, inadequate parenting, and history of school problems and delinquency.

Kavoussi and colleagues (1988), using semistructured interviews, evaluated 58 outpatient adolescent sex offenders aged 13 to 18 years and found that 81% had additional psychiatric diagnoses. The most frequent diagnoses were conduct disorder (48%), substance abuse (18.9%), adjustment disorder with depressed mood (8.6%), attention-deficit hyperactivity disorder (6.9%), and social phobia (5.2%). Becker and associates (1986a, 1986b) found that 63% of adolescent sex offenders presenting for psychiatric assessment were diagnosed as having conduct disorder. In a later study, Becker and colleagues (1991) administered the Beck Depression Inventory to 246 outpatient adolescent sex offenders and noted that 42% could be described as being depressed.

Shaw and colleagues (1993) reported on 26 boys, aged 9 to 14 years, who had been admitted to a residential treatment center for severe sexual offending behavior. Using the Diagnostic Interview Schedule for Children, the authors found that 21 (81%) met the DSM-III-R (American Psychiatric Association 1987) criteria for conduct disorder, 13 (50%) for anxiety disorder, and 9 (35%) for major depression or dysthymia. The younger the child when he committed his first sexual offense, the higher the number of coexisting psychiatric diagnoses (Shaw et al. 1994). When the sexual offending group was compared with a control group matched for conduct disorder, age, and ethnicity, the only significant differences found between the two groups was that the sexual offending group scored significantly lower on the Math subtest of the Wide Range Achievement Test—Revised and manifested more aggressive symptoms. No differences were found between the two groups in terms of psychiatric comorbidity. The authors suggested that sexual offending behavior is strongly linked to conduct disorder and that youths who force sex may not differ from other youths with conduct disorder. It appears that sexual offending behavior in this inpatient sample is an interesting variation on a well-established matrix of antisocial and aggressive behavior. The majority of the boys (65%) had a long-established history of aggressive, antisocial, and criminal behavior. The history of being sexually victimized in these youths (68%) may have facilitated, organized, and consolidated sexual offending as an additional pathway for the expression of antisocial behavior.

It is known that adult sex offenders frequently manifest significant personality disturbances (Packard and Rosner 1985). Shaw and colleagues (1993, 1996), in an effort to explicate personality traits and to unravel the complexity of character pathology among juvenile sex offenders, administered the Structured Clinical Interview for DSM-III-R Personality Disorders (SCID-II; Spitzer et al. 1989), Millon Adolescent Personality Inventory (MAPI; Millon et al. 1984), and Revised Diagnostic Interview for Borderlines (DIB-R; Gunderson and Zanarini 1983) to adolescent sex offenders in a residential center. On the SCID-II, the average sex offender in their sample manifested five personality diagnoses, with 68% of the boys having more than four diagnoses. This finding is congruent with findings from the adult literature, in which it is noted that more than one personality disorder is usually present in severe character pathology. Shaw et al. found a high prevalence of severe personality traits, including conduct-disorder, borderline, and narcissistic behaviors. Ninety-two percent of the boys were diagnosed with conduct disorder, 67% with narcissistic personality disorder, and 72% with borderline personality disorder (BPD). The high prevalence of narcissistic and borderline psychopathology is congruent with histories of severe emotional, physical, and sexual abuse.

On the MAPI, the personality traits that best described this population were asociality, indifference to others, strong-willed traits, social uneasiness, tendency to dominate others, unkindness, impatience with the weaknesses of others, discontent, pessimism, and unpredictability and preference for unpredictable situations. These adolescents presented with egocentricity, low self-esteem, poor self concept, poor sexual acceptance, family discord, self-deprecation, and a readiness to be influenced by others. They manifested poor impulse control, impulsivity without concern for eventual consequences, negative school experiences, and truancy. The general pattern of personality traits in this group of adolescent sex offenders noted on the MAPI was similar to those reported for adolescents with severe behavioral and conduct disorders (Hart 1993; Holcomb and Kashani 1991).

The presence of BPD varied from 35% to 72% depending on the measure. On the DIB-R, 44% of the offenders met the diagnostic criteria for BPD. The younger the age at onset of the sexual offending behavior and the younger the sex offender was at the time of his own sexual victimization, the more likely he was to exhibit borderline symptomatology. Those sex offenders who only abused boys were significantly more impulsive.

Shaw et al.'s findings suggest that sexual offending behavior is strongly linked to core antisocial psychopathology with severe characterological disturbances. Prior nonsexual delinquent behavior in the history of the sex offender has been reported in from 27% to 91% of sex offenders depending on the sample (Awad et al. 1984; Becker et al. 1986a, 1986b; Fehrenbach et al. 1986; Saunders et al. 1986; Schoor et al. 1966). Ryan and colleagues (1996) found that the majority of juvenile sex offenders in a national survey had a history of nonsexual delinquent behavior, including shoplifting (41.4%), theft (30.7%), assault (26.4%), vandalism (20.0%), and cruelty to animals (8.1%). Nonsexual offenses at the time of evaluation were reported in 63% of the offenders, and approximately 30% had committed more than three nonsexual offenses. Ageton (1983) observed that adolescent sex offenders are basically delinquent youth who are not well integrated into the social order or school and are strongly bonded to delinquent peers.

Elliott (1994a), based on the National Youth Survey, a longitudinal study of a national probability sample of 1,725 youths aged 11 to 17 years, with subsequent waves of data, documented that rape is the final step in a progressive sequence of violent criminal activity. He found that aggravated assault precedes rape in 92% of the cases and that robbery precedes rape in 72%. The usual sequence of criminal behavior is from aggravated assault to robbery to rape. The peak age at commission of sexual assault was 17 years. Rapists were found to have committed virtually every form of violent offense. One subset of sexually aggressive offenders is characterized by core antisocial character structure in which the sexual aggression is only one facet of a lifestyle in which the individual opportunistically exploits others for personal gain and gratifications.

A history of prior sexual offenses at the time of the apprehension approximated 60% in two surveys of adolescent sex offenders (Fehrenbach et al. 1986; Smith and Monastersky 1986). Ryan and colleagues (1996), in her national survey of juvenile sex offenders, observed that only 7.5% of the offenders had been previously charged with a sexual offense.

Academic and School Problems

The adolescent sex offender usually presents with a history of academic and school behavior problems and performs less well on tests of academic skills (Awad and Saunders 1989; Awad et al. 1984; Fehrenbach et al. 1986; Kahn and Chambers 1991; Langevin 1992; Lewis et al. 1979; Shaw et al. 1993; Ryan et al. 1996). Awad and Saunders (1989) found that 83% of the adolescent sex offenders in their sample had serious learning difficulties. In their national survey of juvenile sex offenders, Ryan and colleagues (1996) discovered that 60% of sexually abusive youths were known to have a history of truancy, learning disabilities, and learning problems at school. Lewis and associates (1979) reported that a group of violent sex offenders functioned 5.59 years below their age in reading.

Not infrequently, learning deficiencies and vulnerabilities associated with biological substrate and cognitive impairments have compromised the adolescent's capacity to do well in school and to assimilate and integrate complex social information. Langevin (1992) presented evidence of neuropsychological impairment in 40% of a sample of sex offenders.

Social and Family Environment

Adolescent sex offenders manifest impaired social and interpersonal skills. Fehrenbach and colleagues (1986) found that 65% of the offenders in their sample were socially isolated and that 32% did not have a friend. Awad and colleagues (1984) reported that 46% of their sample of adolescent sex offenders were loners. There is some evidence that adolescent sex offenders who are unable to relate to their peer group frequently turn to younger children for companionship (Awad and Saunders 1989; Schoor et al. 1966).

The family environment of adolescent sex offenders is usually characterized by psychosocial adversity manifested by family instability, exposure to violence, emotional neglect, harsh inconsistent parenting, physical and sexual maltreatment, and loss of parental figures through death, divorce, and out-of-home placement (Awad et al. 1984; Becker et al. 1993; Knight and Prentky 1993; Lewis et al. 1979; Ryan et al. 1996; Shaw et al. 1993). Ryan and colleagues (1996) found that 41.8% of the sexual offending youth in their sample had been victims of physical abuse and that 38.1% had been victims of sexual abuse. Approximately 64% had witnessed "family violence in the home." There is increasing evidence that sexual maltreatment and exposure to family violence are contributory to the later onset of sexual offending behavior.

The Role of Sexual Victimization

The evidence of psychosocial adversity in the lives of adolescent sex offenders has been well documented. The cycle of violence and sexual aggression is passed from one generation to the next. Early childhood victimization increases the risk for subsequent delinquent behavior, violent behavior, and criminality (Kobayashi et al. 1995; Widom 1989; see also Hunter and Becker, Chapter 8, this volume). Kobayashi and colleagues (1995) found that physical abuse by father and sexual abuse by males increased sexual aggression by adolescents.

Knight and Prentky (1993) described the intertwining of sexual and physical abuse and neglect in the developmental histories of sexually aggressive juveniles. Although exposure to physical violence and abuse among these boys is high, it is comparable to that generally found among other delinquents (Lewis et al. 1979). More emphasis has been placed on the role of sexual victimization in the history of sex offenders.

The proportion of adolescent sex offenders who were themselves sexually victimized prior to committing their first offense varies from 19% to 82% depending on the sample (Becker et al. 1986b; Fehrenbach et al. 1986; Longo 1982; Ryan et al. 1996; Shaw et al. 1993). Additionally, there is evidence that the younger the child is when he commits his first sexual offense, the more likely it is that that child has been sexually victimized (Johnson 1988). The relationship between childhood sexual victimization and sexually aggressive behavior, along with representative clinical examples, is discussed in Chapter 1 of this volume.

Clinical Vignettes

A number of clinical vignettes are now presented to illustrate the complex relationship between sexual offending behavior and a history of having been sexually victimized.

▶ Case 1

A., a 14-year-old boy, was brought in for treatment after anally so-domizing three younger boys and tying one up with ropes and holding a knife to his throat. He showed little remorse, regret, or victim empathy.

In his therapy he would reveal and openly acknowledge "violent sexual fantasies." He described how he would "seek out" little boys, wishing to "trap them" and wanting "to have control over them." He spoke of the pleasure he derived from "having the power to make anybody I want to do anything I want." He enjoyed his victims being "scared, shaking and cooperative." He coerced them by threatening to cut off their penises or to shoot them in the head.

A. had a history of aggressive and impulsive behavior and had been called a bully because he threw a baseball at a child's face and often kicked and hit other children. He reportedly "sexualized" everybody. He grabbed the breasts of his 60-year-old foster mother. A. had a history of sexually touching younger children.

When asked about his feelings while sexually molesting children, A. responded, "My mother did this to me, and I decided I will do it to them." He reported that in his family "we would have sex together." He claimed that since about 5 years of age, "We would have sex with each other, Mom, Dad, sister, and me." There was a long history of physical abuse, neglect, and abandonment. His mother had been sent to jail for sexually molesting his sister. He was ordered into foster care when he was 7 years of age "based on abandonment and a history of being exposed to deviant sexual behavior." His school record was characterized by behavior problems and poor academic performance in spite of above-average intelligence.

He recalled how when he was a young child, from 3 to 7 years of age, his mother would come home drunk and make him sleep with her, forcing him down upon her, coercing him to have oral sex with her, and laying on top of him trying to get him to stick his penis into her. He described these experiences without affect, minimizing their importance. He spoke of "enjoying the scary moment." It is only with continuing therapy that he began to talk about feeling trapped, his repugnance to her drunken breath, her threats to deprive him of food, and her slapping him and vague threats to castrate him. The mother had a history of being sexually abused by her own father. A. stated that he had a "big problem. . . . If I don't get help I will be doing these things to kids the same that they did to me, get arrested . . . maybe the electric chair."

▶ Case 2

B., a 12-year-old boy, was referred to treatment after being apprehended for sexual assault. He presented with a history of breaking and entering 17 times during the previous year. Although it was initially thought that the infraction was for the purpose of stealing, it became apparent that it was motivated by a wish to molest women as they slept. He would peep through the windows, spying on a woman until she went to sleep. He would then sneak into her room and proceed to uncover her and begin to sexually touch her. He had been caught four times for this behavior and had been placed in juvenile detention for short periods of time with no change in his criminal behavior.

B. reported that since the age of 11 he felt a compulsion to observe women aged 20 to 30 years through windows as they were undressing or taking a shower. As this compulsion became stronger, it became associated with the wish to break into the house in order to sexually touch the women. He had the fantasy that the women would wake up and want to have sex with him. He did not understand the nature of this compulsion and was initially very vague when talking about his sexual activities. B. reported that in kindergarten he was instructed by his teacher to sit under her desk and stroke her legs repetitively, and he recalled moments of sexual arousal and excitement. Upon admission to the residential treatment center he was found to be very depressed and suicidal, with symptoms of insomnia, psychomotor retardation, appetite disturbance, and self-recrimination.

▶ Case 3

C., a 13-year-old boy, was apprehended and brought to treatment after allegations of sexual misconduct with a 4-year-old girl. It was alleged that he had digitally penetrated her anus and vagina and had oral contact with these organs. He admitted to having planned the sexual attack after watching pornographic videotapes. "I started to get ideas, and I started to think that I could get away with it with the little girl. . . . I started to plan it out and reassured myself that I wouldn't get caught. I went down there one day after school. I felt she trusted me and I could get away with it." There was a history of precocious sexual activity with other children from the time he was 5 years of age that included fellatio and penile-anal sex with other boys in a day care center. At age 5, C. and a 6-year-old boy watched a cable television channel with pornographic programming and fondled each other. At age 7 years, C. engaged in mutual masturbation with two other boys. At age 12 years, he fondled, fellated, and performed anal intercourse on a 9-year-old boy.

    C. had a history of voyeurism, exhibitionistic behavior, fire setting, bestiality, and sadism toward animals. He would be cruel to any animal he could get his hands on; he would kick and throw things at them. He had deliberately broken the leg of a dog. C. showed little remorse or empathy. At 2 years of age, he was expelled from day care for his aggressive behavior. He was subsequently diagnosed as having attention-deficit hyperactivity disorder and was treated with various psychostimulants. He would have explosive aggressive outbursts when confronted with his misdeeds. He bullied other children and was described as predatory.

▶ Case 4

D., a 13-year-old boy, was referred for treatment because he had molested his 6-year-old sister, 4-year-old brother, and a 14-year-old boy. He performed vaginal and anal intercourse on his sister. He forced his younger brother to lick his ear while he fondled his buttocks. Another time he had sucked his brother's ear and bellybutton. The mother had been aware that for a prolonged period of time D. had been coercing his brother and sister to suck his ear. After being placed in a detention center, he forced a 14-year-old boy to allow him to place his penis in the boy's ear.

At age 4 years, D. had been sexually molested by an adult female neighbor who would invite him over to play with her little girl. The neighbor reportedly made D. perform vaginal intercourse on her and other sexual acts. He contracted gonorrhea, which was subsequently treated. D.'s mother had a history of drug problems and prostitution, and she subsequently died from AIDS. D. remembered an aunt who would frequently come to the house and who would constantly play with his ears, nibble on them, and lick them, which he found exciting and arousing. This behavior sensitized his own erotic sensitivity to ears. During treatment, D. was perceived as a highly dependent adolescent who yearned for nurturance. He had a poor self-image and feared injury and rejection. Quickly overwhelmed with minor stress, he responded with impulsive aggressive behavior.

▶ Case 5

E., a 13-year-old boy, was brought into treatment after repetitively sexually abusing his 7-year-old sister by forcing her to fellate him and vaginally penetrating her. He showed little remorse or regret. In spite of her protestations and crying, he would persist in his behavior. His family minimized the behavior, noting that he was just being a boy. In the course of therapy, he described his masturbatory fantasy, which graphically illustrates how one's own sexual victimization gets played out over and over again in sexual offending behavior.

In his fantasy, E. reported, "I walk into a small room, there is a girl, 10–11 years of age. She is sitting and writing at a desk. I look around to see if there is anybody around. I look twice. I scream at her to stand up. She looks scared and helpless. She is terrified. I tear off her dress. I begin to fondle her. She fights back. I overpower her. I feel strong. I force her to suck my penis. I stick my penis in her vagina. I interrupt the fantasy. I try to intervene. Suddenly the image turns into my father. I remember my father coming into my room. It is a small room. He begins to fondle me, touching my penis. I remember he tore off my clothes and made me suck his penis, and he stuck his penis into my anus. I felt powerless and afraid. I don't like to feel powerless. It's when I feel powerless that I begin to imagine raping a girl. When I tear off her dress I feel in control." He describes being powerless as meaning "I can't control other people." Further discussion led to his remembering the sexual excitation he felt and his penis becoming erect when his father abused him. He had two feelings. He felt scared, helpless, and terrified, but he also had the feeling of sexual excitement. He didn't understand why he was sexually aroused. He felt guilty about the sexual excitement.

Treatment Considerations

The natural course of adolescent sexual offending behavior is not well known. Dorshay (1943) found very little recidivism among 256 juvenile sex offenders treated in New York Court Clinic. Marshall and Barbaree (1988) estimated that the recidivism rate for untreated sexual offenders is 40%. In an 8-year follow-up of 19 sexually assaultive male adolescents, Rubenstein and colleagues (1993) found that 37% had sexually reoffended and that 89% had committed other acts of violence.

It is a social imperative that the population of adolescent sex offenders who will be the adult sex offenders of tomorrow be the focus of prevention-intervention strategies today. As therapists, our first task is to protect the community. There is encouraging evidence that a high percentage of these offenders will respond to therapeutic intervention. In contrast to the pessimism usually articulated by laypeople regarding treatment of the adolescent sex offender, the empirical evidence indicates that this is a population that responds well to treatment interventions (Becker 1994; Bremer 1992; Dwyer 1997). There are several reasons why the adolescent offender is more amenable to treatment than the adult sex offender:

1. The adolescent offender's deviant pattern of sexual offending behavior is less deeply ingrained.
2. The adolescent is still exploring alternative pathways to sexual gratification.
3. The adolescent's central masturbatory fantasy is still evolving and is not fully consolidated.
4. The adolescent is more amenable to learning more effective interpersonal and social skills.

There is general agreement that the recidivism rate for effective treatment programs is in the range of 5% to 15% (Knopp 1991). In a follow-up of 285 adolescent sex offenders, aged 12 to 18 years, at an average of 3 years of "time from release to follow-up," Bremer (1992) found a 6% recidivism rate based on sexual offense conviction. When the subjects were interviewed, the recidivism rate rose to 11% based on self-report. Schram, as cited by Becker and Hunter (1993), reported on a 6.8-year follow-up of 197 treated adolescent sex offenders and observed that 10% had been convicted of sexual offenses. Smith and Monastersky (1986) found that 14.3% of their 112 adolescents had reoffended within a period of 17 to 49 months following discharge from a community-based adolescent sex offender program. O'Brien, as cited in Bremer (1992), noted a 9.2% recidivism rate among 69 adolescents within 12 to 30 months after release from the program.

In spite of the number of studies suggesting a low recidivism rate among treated juvenile sex offenders, questions remain. Critical commentary of treatment studies has focused on methodological flaws, and specifically the lack of random assignment, controls, and post-test design only paradigms (Furby et al. 1989; Miner 1997). Maletzky (1997) suggests, however, that few would argue for untreated control groups of juvenile sex offenders. It is unethical to withhold treatment for those who want treatment and unethical to fail to protect the community by failing to intervene with juvenile sex offenders. In spite of the lack of empirical rigor, there is considerable evidence that treatment interventions are effective in interrupting the course of sexually abusive behavior. Hall (1995), in a meta-analysis of 12 studies, found a small but significant effect of treatment over no treatment.

Treatment of the adolescent sex offender has generally focused on a number of different goals, outlined by Becker (1988, 1994), that are thought to be integral to ending sexually aggressive behavior:

1. Confronting the offender's denial
2. Decreasing deviant sexual arousal
3. Facilitating nondeviant sexual interests
4. Promoting victim empathy
5. Providing sex education
6. Enhancing social and interpersonal skills
7. Using values clarification
8. Incorporating cognitive restructuring
9. Teaching the adolescent to recognize the internal and external antecedents of sexual offending behavior with appropriate intervention strategies
10. Implementing family therapy

The level of therapeutic intervention is determined by the frequency and aggressivity of the sexual offense, psychiatric comorbidity, individual acknowledgments of the sexual crime, motivation for treatment, capacity for empathy, social and interpersonal relatedness, and appropriate intellectual, psychological, and social support systems (Groth et al. 1981; Shaw et al. 1994).

Nevertheless, it is evident that not all adolescent sex offenders are treatable. A careful assessment and diagnostic procedure is instrumental to any treatment program and should include psychosocial, educational, and medical-psychiatric evaluations. Treatability depends on a number of factors (Smith and Monastersky 1986; Shaw et al. 1994):

1. Understanding of the seriousness of the offense
2. Motivation for change
3. Capacity for empathy and human relatedness
4. Severity of psychopathology
5. Deviant sexual arousal patterns
6. Type and frequency of sexual offending behavior
7. Aggressivization of the sexual offense
8. Degree of characterological impairment of personality functioning
9. Nature of the treatment program

As a group, adolescent sex offenders have generally experienced considerable psychosocial adversity, including exposure to violence and coercive sexuality, psychological neglect, inconsistent and harsh and often cruel punishment, family instability, and a lack of a predictable caring and nurturing environment. Many of these individuals have been sexually and physically abused. Frequently, they have experienced the losses of significant loved ones through separations, divorce, violence, and death. Family instability and family insensitivity to societal norms have often exposed these children at a very early age to explicit and coercive sexuality and pornography, including X-rated films. These youths emerge out of these experiences with little capacity for empathy and compassion. They are opportunistic and exploitative and have little respect for or appreciation of societal norms and expectations.

The spectrum of emotional, behavioral, and developmental problems presented by these young people requires a complex, multimodality, and multidimensional treatment program. Treatment approaches may include the following:

1. *Group therapy*, which is the preferred intervention for sex offenders and is usually the format through which psychoeducational, behavioral, and relapse prevention models are implemented
2. *Behavioral management techniques* that attempt to decrease deviant sexual arousal patterns and encourage and reward appro-

priate peer-related social behavior, impulse control, modulation of victimization behavior, and respect for the rules of group life

3. *Psychoeducational modules* that provide information and instruction regardng victim empathy, anger management, cognitive restructuring, sex education, anxiety managment techniques, and social skills

4. *Relapse prevention techniques* that stress the importance of understanding cognitive distortions, the antecedents and contextual factors that trigger sexually aggressive fantasies and behavior, and the development of coping strategies with which to interrupt the sexual offending

5. *Peer-related group therapy* to facilitate interpersonal relatedness and the capacity to work with others in a shared task

6. *Individual therapy*, which, with its emphasis on understanding the offender's individual distress, provides an opportunity to work through earlier childhood experiences and history of child maltreatment or sexual victimization and facilitates the development of a therapeutic alliance, increasing the receptivity of the offender to other aspects of the treatment

7. *Specialized educational programs*, with an emphasis on academic and learning deficiencies that are invariably present in the lives of adolescent offenders

8. *Psychopharmacological interventions*, when necessary, to address compulsive and obessional sexual preoccupations and the spectrum of emotional and behavioral problems that are frequently comorbid with the sexual offending

9. *Family therapy* to facilitate the resolution of family conflict and, when applicable, to prepare for the reintegration of the adolescent sex offender back into the home

Nevertheless, in spite of our best efforts, there will be individuals who are so psychologically and neurologically damaged and without social conscience or respect for others that they will not respond to our treatment armamentarium as it now exists. These individuals will continue to be a threat to society, and it will be necessary to incarcerate them for the protection of the community.

References

Abel GG, Osborn C: The paraphilia, the extent and nature of sexually deviant and criminal behavior. Psychiatr Clin North Am 15 (suppl 3): 675–687, 1992

Abel GG, Mittelman M, Becker JV: Sex offenders: results of assessment and recommendations for treatment, in Clinical Criminology: The Assessment and Treatment of Criminal Behavior. Edited by Ben-Aron M, Hucker SJ, Webster CD. Toronto, M & M Graphics, 1985, pp 191–205

Abel GG, Rouleau J, Cunningham-Rathner J: Sexually aggressive behavior, in Psychiatry and Psychology: Perspectives and Standards for Interdisciplinary Practice. Edited by Curran W, McGarry A, Shah S. Philadelphia, PA, FA Davis, 1986, pp 289–314

Ageton SS: Sexual Assault Among Adolescents. Lexington, MA, Lexington Books, 1983

American Psychiatric Association: Diagnostic and Statistical Manual of Mental Disorders, 3rd Edition, Revised. Washington, DC, American Psychiatric Association, 1987

American Psychiatric Association: Diagnostic and Statistical Manual of Mental Disorders, 4th Edition. Washington, DC, American Psychiatric Association, 1994

Araji SK: Sexually Aggressive Children. Thousand Oaks, CA, Sage Publications, 1997

Awad GA, Saunders EB: Adolescent child molesters: clinical observations. Child Psychiatry Hum Dev 19:195–206, 1989

Awad GA, Saunders EB, Levene J: A clinical study of male adolescent sex offenders. International Journal of Offender Therapy and Comparative Criminology 28 (suppl 2):105–116, 1984

Becker JV: Adolescent sex offenders. Behavior Therapist 11:185–187, 1988

Becker JV: Offenders: characteristics and treatment. Future Child 4:176–197, 1994

Becker JV, Hunter JA: Aggressive sex offenders. Child Adolesc Psychiatr Clin North Am 2:477–487, 1993

Becker JV, Cunningham-Rathner J, Kaplan MS: Adolescent sex offenders. Journal of Interpersonal Violence 1:431–445, 1986a

Becker JV, Kaplan MS, Cunningham-Rathner J, et al: Characteristics of adolescent incest sexual perpetrators: preliminary findings. Journal of Family Violence 1:85–97, 1986b

Becker JV, Kaplan MS, Tenke CE, et al: The incidence of depressive symptomatology in juvenile sex offenders with a history of abuse. Child Abuse Negl 15:531–536, 1991

Becker JV, Harris CD, Sales BD: Juveniles who commit sexual offenses: a critical review of research, in Sexual Aggression. Edited by Nagayama Hall GC, Hirschman R, Graham JR, et al. Washington, DC, Taylor & Francis, 1993, pp 215–228

Bremer JF: Serious juvenile sex offenders: treatment and long term follow-up. Psychiatric Annals 22:327–332, 1992

Davis GE, Leitenberg H: Adolescent sex offenders. Psychol Bull 101:417–427, 1987

Davis TC, Peck GQ, Storment JM: Acquaintance rape and the high school student. J Adolesc Health 14:220–224, 1993

Deisher RW, Wenet GA, Paperny DM, et al: Adolescent sexual offense behavior: the role of the physician. Journal of Adolescent Health Care 2:279–286, 1982

Dorshay LJ: The Boy Sex Offender and His Later Career. New York, Grune & Stratton, 1943

Dwyer SM: Treatment outcome study: seventeen years after sexual offender treatment. Sexual Abuse: A Journal of Research and Treatment 9:149–160, 1997

Elliott D: The developmental course of sexual and non-sexual violence: results from a national longitudinal study. Paper presented at the annual meeting of the American Association for the Treatment of Sexual Abusers, San Francisco, CA, November 1994a

Elliott D: Serious violent offenders: onset, developmental course, and termination—the American Society of Criminology 1993 Presidential Address. Criminology 32 (suppl 1):1–21, 1994b

Elliott D: Youth Violence: An Overview (F-693). Boulder, CO, Center for the Study and Prevention of Violence. University of Colorado, Boulder Institute for Behavioral Sciences, March 1994c

Epps KJ, Haworth R, Swaffer T: Attitudes toward women and rape among male adolescents convicted of sexual versus nonsexual crimes. J Psychol 127:501–506, 1994

Fehrenbach PA, Smith W, Monastersky C, et al: Adolescent sexual offenders: offender and offense characteristics. Am J Orthopsychiatry 56:225–233, 1986

Furby L, Weinrott M, Blackshaw L: Sex offender recidivism: a review. Psychol Bull 105(1):3–30, 1989

Groth AN, Hobson WF, Lucey KP, et al: Juvenile sex offenders: guidelines for treatment. International Journal of Offender Therapy and Comparative Criminology 25 (suppl 2):265–272, 1981

Gunderson JG, Zanarini MC: Revised Diagnostic Interview for Borderlines (DIB-R). Belmont, MA, McLean Hospital, 1983

Hall GCN: Sexual offender recidivism revisited: a meta-analysis of recent treatment studies. J Consult Clin Psychol 63:802–809, 1995

Hart LR: Diagnosis of disruptive behavior disorders using the Millon Adolescent Personality Inventory. Psychol Rep 73:895–914, 1993

Holcomb WR, Kashani JH: Personality characteristics of a community sample of adolescents with conduct disorder. Adolescence 26:579–586, 1991

Johnson TC: Child perpetrators—children who molest other children: preliminary findings. Child Abuse Negl 12:219–229, 1988

Kahn TJ, Chambers HJ: Assessing reoffense risk with juvenile sex offenders. Bulletin of the Child Welfare League of America 70:333–345, 1991

Kavoussi RJ, Kaplan M, Becker JV: Psychiatric diagnoses in adolescent sex offenders. J Am Acad Child Adolesc Psychiatry 27:241–243, 1988

Knight RA, Prentky RA: Exploring characteristics for classifying juvenile sex offenders, in The Juvenile Sex Offender. Edited by Barbaree HE, Marshall WL, Hudson SM. New York, Guilford, 1993, pp 45–83

Knopp FH: The Youthful Sex Offender: The Rationale and Goals of Early Intervention and Treatment. Orwell, VT, Safer Society Press, 1991

Kobayashi J, Sales BD, Becker JV, et al: Perceived parental deviance, parent child bonding, child abuse and child sexual aggression. Sexual Abuse: A Journal of Research and Treatment 7:25–44, 1995

Langevin R: Biological factors contributing to paraphiliac behavior. Psychiatric Annals 22:307–314, 1992

Levin SM, Stava L: Personality characteristics of sex offenders: a review. Arch Sex Behav 16 (suppl 1):57–79, 1987

Lewis DO, Shankok SS, Pincus JH: Juvenile male sexual assaulters. Am J Psychiatry 136 (suppl 9):1194–1196, 1979

Longo RE: Sexual learning and experience among adolescent sex offenders. International Journal of Offender Therapy and Comparative Criminology 26 (suppl 3):235–241, 1982

Longo RE, Groth AN: Juvenile sexual offenses in the histories of adult rapists and child molesters. International Journal of Offender Therapy and Comparative Criminology 27:50–55, 1983

Maletzky BM: Editors Note. Sexual Abuse: A Journal of Research and Treatment 9:147, 1997

Marshall W, Barbaree H: An outpatient treatment program for child molesters. Ann N Y Acad Sci 528:205–214, 1988

Millon T, Green CJ, Meagher RB: Millon Adolescent Personality Inventory Manual, Interpretive Scoring Systems. Minneapolis, MN, 1984

Miner MH: How can we conduct treatment outcome research. Sexual Abuse: A Journal of Research and Treatment 9:95–110, 1997

National Task Force on Juvenile Sex Offending: Revised report. Juvenile and Family Court Journal 44(4):5–120, 1993

Office of Juvenile Justice and Delinquency Prevention. Juveniles and Violence (Fact Sheet 19). Washington, DC, U.S. Department of Justice, Office of Justice Programs, November 1994

Packard WS, Rosner R: Psychiatric evaluations of sexual offenders. J Forensic Sci 30:715–720, 1985

Rubenstein M, Yeager C, Goodstein C, et al: Sexually assaultive male juveniles: a follow-up. Am J Psychiatry 150:262–265, 1993

Ryan G, Miyoshi TJ, Metzner JL, et al: Trends in a national sample of sexually abusive youths. J Am Acad Child Adolesc Psychiatry 34 (suppl 1): 17–25, 1996

Saunders EB, Awad GA, White G: Male adolescent sexual offenders: the offender and the offense. Can J Psychiatry 31:542–549, 1986

Schoor M, Speed MH, Bartelt C: Syndrome of the adolescent child molester. Am J Psychiatry 122:783–789, 1966

Shaw JA, Campo-Bowen AE, Applegate B, et al: Young boys who commit serious sex offenses: demographics, psychometrics and phenomenology. Bulletin of the American Academy of Psychiatry and the Law 21:399–408, 1993

Shaw JA, Roth E, Applegate B, et al: Psychopathology in adolescent sex offenders. Paper presented at the annual meeting of the American Association for the Treatment of Sex Abusers, San Francisco, CA, November 1994

Shaw JA, Applegate B, Roth E: Psychopathology and personality disorders in adolescent sex offenders. Am J Forensic Psychiatry 17(4):19–38, 1996

Smith WR, Monastersky C: Assessing juvenile sexual offender's risk for reoffending. Criminal Justice and Behavior 13 (suppl 2):115–140, 1986

Spitzer RL, et al: Structured Clinical Interview for DSM-III-R Personality Disorders (SCID II). New York, New York State Psychiatric Institute, Biometrics Research, 1989

Tartar RE, Hegedus AM, Alterman AI, et al: Cognitive capacities of juvenile, non-violent and sexual offenders. J Nerv Ment Dis 171:364–367, 1983

Wasserman J, Kappel S: Adolescent Sex Offenders in Vermont. Burlington, VT, Vermont Department of Health, 1985

White JW, Koss MP: Adolescent sexual aggression within heterosexual relationships: prevalence, characteristics, and causes, in The Juvenile Sex Offender. Edited by Barbaree HE, Marshall WL, Hudson SM. New York, Guilford, 1993, pp 182–202

Widom CS: The cycle of violence. Science 244:160–166, 1989

7

Female Sex Offenders

Arthur H. Green, M.D.

Prevalence of Child Sexual Offending by Females

Despite the fact that significant numbers of females molest children, most of the clinical observations and research dealing with sex offenders against children have focused on male adult and juvenile perpetrators. Although males are responsible for the majority of child sexual abuse, case report studies indicate that 14% to 24% of boys and 6% to 14% of girls who are molested are molested by women (American Humane Association 1981; National Center for Child Abuse and Neglect 1981). In a college student sample, as reported by Finkelhor (1979), 16% of male victims and 6% of female victims were molested by women. Some self-report studies reveal that 44% to 60% of young adult males have been sexually victimized by women (Fritz et al. 1981; Johnson and Schrier 1987).

Finkelhor and Russell (1984) speculated on the existence of intrinsic and culturally determined characteristics of women that might determine their decreased potential for child molesting compared with men. Among these are their disinclination to sexualize relationships and to initiate sexual activity, their tendency to prefer older and more powerful sexual partners, their stronger bonding with children, and the greater acceptance of sexual contact with children within the male subculture.

Data regarding childhood molestation in the histories of convicted male sex offenders provide an additional perspective regarding the frequency and impact of sexual offenses committed by women. Allen (1991) found that 45% of the molesters of a sample of 75 male sex offenders were female. Groth (1979) observed that among 348 convicted adult male rapists and child molesters, 38% of the rapists and 18% of the child molesters reported childhood (under the age of 16) sexual victimization by adult females. Burgess and colleagues (1987) found that 56% of their sample of 41 male rapists had been sexually abused in childhood and that 40% of the incidents of molestation were perpetrated by females. Petrovich and Templer (1984) found that 59% of 83 incarcerated rapists had been molested by females in childhood. One might speculate about how sexual abuse by a female during the childhood of a male sex offender might predispose that individual toward sexual violence against women.

Using U.S. Census Bureau figures, Allen (1991) estimated that approximately 1.6 million males are abused by women (7% of males sexually abused in childhood; 20% abused by females) and 1.5 million females are sexually abused by women (23% of females sexually abused in childhood; 5% abused by females). Allen suggests that the comparatively low incidence rates of sexual abuse by females should not mask the absolute numbers of occurrences.

Demographic Data

The few studies of female child molesters yielding demographic data (Allen 1991; Faller 1987; Mathews et al. 1989; Wolfe 1985) described predominantly white, lower-socioeconomic-class populations of women who either were unemployed or had unstable work histories. Except for Allen's (1991) study, in which 75% of his sample were high school graduates, the majority of the molesters had dropped out of high school. The victims of these female perpetrators were most likely to be their biological children or stepchildren (56%–85% of the offenses), and girls were more likely to be victimized than boys, except for Allen's sample, in which the reverse was true. The female molesters collaborated with a male coperpetrator in about half of the cases cited, and genital fondling was the most common sexual activity, followed by vaginal intercourse and oral sex.

Allen (1991), in the only comparative study of male and female child molesters, examined demographic variables in 65 female and 75 male offenders. The female offenders were significantly younger than the male offenders (mean ages of 32.8 and 41.5 years, respectively) and reported making less than half of the mean income of the male offenders ($7,250 vs. $18,700). The female offenders were more likely to be unemployed and were more geographically mobile than their male counterparts. There were no ethnic differences, with over 90% of each sample consisting of non-Hispanic Whites. With respect to family of origin, the marital relationships of the parents of the female offenders were less stable than those of the male offenders' parents. Female offenders more often reported having been subjected to parental physical abuse during adolescence and to sexual abuse than did male offenders and were more likely to have run away from home during adolescence. Only 37% of the female offenders and 35% of the male offenders had just one marital partner. Female offenders reported having more sexual partners than did the male offenders. They also reported having less marital satisfaction with their partner than did the male offenders. The female perpetrators also reported more physical abuse by their partners than did the male offenders. More than half of the victims of the female and male offenders were the offenders' own natural, adopted, step-, or foster children. The female offenders were less likely to admit their child molesting and were less likely to acknowledge their guilt.

Abnormal Characteristics of Female Child Molesters

Psychiatric Impairment

A high incidence of psychiatric impairment has been documented in the few existing studies of female child molesters; however, the exact nature of the psychopathology was not determined, and there was a failure to utilize control groups. For example, 48% of O'Connor's sample (1987) had a previous history of psychiatric disorder, 77% of the female incest offenders in Mayer's (1983) sample manifested "infantile or psychotic behavior," and 50% of the female sex offenders in McCarty's (1986) sample were described as experiencing "severe emotional disturbance." Faller (1987) reported that 47% of her sample of female molesters had a history of mental illness; 32% of the mentally disturbed group were reported to have mental retardation or brain damage, while 17% had a history of psychosis.

Green and Kaplan (1994) used standardized instruments to diagnose psychiatric disorders in 11 incarcerated female child molesters and compared them with a control group of 11 women who were serving time in jail for nonsexual crimes. The subjects were assessed with the Structured Clinical Interview for DSM-III-R, Outpatient Version (SCID-OP); the Structured Clinical Interview for DSM-III-R Personality Disorders (SCID-II); and the Harvard Upjohn Post-Traumatic Stress Disorder Interview. The molesters had a mean of 4.8 Axis I psychiatric diagnoses per subject, whereas the control subjects had a mean of 6.4 per subject. The higher number of Axis I diagnoses among the control subjects was due to the higher incidence of substance abuse disorders in that group. The molesters had a mean of 3.6 personality disorders per subject, whereas the control subjects had a mean of 2.4 per subject. A majority of the molesters and the control group met the lifetime DSM-III-R criteria for major depression and posttraumatic stress disorder (PTSD). However, in all of the molesters with PTSD the PTSD was associated with sexual or physical assault during childhood, whereas in slightly more than half of the control group the PTSD was linked to childhood assault. The molesters were more frequently diagnosed as having avoidant and dependent personality disorders, while the control subjects were more often diagnosed as having antisocial personality disorder. As a group, the molesters were more psychiatrically impaired than the control subjects as assessed by the Global Assessment of Functioning (GAF) Scale in the SCID-OP. The molesters received a lower mean GAF Scale score compared with the control group (60 vs. 72).

Substance Abuse

A varying incidence of substance abuse has been found in the histories of female child molesters. Faller (1987) reported a 55% incidence of substance abuse in her sample of female offenders, and Allen (1991) found that 17% of his sample of female offenders suffered from alcoholism and 26% abused drugs. McCarty (1986) reported substance abuse in 40% of her sample, while Green and Kaplan (1994) documented a 73% incidence of substance abuse in an incarcerated sample of female child molesters. Substance abuse might be a risk factor for sexual offending in females. For example, some of the subjects in Green and Kaplan's (1994) sample used substances while molesting their victims.

Frequent Childhood Victimization

Childhood victimization in the form of sexual and/or physical abuse has been frequently reported in the family background of female child molesters. McCarty (1986) reported that 95% of her sample had been physically or sexually abused during childhood. Allen (1991) found that 72% of female offenders had been sexually abused during childhood, while about half of them had been physically abused. Faller (1987) found that nearly half (47.5%) of the female offenders in her sample had been victims of child sexual abuse, and Fehrenbach and Monastersky (1988) described a childhood history of sexual abuse in 50% of a sample of female adolescent sex offenders.

Green and Kaplan (1994) reported that 82% of their sample of female offenders had been sexually abused and 73% had been physically abused during childhood. In all cases, the childhood abuse had been inflicted by family members and was frequently associated with PTSD. The majority of the female molesters who had been sexually abused during childhood were victimized by older males within the family setting.

Deviant Sexual Behavior

Mathews and colleagues (1989) found that the female child molesters in their sample had been promiscuous with men prior to their offending. However, these women reported that they did not enjoy sexual relations and felt exploited by their male partners. They remained in these unrewarding relationships because of their strong dependency needs. Allen (1991), on the other hand, reported that 82% of his sample of female child molesters were moderately or extremely satisfied with their sexual relationships with their partners.

Kaplan and Green (1995) found that incarcerated female child molesters reported a later onset of sexual activity, as assessed by measures such as age at first masturbation and first orgasm, compared with a nonoffender control group of incarcerated women. This finding suggested an inhibition of childhood and adolescent sexuality in the female sex offenders. Sixty-four percent of the offenders, compared with 73% of the control subjects, had engaged in consensual intercourse during adolescence.

Hunter and colleagues (1993) described deviant sexual arousal patterns in female adolescent sex offenders. The majority of these adolescents acknowledged having had sexual fantasies about younger children prior to their first sexual offense. These young perpetrators also reported having been sexually aroused during their own previous sexual molestation during childhood.

Matthews and colleagues (1991) reported either sexual arousal or sexual fantasies in 11 of 16 female child molesters. These perpetrators described fantasizing specifically about their victims, not about children in general. Most reported that their arousal during their perpetration of the molestation was associated with imagining that the children were adult males or with having power in relationships. Those perpetrators who reported that they molested exclusively when coerced by a male denied sexual arousal or fantasies while committing their sexual offenses.

Typology of Child Sexual Abuse by Females

Mathews and colleagues (1989) devised a typology of female child molestation consisting of 1) an *exploration/exploitation* type, in which a teenager fondles a younger child; 2) a *predisposed* type, in which a woman with a severe history of physical or sexual abuse molests her own child or a child she knows; 3) a *teacher-lover* type, in which a woman "falls in love" with a teenage male; 4) a *psychologically disturbed* type, in which, for example, a woman with severe psychiatric impairment and/or substance abuse who is psychologically unstable abuses a child; and 5) a *male coerced* type, in which a dependent women participates in the molestation of a child or children initiated by her husband or boyfriend.

Faller (1987) reported that 72.5% of 40 female offenders molested children in polyincestuous family situations involving at least two perpetrators and two or more victims, with the sex acts usually initiated by a male offender. The victims were the children of the female offenders in 75.6% of these cases. Additional types of female molestation reported by Faller are abuse by a single parent (15%), a psychotic individual (7.5%), and an adolescent (7.5%).

McCarty (1986) described a typology consisting of 1) *independent offenders* of average intelligence, acting alone and usually victimizing a daughter, 2) *co-offending mothers*, often with borderline intelligence and strong dependency needs, in many cases acting in concert with a dominant male, and 3) *accomplices* with average intelligence and strong dependency needs who do not have actual sexual contact with the victims, who are usually girls.

Sarrel and Masters (1982) described four types of female perpetration of molestation of males: 1) *forced assault*, characterized by the use of physical restraints and/or threats of violence, 2) *"baby sitter" abuse*, in which the victim is an unrelated young boy, 3) *incestuous abuse*, in which a boy is seduced by an older female relative, and 4) *dominant woman abuse*, in which an adult male is intimidated by an aggressive sexual approach that does not involve direct physical force.

The major variables emerging from the most common types of female sexual offenses against children are

1. Sole offending versus dependency on a dominant male co-offender
2. Genital contact versus no contact
3. Incestuous versus nonincestuous molestation
4. Intense loving attachment with victim versus angry interaction
5. Male versus female victim

More than one of these variables can, and usually do, apply to any given case.

The variables contributing to the two most common and most distinct patterns of sexual victimization are *sole versus co-offending* and *contact versus noncontact offending*. These two patterns of sexual offending have been described in detail by Green and Kaplan (1994). In the first pattern, the female offender initiates "hands on" sexual activity with a child, often her own, after perceiving the child as sexually exciting or seductive. The victim is often the same age as the offender when she herself had first been molested. These offenders usually deny the seriousness of their deviant behavior and its impact on the child. Some of these women are able to acknowledge a link between the sexual excitement experienced during their own childhood sexual abuse and their sexual arousal while molesting their child victims.

Case Example

A., a 34-year-old unmarried mother, had intercourse with her 11-year-old son after becoming sexually aroused while watching him take a bath. She got on top of him and had orgasms while fantasizing having sex with her father, who had molested her when she was about the same age as her son. She also physically abused and scapegoated this child because he reminded her of his father, whom she hated. A. had been physically abused and rejected by her alcoholic mother, who favored her younger brothers. Even though she was molested by her father, she preferred him to her mother because he gave her attention. Her subsequent relationships with men were negative, and she turned to women as sexual partners. However, she required fantasies of having sex with her father in order to have an orgasm.

A. identifies with her sexually abusive father and with her physically abusing and rejecting mother as she reenacts the sequence of physical and sexual abuse with her son. A.'s son also serves as a target for her displaced aggression toward his father and toward her brothers, who were preferred by her mother. She also identifies with her son as the victim of physical and sexual abuse and scapegoating. A.'s ambivalence toward her father is expressed in her simultaneous hatred of him and her dependence on the incest fantasy for sexual pleasure.

In the second pattern, the female offender does not initiate sexual contact with her victim but is coerced or influenced by another adult, usually a male sexual partner, to participate either directly or indirectly. The woman assists while her more aggressive partner performs sexual acts with the victim, who is usually a girl. The woman either engages in sexual activity with the partner in the child's presence or joins him in molesting the child. The woman identifies with her own nonprotective mother and appears to reenact the nonprotective or facilitating role that her mother played in her own sexual abuse. The woman often has a diagnosis of dependent personality disorder.

Case Example

B., a 37-year-old unmarried woman, allowed a male accomplice to have vaginal, anal, and oral sex with a 6-year-old girl under her care. B. took the child to the perpetrator's apartment, and she was paid by him, but she did not have direct sexual contact with the child. She took photographs of the sexual activity and performed fellatio on her accomplice in view of the child. B. claimed that she was using "crack" at the time and was threatened with harm if she did not comply with the partner's wishes. B. minimized the seriousness of the child's victimization, insisting that the girl had not been penetrated. B. had been forced to perform fellatio on an older male cousin from the ages of 8 through 17 years. When she reported the molestation to her mother, she was either ignored or told that she was overreacting.

B. reenacted her childhood sexual victimization by arranging to have a young girl serve as a sexual object for a male accomplice, while identifying with the victim. She re-created the specific sexual act perpetrated by her cousin when she performed fellatio on the perpetrator while the girl looked on. B. simultaneously identified with her nonprotective mother by facilitating the sexual abuse of the child.

Psychodynamic Issues in Female Child Molesters

The predominantly unhappy, negative childhood experiences of the vast majority of female sex offenders, compounded by sexual and/or physical abuse and rejection, contributed to the development of pathological internalized object relationships with primary caretakers. These women's fathers were usually sexually and/or physically abusive, while their mothers, when not abusive themselves, failed to protect them from the sexual advances of their fathers or father-surrogates. Their mothers often did not believe their accusations of sexual abuse. When the mothers were psychologically unavailable, the incestuous fathers or father-surrogates often satisfied the daughters' hunger for love and nurturance, which then became associated with sexual excitement. The negatively charged perception of an abusing/neglecting parent–abused child dyad was retained as a model for subsequent relationships with significant objects.

Green and Kaplan (1994) observed that the female offenders in their sample had initially reenacted their victimization in a passive manner, choosing boyfriends or husbands who were physically assaultive. On the other hand, the molesters subsequently assumed a sadistic and aggressive role with their child victims. This active reenactment of their own victimization might represent a belated attempt to master a passively endured trauma.

Green and Kaplan (1994) cited the following pathological defense mechanisms used by female sex offenders:

- Identification with the aggressor (e.g., identification with their own sexual abuser)
- Identification with their child victim (e.g., often choosing a child victim the same age as the women were when they had been molested)
- Identification with their nonprotective mothers, especially in cases in which the women offended with male co-offenders
- Denial (e.g., denying their offense or trivializing the consequences to their victim)
- Projection, in which the offender attributed a sexual mo-

tivation or seductiveness to their child victims, which was then used as a rationalization for the molestation

Matthews and colleagues (1991) reported that the women in their sample who molested boys regarded them as substitutes for adult males. One might hypothesize that many women who molest children have difficulty in relating to adult sexual partners because of their low self-esteem and social immaturity. The frequent occurrence of avoidant and dependent personality disorders among female offenders in Green and Kaplan's (1994) sample would tend to confirm this theory.

Wolfe (1985) maintains that sexual abuse of children by females is often a violent response to feelings of powerlessness. She describes how these offenders frequently inflict severe physical and emotional abuse on their victims in the context of their own sexual assault.

Risk Factors in
Female Child Molestation

Prior research carried out with adolescent males who have committed sexual offenses against children might be relevant in providing clues to risk factors in female child molestation. Becker (1988) described an etiological model for the development of deviant sexual behavior in which a series of risk factors operating within the individual, the family, and the social environment might act as precursors to the first deviant sexual act. Individual risk factors include an impulse-control or conduct disorder or a history of physical or sexual abuse. Family risk factors include parents who engage in coercive physical or sexual behavior or use poor parenting techniques. Environmental risk factors include identification with social isolation or involvement with a peer group engaging in antisocial behavior. According to Becker, the adolescents who reoffended were likely to be those who found the act to be pleasurable, experienced minimal negative consequences in relation to the sexual crime, experienced reinforcement of the deviant sexual behavior through masturbatory activity and fantasy, and were deficient in peer relationships. Adolescents who had supportive parents and had received protection and treatment after being molested during childhood were less likely to reenact their victimization with others.

When this model is applied to female child molesters, their coercive sexual behavior with children could be viewed, in part, as a reenactment of their childhood sexual victimization. However, since many female children are victims of sexual abuse and relatively few become child molesters, the presence of additional individual risk factors such as psychiatric impairment, substance abuse, cognitive deficits, lack of social competency associated with personality disorders, low self-esteem, and conditions contributing to impulsivity might be necessary to catalyze the tranformation of victim to victimizer. This process might be further potentiated by the presence of environmental reinforcers such as dependency on co-offenders and the lack of punishment and by the reinforcement associated with sexual excitement and pleasure. In addition, female child molesters might have experienced as children sexual and physical abuse of greater severity, longer duration, and a higher frequency of victimization by family members than that experienced by female survivors of physical and sexual abuse who do not become molesters. These more severe types of victimization are more likely to be associated with PTSD and result in dissociative responses that would render these traumata less accessible to retrieval, integration, and working through.

Interventions With Female Child Molesters

There are very few references to the treatment of female child molesters in the sex offender literature, and no treatment outcome studies have appeared. Based on the male sex offender literature (Abel et al. 1985; Becker and Kaplan 1988), confrontational cognitive-behavioral interventions focusing on eliminating deviant patterns of sexual arousal and perpetrator denial have been used with female child molesters. These interventions include satiation, covert sensitization, cognitive restructuring, social skills training, and relapse prevention. However, according to Travin and colleagues (1990) and Matthews and associates (1991), the use of such confrontational techniques might interfere with the establishment of a therapeutic relationship with the female offender. These clinicians stress the need for an additional psychotherapeutic focus designed to deal with the offender's childhood victimization experiences and the concomitant depression, low self-esteem, shame and guilt, and PTSD. This nurturing, nonjudgmental approach, which takes into account the dual nature of these offenders as victims and victimizers, combined with cognitive-behavioral techniques, is believed to offer the most promise for rehabilitation. One hopes that with the growing awareness of the problem of child sexual abuse by females, much-needed research on effective treatment strategies will be carried out.

Summary

Child sexual abuse by females appears to be more widespread than previously believed. Female child molesters demonstrate significant psychopathology in terms of extensive psychiatric impairment, substance abuse, and deviant sexual behavior, often attributable to a high incidence of childhood victimization (e.g., parental physical abuse, sexual abuse, and neglect).

Compared with male child molesters, female offenders seem to have lower income and higher rates of unemployment, more unstable families of origin, and a higher incidence of childhood and spousal victimization and express less marital satisfaction. The female offenders are also more likely to molest a child with an accomplice and are less likely to acknowledge their guilt. It is likely that female child molesters have more impairment than their male counterparts.

The following variables have been identified as being relevant in attempts to establish a typology of female child molesters: contact versus noncontact offenses, individual offending versus offending with an accomplice, incest versus extrafamilial offending, intense loving attachment with victim versus angry interaction, and male versus female victims. Efforts at describing a valid typology must be considered preliminary at this time.

Potential risk factors predisposing females to molest children are severe childhood victimization experiences, psychiatric impairment, cognitive deficits, abnormal sexual behavior, impaired social skills, and conditions that increase impulsivity, such as substance abuse or central nervous system impairment.

Major psychodynamic issues in the female offenders include their tendency to reenact in subsequent relationships (e.g., with peers, sexual partners, and children) their pathological object relationships derived from exposure to negatively perceived primary caretakers. Defense mechanisms commonly used by these women are identifications with the aggressor, the child victim, and the non-protective mother; denial; and projection.

Future Directions and Potential Areas of Research

More extensive clinical investigation of female child molesters is clearly needed. Research should be directed toward measuring current and past psychopathology and psychological deviancy with standardized instruments in cohorts of female child molesters compared with nonoffender control groups. Quantitative measures should be developed to assess the severity of childhood victimization experiences that appear to be risk factors for female child molesting. In order to identify a hierarchy of risk factors predisposing women toward child molesting, it would be helpful to design research utilizing comparison groups of female sex offenders with and without a history of childhood victimization and women who had been victimized during childhood but who did not go on to commit sexual offenses against children.

Comparative studies of female offenders acting alone or with accomplices, engaging in contact versus noncontact offenses, molesting their own versus unrelated children, and molesting boys versus girls that assess their sexual responsiveness would contribute to the establishment of a valid typology of women who molest children. When the family experiences, psychopathology, sexual deviancy, and other potential risk factors in female child molestation are better known, and a workable typology is in use, it will be possible to design effective prevention and treatment strategies for this population. It is likely that important modifications of current treatment designed for male sex offenders will be necessary to accommodate the specific needs of the female sex offenders. Treatment outcome studies with female child molesters should receive the highest priority.

References

Abel GG, Mittelman M, Becker JV: Sex offenders: results of assessment and recommendations for treatment, in Clinical Criminology: The Assessment and Treatment of Criminal Behavior. Edited by Ben-Aron M, Hucker SJ, Webster CD. Toronto, M & M Graphics, 1985, pp 191–205

Allen CM: Women and Men Who Sexually Abuse Children: A Comparative Analysis. Orwell, VT, Safer Society Press, 1991

American Humane Association: National Study on Child Neglect and Abuse Reporting. Denver, CO, American Humane Association, 1981

Becker JV: The effect of child sexual abuse on adolescent sex offenders, in The Lasting Effects of Child Sexual Abuse. Edited by Wyatt G, Powell G. Beverly Hills, CA, Sage Publications, 1988, pp 193–207

Becker JV, Kaplan MS: Assessment and treatment of the male sex offender, in Child Sexual Abuse: A Handbook for Health Care and Legal Professionals. Edited by Schetky DH, Green AH. New York, Brunner/Mazel, 1988, pp 136–149

Burgess AW, Groth AN, Holmstrom LL, et al: Sexual Assault of Children and Adolescents. Lexington, MA, Lexington Books/DC Heath, 1987

Faller KC: Women who sexually abuse children. Violence and Victims 2:263–276, 1987

Fehrenbach PA, Monastersky C: Characteristics of female adolescent sex offenders. Am J Orthopsychiatry 58:148–151, 1988

Finkelhor D: Sexually Victimized Children. New York, Free Press, 1979

Finkelhor D, Russell D: Women as perpetrators, in Child Sexual Abuse: New Theory and Research. Edited by Finkelhor D. New York, Free Press, 1984

Fritz G, Stoll K, Wagner N: A comparison of males and females who were sexually molested as children. J Sex Marital Ther 7:54–59, 1981

Green AH, Kaplan M: Psychiatric impairment and childhood victimization experiences in female child molesters. J Am Acad Child Adolesc Psychiatry 33:954–961, 1994

Groth AN: Men Who Rape. New York, Plenum, 1979

Hunter JA, Lexier LJ, Goodwin BA, et al: Psychosexual attitudinal and developmental characteristics of juvenile female sexual perpetrators in a residential treatment setting. Journal of Child and Family Studies 2:317–326, 1993

Johnson RL, Schrier D: Past sexual victimization by females of male patients in an adolescent medicine clinic population. Am J Psychiatry 144:650–662, 1987

Kaplan MS, Green AH: Incarcerated female sex offenders: a comparison of sexual histories with eleven female nonsexual offenders. Sexual Abuse: A Journal of Research and Treatment 9:287–300, 1995

Matthews J, Mathews R, Speltz K: Female sex offenders: a typology, in Family Sexual Abuse: Frontline Research and Evaluation. Edited by Patton MQ. Newbury Park, CA, Sage Publications, 1991, pp 199–219

Mayer A: A Treatment Manual for Therapy With Victims, Spouses, and Offenders (Publ No 21-19). Holmes Beach, FL, Florida Learning Publications, 1983

McCarty L: Mother-child incest: characteristics of the offender. Child Welfare 65:457–458, 1986

National Center for Child Abuse and Neglect: Study Findings: National Study of Incidence and Severity of Child Abuse and Neglect (DHEW Publ No OHDS 81-30325). Washington, DC, Department of Health, Education and Welfare, 1981

O'Connor A: Female sex offenders. Br J Psychiatry 150:615–620, 1987

Petrovich M, Templer D: Heterosexual molestation of children who later became rapists. Psychol Rep 54:810, 1984

Sarrel P, Masters W: Sexual molestation of men by women. Arch Sex Behav 11:117–131, 1982

Travin S, Cullen K, Protter B: Female sex offenders: severe victims and victimizers. J Forensic Sci 35:140–150, 1990

Wolfe F: Twelve female sex offenders. Paper presented at the Next Steps in Research on the Assessment and Treatment of Sexually Aggressive Persons Conference, St Louis, MO, March 1985

8

Motivators of Adolescent Sex Offenders and Treatment Perspectives

John A. Hunter, Jr., Ph.D., and Judith V. Becker, Ph.D.

It is currently believed that juveniles, particularly adolescent males, account for a relatively high percentage of the sexual assaults committed against children and women in our society. Studies suggest that juveniles are responsible for 30% to 60% of the cases of child sexual abuse and 20% to 30% of the rapes that are committed in this country each year (Brown et al. 1983; Fehrenbach et al. 1986). Furthermore, consistent with an overall trend of increased violent crime committed by juveniles during the past decade, there has been a steady rise in the number of juveniles arrested for sexual offenses (Snyder and Sickmund 1995). Growing public and professional cognizance of the seriousness of juvenile sexual offending has provided impetus for the development of treatment programs for youthful perpetrators.

Patterns of Sexual Offending

Adolescent males have been found to account for a greater proportion of the perpetrations of molestation of young male children than
young female children (Hunter 1991; Rogers and Terry 1984). This
finding appears to reflect both the high numbers of female children
who are molested by a father or stepfather and the greater fluidity in
the patterns of sexual offending of juveniles than adults (Hunter
1991). With regard to the latter, juveniles who target child victims
are less likely than adults to display gender specificity in their selection of victims and are more likely to have engaged in multiple
paraphiliac behaviors (e.g., child molestation and exhibitionism)
(Hunter et al. 1994). Approximately one-fourth of juvenile child molesters have only male victims, slightly less than one-half have only
female victims, and one-fourth to one-third have victims of both gen-
ders (Hunter et al. 1994; Mathews et al. 1997). In contrast to juvenile child molesters, the vast majority of juveniles who target peers
or adults exclusively offend against females (Hunter et al., in press).

The distinction between incestuous and extrafamilial sexual offending does not appear to be as pronounced in juveniles as in adults.
Unlike their adult counterparts, incestuous juvenile child molesters
do not evidence on phallometric assessment less sexual arousal to
stimuli depicting deviant sexual activity than do extrafamilial offenders; nor do they have fewer victims or begin offending at an
older age (Hunter et al. 1994; Marshall et al. 1991). Recent research
does suggest that juveniles who offend within their families may
utilize different modus operandi in attempting to gain the cooperation of their victims. Specifically, they may rely more on bribes and
enticements (e.g., giving gifts, love and attention) than do juveniles
who select children from outside of their home and family environments (Kaufman et al. 1996).

Data suggest that patterns of sexual offending that emerge during adolescence may signify more chronic proclivities. Studies reveal
that as many as 60% of adult sex offenders report a juvenile onset
to the behavior, and in many cases there appeared to be a progression
from less serious to more serious sexual offending over time (Abel
et al. 1987). With regard to child molestation, a juvenile onset to

the offending behavior has been observed far more frequently among extrafamilial than among solely intrafamilial offenders, with the earliest average age at onset found in males who develop patterns of same-gender pedophilia (Marshall et al. 1991). More recent data suggest that rapists also frequently begin to offend during adolescence, with one longitudinal study showing that the average age at onset in this population was 16 years (Elliott 1994). While there is clear evidence that juvenile sexual offending may portend a continuation of such behavior into adulthood, the likelihood of this occurring is unknown. It is noted that the majority of studies that have been conducted on this issue have been retrospective in nature. The above-referenced longitudinal study (Elliott 1994) suggested that approximately 80% of the tracked adolescent rapists ceased engaging in this behavior by the time they reached adulthood.

Developmental and Familial Characteristics

The study of male juvenile sex offenders has led to exploration of etiological factors that help explain the developmental origin of child molestation and rape. Factors that have received empirical and clinical attention in the literature to date include 1) childhood maltreatment experiences and exposure to aggressive role models, 2) substance abuse, and 3) exposure to pornography. Each of these factors is briefly reviewed in the following.

Childhood Maltreatment and Aggressive Role Models

Childhood maltreatment, including both physical and sexual abuse experiences, has been frequently cited as playing a prominent role in the emergence of patterns of sexual perpetration in juveniles (Paperny and Deisher 1983; Rogers and Terry 1984; Ryan 1989). Interest in the influence of maltreatment on the male child's potential for engaging in sexually exploitive behavior stems from the observation that a relatively high percentage of juvenile sex offenders report that they were sexually and/or physically abused prior to ever having engaged in acts of sexual perpetration. In this regard, a reported history of sexual abuse has been found in approximately 40% to 80%, and a history of physical abuse in 25% to 50%, of adolescent sex offenders in various study samples (Kahn and Chambers 1991; Ryan et al. 1987; Smith 1988). Generally, higher incidence rates of sexual victimization have been found in samples of younger and more psychosexually and psychiatrically disturbed juvenile sex offenders (Hunter and Becker 1994).

The influence of maltreatment on a young male's potential for sexual perpetration has been discussed from a number of theoretical and diagnostic perspectives. It has been suggested that the sexual acting-out of the majority of prepubescent children is in reaction to their own abuse histories and associated with posttraumatic stress disorder (PTSD) phenomenology (Gil and Johnson 1993). These children appear to be prone to engagement in repetition–compulsion phenomena that can be interpreted as their attempt to gain mastery over painful inner affects and cognitions stemming from abuse-generated trauma. Residual PTSD symptomatology has been clinically observed by the present authors in a number of older adolescent offenders. The authors hypothesize that untreated PTSD in young males may ultimately lead to more characterological disturbances in later adolescence manifested by attachment problems, deficits in empathy, eroticization, and impulse regulation dysfunction.

The manner in which early maltreatment experiences can create a greater propensity for later sexual aggression has also been discussed from the perspective of social-learning theory and the influence of modeling (Becker et al. 1989; Freeman-Longo 1986). It is believed that abused children may imitate the sexually aggressive behavior of the perpetrator of the abuse in their subsequent interactions with others. It can be speculated that the likelihood of this occurring is amplified when the youths' home environment is devoid of a healthy male role model with whom they can identify. Such formulations are also consistent with an evolutionary psychological model which posits that sexual and aggressive behavior in males is learned primarily through interaction with other males, including male relatives, during critical developmental periods (Hunter and Figueredo, in press).

A study by Kobayashi and colleagues (1995) provides empirical support to the above-discussed salience of maltreatment experiences and modeling in the etiology of sexual aggression in juvenile males. Using structural equation modeling, these investigators demonstrated that increased sexual aggressiveness in juvenile sex offenders could be predicted by histories of physical abuse by the father and sexual abuse by males. In support of the relevance of the parent–child attachment, higher adolescent ratings of importance placed on bonding to the mother were found to be predictive of lower levels of sexual aggressiveness.

In yet another study, Hunter and Figueredo (in press) utilized structural equation modeling to investigate the relationship between sexual victimization, personality and adjustment, and family support variables in the prediction of patterns of sexual perpetration in adolescent males. Perpetrators with a history of prior sexual victimization were compared with those who had been sexually victimized but had no history of sexual perpetration. Results demonstrated that a younger age at time of victimization, a greater number of incidents, a longer period of waiting to report the abuse, and a lower level of perceived family support postrevelation of the abuse were predictive of perpetrator classification.

In addition to the above-cited studies, other researchers have examined the potential link between exposure to violence during childhood and subsequent aggressive and sexual acting-out. Studies of children who have witnessed domestic violence have shown that male children, in particular, are prone toward engaging in externalizing behaviors, including acts of aggression toward others (Hughes 1988; Jaffe et al. 1986; Stagg et al. 1989). Other studies have established that exposure to domestic violence is a correlate of both the likelihood of sexually perpetrating as a juvenile and the severity of psychosexual disturbance (Fagan and Wexler 1988; Smith 1988). Studies have also consistently demonstrated an association between juvenile delinquency and poor parent–child emotional bonding (Loeber and Stouthamer-Loeber 1986; Patterson et al. 1992), as well as the prevalence of histories of problematic father–son relationships among sexually aggressive adult males (Hazelwood and Warren 1989; Lisak 1994; Lisak and Roth 1990).

Substance Abuse

Whereas the literature is replete with studies demonstrating an association between violent crime and alcohol use, the connection between sexual acting-out and substance abuse has not been as well established (Davis and Leitenberg 1987; Lightfoot and Barbaree 1993). Lightfoot and Barbaree (1993) point out that there appears to be little agreement as to the extent of alcohol/drug abuse among juvenile sex offenders. Furthermore, the self-reports of juvenile sex offenders with histories of alcohol or drug use suggest that the majority do not believe that the drugs or alcohol had any effect on their sexual arousal (Becker and Stein 1991).

Pornography

The influence of pornography on the developing male's potential for sexually offending has, as with substance abuse, been an issue of some controversy. A number of experimental studies, involving non-offender male volunteers, have demonstrated that the viewing of films depicting violence toward women and sexual aggression can adversely affect attitudes toward women and increase acceptance of interpersonal violence (Linz et al. 1989; Weisz and Earls 1995). However, relatively few studies have examined the use and role of pornography in identified populations of sex offenders.

In one of the few available studies, Ford and Linney (1995) found that juvenile sex offenders were exposed to pornographic magazines at younger ages on the average (between ages 5 and 8 years) than were status offenders or violent non–sex-offending youths. Furthermore, these investigators found that juvenile sex offenders were more likely than the other two groups to have been exposed to "hard-core" sex magazines. Becker and Stein (1991) found that the majority of juvenile sex offenders in their sample (89%) acknowledged the use of sexual erotica (e.g., magazines, videos) and stated that the sexually explicit material increased their sexual arousal.

Clinical Characteristics

The clinical characteristics typically ascribed to juvenile sex offenders are those that have been identified primarily through clinical observation, as opposed to empirical investigation. Furthermore, as will be discussed in the next section, professional perception of juvenile sex offenders and their treatment needs has been heavily influenced by the study and treatment of adult sex offenders. Consequently, there is growing cognizance in the field of the need to empirically validate common clinical assumptions and modify diagnostic conceptualizations and treatment approaches as necessary. The more salient clinical characteristics traditionally ascribed to juvenile sex offenders, as well as supportive empirical data for each, are reviewed in this section.

A considerable body of literature exists on the role of sexual deviancy in male sexual offending, including the presence of deviant sexual arousal and distorted cognitions regarding the acceptability of sexual aggression and sexual relations with children. Support for the validity of deviant sexual arousal as a major motivator of sexual acting-out comes largely from the adult sex offender literature and, specifically, phallometric study of the arousal patterns of pedophiles versus incest offenders and non-offending control subjects. A number of such studies have shown that pedophiles typically show more pronounced arousal to sexual stimuli depicting children than the last-mentioned two groups and that the highest ratios of deviant to nondeviant arousal are found among adult pedophiles who molest children of the same gender (Marshall et al. 1991). Data have not been so compelling in supporting the relevance of deviant arousal to an understanding of why men rape (Barbaree et al. 1994; Baxter et al. 1986).

As a result of the research on adult child molesters described above, momentum has steadily developed in recent years for evaluation and treatment of patterns of deviant sexual arousal in male juvenile sex offenders. As evidence of this trend, a survey conducted by the Safer Society in 1992 revealed that more than 165 practitioners in the United States were using phallometric assessment in their evaluation of juvenile sex offenders (Safer Society, personal communication, July 25, 1995).

It has been empirically established that juvenile sex offenders produce reliable patterns of arousal upon phallometric assessment and that such patterns can be differentiated according to erection profile characteristics: nonresponder and minimal responder, non-discriminator, and child, peer, or adult–child responder (Becker et al. 1992, 1992b). However, as a result of recent investigation, questions have been raised about the relevance of deviant sexual arousal in general, and the ratio of deviant to nondeviant arousal in particular, to understanding the majority of cases of juvenile sexual offending. Research suggests that there is greater fluidity in the arousal patterns of juvenile compared with adult sex offenders and generally less correspondence between phallometrically measured arousal patterns and offense characteristics. This research suggests that deviant sexual arousal may be most valid in understanding cases of juvenile sexual offending against young male victims or cases of early-onset same-gender pedophilia (Hunter et al. 1994).

Similarly, it has not yet been empirically established that adolescent sex offenders are more likely than non–sexually offending control subjects to endorse distorted cognitions or beliefs regarding sexual misbehavior (Hunter et al. 1991). However, this construct has received only limited research attention in the juvenile sex offender literature, and there are no known studies examining this variable across different juvenile sex offender subgroups. In study of adult sex offenders, Hayashino and colleagues (1995) found that extrafamilial child molesters were more likely than incestuous offenders or rapists to endorse distorted cognitions. Interestingly, the last-mentioned two offender groups did not score significantly higher on a measure of cognitive distortions than a group of non-offending control subjects.

Psychopathy, or the presence of antisocial personality traits and criminal tendencies, has also received theoretical attention in the attempt to explain why some juveniles sexually offend. Interest in this variable has been relatively long-standing (Doshay 1943) and centers on the question of whether juvenile sex offenders are inherently different from non–sexually offending juveniles who exhibit delinquent behavior. It has been suggested that all socially deviant behavior, including sexual offending, can be accounted for by a common criminologic trait of low self-control (Gottfredson and Hirschi 1990).

In support of a general delinquency factor, several studies have documented that juvenile sex offenders share a number of similarities with non–sexually offending delinquent youths, including family background variables and abuse histories, histories of academic problems, and tendencies to engage in a wide variety of antisocial behaviors (Awad and Saunders 1989; Awad et al. 1984). With regard to the last variable, a number of investigators have documented that in nonforensic samples of juvenile sex offenders, 40% to 50% have histories of having engaged in nonsexual legal offenses. Such histories are even more prevalent in samples of incarcerated juvenile sex offenders (Amir 1971; Becker et al. 1986; Fehrenbach et al. 1986; Van Ness 1984).

Data contradicting a general delinquency theory for explaining juvenile sexual offending come from a number of studies showing that in only about one-half of juvenile sex offenders can the diagnostic criteria for a conduct disorder be met. Juvenile sex offenders also show more deficits in emotional functioning and peer relationships and have more extensive histories of physical and sexual abuse than do other types of juvenile offenders (Becker et al. 1986; Blaske et al. 1989; Ford and Linney 1995). France and Hudson (1993) point out that nonsexual delinquency is more likely to be found in the histories of "hands on" aggressive sex offenders than in nonaggressive offenders and that juvenile sex offenders without conduct disorder may be quite different from their more delinquent and aggressive counterparts.

Adolescent sex offenders have also been characterized as suffering from deficits in social competency, self-esteem, and empathy that hamper their ability to form and maintain healthy peer relationships and successfully resolve interpersonal conflicts (Becker and Abel 1985; Blaske et al. 1989; Figia et al. 1987). Closely associated with these deficits are ascribed fears of emotional intimacy and pronounced feelings of loneliness and social alienation (Awad and Saunders 1989; Fehrenbach et al. 1986). Until recently, however, there had been no studies in which juvenile sex offenders were compared with other populations of adolescents on these variables. Ford and Linney (1995) found that juvenile child molesters manifested a greater need for control and inclusion in interpersonal relationships than did juvenile rapists, non–sexually offending violent offenders, and status offenders. The juvenile rapists showed more emotional detachment than did the child molesters. Although the differences were not statistically significant, the group of child molesters evidenced more problems with self-esteem (e.g., physical appearance, popularity) and more dysphoria and anxiety than did youths in the other comparison groups.

Hunter and Figueredo (1995) found that adolescent child molesters evidenced deficits in self-sufficiency and had more pessimistic explanatory styles than did the non–sexually offending control group of offenders. Self-sufficiency was defined as reflecting attitudes of self-confidence, independence, assertiveness, and self-satisfaction. With regard to pessimism, the sexually offending youths showed a greater tendency than control subjects to assign internal, stable, and global attributions for the occurrence of negative events in their lives. The results of this study were interpreted as supporting a conceptualization of juvenile child molesters as youths who are lacking in social competencies and who are perhaps competitively disadvantaged relative to their peers.

In addition to the purported causal factors described above, a number of other clinical characteristics have been found to be associated with juvenile sex offenders. Learning disabilities and/or poor academic performance have been found in 30% to 60% of samples of adolescent sex offenders (Awad and Saunders 1991; Fehrenbach et al. 1986; Hunter and Goodwin 1992). Impulse-control problems and associated difficulties with disinhibition have also been frequently clinically observed (Smith et al. 1987), although there are no known experimental studies comparing juvenile sex offenders with control subjects on neurological or neuropsychological function related to these impulse-control difficulties.

The index of psychiatric comorbidity in samples of juvenile sex offenders is relatively high, particularly in those samples derived from residential treatment settings. Aside from the diagnosis of conduct disorder, the most frequently observed psychiatric condition in juvenile sex offenders is depression. Depressive symptomatology appears prevalent in both residential and outpatient samples of juvenile sex offenders, with one study finding that 42% of an outpatient sample of youthful perpetrators of sexually offending behavior met the clinical criteria for diagnosis of depression as established by the Beck Depression Inventory (Becker et al. 1991).

Treatment Approaches

Very few treatment programs were available for juvenile sex offenders prior to the 1980s. Since that time there has been a steady proliferation of both outpatient and residential treatment programs for youthful offenders. As evidence of the rapid growth in the field, a survey by the Safer Society found that the number of treatment programs for juvenile sex offenders in the United States increased from 346 in 1986 to 755 in 1992. Of the existing programs, approximately 80% were outpatient and 20% were residential (Safer Society, personal communication, July 25, 1995).

Historically, approaches to the treatment of juvenile sex offenders have been heavily influenced by both adult sex offender treatment models and the philosophy of the juvenile criminal justice system. With regard to the latter, most practitioners have developed an appreciation for the value of prosecution in holding sex offenders accountable for their behavior. It is currently the consensus of most experts in the field that the placement of legal contingencies on juvenile sex offenders enhances their amenability to treatment and helps ensure that standards of public safety will be maintained (National Task Force on Juvenile Sexual Offending 1993).

Theoretical Influences

Although a number of theoretical conceptualizations have been drawn upon in explaining the etiology of sexual offending in juveniles and the treatment needs of this population, cognitive-behavioral approaches have perhaps been most often endorsed and adopted (Hunter and Becker 1994). Theorists and practitioners working from this framework have utilized conditioning and social-learning theory models to explain the onset and maintenance of deviant sexual behavior and have developed interventions aimed at diminishing aberrant sexual interest and arousal patterns, improving cognitive con-

trols, correcting faulty belief systems, and teaching prosocial and relapse prevention skills (Becker 1994). This school of thought has also
been influential in encouraging the use of objective assessment instruments and the conducting of empirical research on the efficacy
of intervention methodologies.

Other theoretical influences on the treatment of juvenile sex
offenders include psychodynamic and developmental, biological,
family systems, and feminist models. Practitioners influenced by
psychodynamic and developmental theory have fostered greater
cognizance of the importance of examining and treating the juvenile's psychosexual problems in a holistic manner with an appreciation of his or her overall emotional and psychological needs. These
practitioners have also brought attention to the importance of examining the manner in which early maltreatment and deprivation
experiences disrupted normal developmental and attachment processes and left these youths with deficits in capacity for empathy
and healthy relationship functioning (Bremer 1992; Ryan and Lane
1991; Steele 1985).

Biologically oriented practitioners have pointed to the potential
utility of pharmacological therapies in the treatment of juvenile
sex offenders. Such approaches include consideration of the use of
serotonin reuptake inhibitors with youths who show evidence of
depression and obsessive-compulsive spectrum disorders, and hormonal agents (e.g., medroxyprogesterone acetate) with more seriously disturbed older adolescents who experience persistent and
pronounced deviant sexual arousal and interests (e.g., sexual sadism)
(Bradford 1993) (see also Chapter 11, this volume).

Family systems therapists have emphasized the importance of
1) understanding the juvenile sex offender's behavior in the context
of the larger familial and community systems in which he functions
and 2) effecting systems changes that support the long-term maintenance of more adaptive styles of relating to others (Blaske et al.
1989; Henggeler 1989). Proponents of feminist theory have raised
awareness as to the relationship between the perpetration of sexual
aggression toward females and larger societal attitudes and practices
that support the oppression of women (Brownmiller 1975; Herman
1990).

Continuum of Care

Clinical and research data suggest that juvenile sex offenders are a heterogeneous clinical population with a variety of types and levels of sexual and nonsexual disturbances represented. As such, a continuum of care needs to be established to meet their differential treatment needs. This continuum ranges from intensive and comprehensive residential services for more severely psychosexually and psychiatrically impaired youths to community-based treatment programs for less maladjusted youths. There also appears to be a need for the availability of correctional options for more characterologically and less therapeutically motivated adolescents.

Specialized residential treatment programs provide a structured and secure environment for the treatment of those juvenile sex offenders who cannot be safely or effectively treated on a community-based level because of the magnitude of their psychosexual and/or other emotional and behavioral problems. Although there is considerable variability in the level of professional care provided in residential programs across the United States, the more intensively clinically staffed programs offer a comprehensive array of specialized and more traditional psychiatric and psychological treatment services to sexually abusive youths, including 1) psychiatric assessment and treatment, 2) individual, group, and family therapy, 3) educational and vocational programming, 4) independent living skills programming, 5) medical care, 6) milieu therapy, 7) and adjunctive therapies (e.g., art, music). Ideally, youths placed in such programs can make the transition from a highly structured living environment to less-structured environments (e.g., group home) in which they have increased opportunity for interfacing with the community prior to discharge.

Community-based treatment programs are most appropriate for less seriously psychosexually, psychiatrically, and characterologically disturbed youths. Typically, these are youths whose sexual acting-out has not been of a long-standing nature and has not involved a high level of aggression or violence. Furthermore, these are youths who do not appear to be primarily delinquent or seriously characterologically disturbed and are capable of being maintained in home, school, and community environments without constant supervision. For such youths, early intervention of a specialized nature may help stem the development of more serious sexual problems. Programming for these juvenile sex offenders typically involves participation in weekly group therapy of a specialized nature, supplemented by family and individual therapies. Additionally, in many cases the parents of these youths participate in a supportive educational program.

Some youths in community-based programming may also require psychiatric consultation and support, especially when the individual has a concomitant psychiatric problem that has a direct or indirect impact on his or her sexual behavior and ability to exercise appropriate judgment and impulse control. Some youths also require supplemental services in the form of in-home services, evening and after-school programs, or group home placement. Youths who have sexually offended against younger siblings typically require removal from the home (e.g., placement in a group home or with a relative) until significant progress has been attained and it has been determined that the youth's return to the home will not jeopardize the physical or emotional well-being of younger siblings or other family members.

Unfortunately, there appears to be a subset of juvenile sex offenders who are not amenable to treatment because of a high level of character pathology. Such individuals may present as highly psychopathic and/or narcissistic and show little remorse for their offending behavior and little empathy or concern for others. Many of these individuals present with relatively lengthy histories of antisocial behavior, beginning early in childhood, and have been refractory to treatment interventions. Confinement in a correctional setting may be the most appropriate disposition for this group of juvenile sex offenders. More limited treatment services are available in a number of such settings for those juveniles who show some motivation to change.

Program Evaluation and Outcome Data

Presently, there is a dearth of empirically conducted treatment outcome studies on juvenile sex offenders. It is hoped that with the increased attention that this subject has received in recent years, and the rapid growth in number of treatment programs for juvenile sex offenders across the country, there will be a commensurate rise in outcome research activity in the near future. The currently available, and more empirically sound, reports on juvenile sex offender treatment outcome are reviewed below.

Borduin and colleagues (1990) compared "multisystemic therapy" with individual therapy in the outpatient treatment of 16 adolescent sex offenders. Multisystemic therapy was defined by the investigators as a systems approach that attempted to decrease denial and cognitive distortions, enhance empathy, strengthen family and peer relationships, and improve academic performance. Youths were randomly assigned to one of the two treatment conditions, with youths in each group receiving approximately the same number of hours of therapeutic contact. With rearrest records used as a measure of recidivism (sexual and nonsexual), the two groups were compared at a 3-year follow-up interval. Results revealed that the youths receiving multisystemic therapy had recidivism rates of 12.5% for sexual offenses and 25% for nonsexual offenses, whereas those receiving individual therapy had recidivism rates of 75% for sexual offenses and 50% for nonsexual offenses.

For a sample of 80 juvenile sex offenders who had been treated as outpatients, Becker (1990) reported an 8% sexual recidivism rate over a follow-up period of up to 2 years. These youths had participated in a cognitive-behavioral treatment program that focused on reducing deviant sexual thoughts and arousal, correcting faulty beliefs regarding the acceptability of sexual aggression or sexual relations with children, improving impulse control and judgment, and increasing social skills and sexual knowledge. Recidivism data were gathered through interviewing the youths, their families, and referral sources. No control groups were included in this study.

Kahn and Chambers (1991) conducted a retrospective study of 221 juvenile sex offenders (95% male; 5% female) who entered 1 of 10 treatment programs in Washington State over a 10-month period during 1984. Eight of these treatment programs were outpatient programs, and two were institution-based correctional programs. Posttreatment conviction records were reviewed over an average follow-up period of 20 months. Results showed that although the overall rate of recidivism (any type of offense) was high (44.8%), the sexual recidivism rate was relatively low (7.5%). High rates of sexual recidivism were found among those youths who used verbal threats in the commission of their offenses and among those who blamed the victim for the offense. This study did not compare the rates of recidivism between "hands on" and "hands off" offenders or examine outcome according to therapeutic approach, length of treatment, whether treatment had been completed, or gender of the perpetrator.

Schram and colleagues reported the results of an extended follow-up study of 197 male juvenile sex offenders who participated in the above-referenced Washington State treatment outcome project (D. D. Schram, C. D. Miloy, W. E. Rowe, unpublished manuscript, 1991). These investigators extended the length of follow-up by 5 years. Results revealed that the rate of arrest for new sexual offenses remained relatively low (12.2%) in comparison to that for nonsexual offenses (50.8%). Sexual recidivism was found to be associated with a history of truancy, thinking errors (including blaming the victim), a prior conviction for a sexual offense, and higher deviant sexual arousal. In this study, deviant sexual arousal was identified via therapist assessments rather than through phallometric measurement.

A relatively low rate of sexual recidivism in residentially treated juvenile sex offenders was also found by Bremer (1992). Bremer reported that only 6% of the treated youths were convicted of new sexual offenses following release from the residential program. Survey data indicated that the sexual recidivism rate rose to 11% if self-report of reoffending was included. The length of follow-up in this study ranged from less than 6 months to 8.5 years.

Although the above-described studies suggest that the rate of sexual recidivism among treated juvenile sex offenders is relatively low and thus provide reason for optimism about the amenability of this clinical population to focused intervention, many questions remain unanswered. To date, there have been no large, experimentally well controlled outcome studies that assess the rate of sexual recidivism in treated versus untreated juvenile sex offenders or the relative efficacy of differential therapeutic approaches, including incarceration alone. Furthermore, there are currently few data on differential recidivism rates based on type of juvenile sex offender or data on increased risk of recidivism as a function of program failure or length of period of follow-up.

Future Directions

Because juvenile sex offenders represent a heterogeneous clinical population with various programming needs, it is vital that an empirically validated typology be developed to help guide dispositional and intervention planning efforts. A nosological description of juvenile sex offenders would potentially permit the delineation of various subtypes of juvenile sex offenders according to etiology, clinical manifestations, response to treatment, and risk of recidivism.

At present, both mental health practitioners and the juvenile criminal justice system are dependent on the largely subjective assessment of each juvenile sex offender's amenability to treatment and his appropriateness for alternative community-based programming versus incarceration or residential placement. As a result, there is an incurred vulnerability to making errors of judgment. Potential errors include placement of high-risk youths in community-based programs where public safety is compromised and limited local court and mental health dollars are inefficiently utilized. Conversely, errors can also be made in committing low- to moderate-risk youths to correctional centers, an approach that exacerbates the problem of institutional overcrowding, contributes to the soaring cost of operation of such programs, and deprives the youths of normalizing familial and community socialization experiences.

The absence of an effective classification system also makes treatment planning a less-than-precise endeavor and contributes to the tendency to provide all juvenile sex offenders with the same program of intervention. The development of a typology would assist in the identification of characteristics common to all or most juvenile sex offenders as well as those that permit offender differentiation. Attainment of a more in-depth understanding of the salient clinical characteristics of major subtypes of juvenile sex offenders and their etiological derivatives would ultimately allow for the development of more refined and prescriptive programs of intervention.

Emerging data on the etiology of juvenile sexual offending, particularly the role of early maltreatment and familial dysfunction, point to the potential for the development of early-identification prevention programs. Maltreated individuals who go on to perpetrate appear to be not only those who were severely traumatized as children but also those who were never afforded opportunities for psychosocial recovery because of inadequate familial and community support systems. It would appear that both the short- and long-term sequelae of childhood trauma could be attenuated, and thus the risk of later delinquency and sexual offending diminished, if children at high risk of becoming sex offenders, as well as their families, could be identified and provided with supportive services.

References

Abel GG, Becker JV, Cunningham-Rathner J, et al: Self-reported sex crimes of nonincarcerated paraphiliacs. Journal of Interpersonal Violence 2:3–25, 1987

Amir M: Patterns of Forcible Rape. Chicago, IL, University of Chicago Press, 1971

Awad GA, Saunders EB: Adolescent child molesters: clinical observations. Child Psychiatry Hum Dev 19:195–206, 1989

Awad GA, Saunders EB: Male adolescent sexual assaulters: clinical observations. Journal of Interpersonal Violence 6 (suppl 4):446–460, 1991

Awad GA, Saunders E, Levene J: A clinical study of male adolescent sex offenders. International Journal of Offender Therapy and Comparative Criminology 28:105–116, 1984

Barbaree HE, Seto MC, Serin RC, et al: Comparisons between sexual and nonsexual rapist subtypes: sexual arousal to rape, offense precursors, and offense characteristics. Criminal Justice and Behavior 21 (suppl 1):95–114, 1994

Baxter DJ, Barbaree HE, Marshall WL: Sexual responses to consenting and forced sex in a large sample of rapists and nonrapists. Behav Res Ther 24:513–520, 1986

Becker JV: Treating adolescent sexual offenders. Professional Psychology: Research and Practice 21 (suppl 5):362–265, 1990

Becker JV: Offenders: characteristics and treatment. Future Child 4 (suppl 2):176–197, 1994

Becker JV, Abel GG: Methodological and ethical issues in evaluating and treating adolescent sexual offenders, in Adolescent Sex Offenders: Issues in Research and Treatment (DHHS Publ No ADM-85-1396). Edited by Otey EM, Ryan GD. Rockville, MD, U.S. Department Of Health and Human Services, 1985, pp 109–129

Becker JV, Stein RM: Is sexual erotica associated with sexual deviance in adolescent males? Int J Law Psychiatry 14:85–95, 1991

Becker JV, Kaplan MS, Cunningham-Rathner J, et al: Characteristics of adolescent incest sexual perpetrators: preliminary findings. Journal of Family Violence 1:85–97, 1986

Becker JV, Hunter JA, Stein RM, et al: Factors associated with erection in adolescent sex offenders. Journal of Psychopathology and Behavioral Assessment 11 (suppl 4):353–363, 1989

Becker JV, Kaplan MS, Tenke CE, et al: The incidence of depressive symptomatology in juvenile sex offenders with a history of abuse. Child Abuse Negl 15:531–536, 1991

Becker JV, Hunter JA, Goodwin DW, et al: Test-retest reliability of audiotaped phallometric stimuli with adolescent sexual offenders. Annals of Sex Research 5:45–51, 1992a

Becker JV, Kaplan MS, Tenke CE: The relationship of abuse history, denial and erectile response: profiles of adolescent sexual perpetrators. Behavior Therapy 23:87–97, 1992b

Becker JV, Harris CD, Sales BD: Juveniles who commit sexual offenses: a critical review of research, in Sexual Aggression: Issues in Etiology and Assessment, Treatment, and Policy. Edited by Nagayama Hall GC, Hirschman R, Graham J, et al. Washington, DC, Taylor & Francis, 1993, pp 215–228

Blaske DM, Borduin C, Henggeler S, et al: Individual, family, and peer characteristics of adolescent sex offenders and assaultive offenders. Dev Psychol 25:846–855, 1989

Borduin CM, Henggeler SW, Blaske DM, et al: Multisystemic treatment of adolescent sexual offenders. International Journal of Offender Therapy and Comparative Criminology 34 (suppl 2):105–114, 1990

Bradford JM: The pharmacologic treatment of the adolescent sex offender, in The Juvenile Sex Offender. Edited by Barbaree HE, Marshall WL, Hudson SM. New York, Guilford, 1993, pp 278–288

Bremer JF: Serious juvenile sex offenders: treatment and long-term follow-up. Psychiatric Annals 22 (suppl 6):326–332, 1992

Brown EJ, Flanagan T, McLeod M (eds): Sourcebook of Criminal Justice Statistics. Washington, DC, U.S. Department of Justice, Bureau of Justice Statistics, 1983

Brownmiller S: Against Our Will: Men, Women, and Rape. New York, Simon & Schuster, 1975

Davis GE, Leitenberg H: Adolescent sex offenders. Psychol Bull 101 (suppl 3):417–427, 1987

Doshay LJ: The Boy Sex Offender and His Later Career. New York, Grune & Stratton, 1943

Elliott D: The developmental course of sexual and non-sexual violence: resulting from a national longitudinal study. Paper presented at the annual meeting of the American Association for the Treatment of Sexual Abusers, San Francisco, CA, November 1994

Fagan J, Wexler S: Explanations of sexual assault among violent delinquents. Journal of Adolescent Research 3:363–385, 1988

Fehrenbach PA, Smith W, Monastersky C, et al: Adolescent sexual offenders: offender and offense characteristics. Am J Orthopsychiatry 56 (suppl 2):225–233, 1986

Figia NA, Lang RA, Plutchik R, et al: Personality differences between sex and violent offenders. International Journal of Offender Therapy and Comparative Criminology 31:211–226, 1987

Ford ME, Linney JA: Comparative analysis of juvenile sexual offenders, violent nonsexual offenders, and status offenders. Journal of Interpersonal Violence 10 (suppl 1):56–70, 1995

France KG, Hudson SM: The conduct disorders and the juvenile sex offender, in The Juvenile Sex Offender. Edited by Barbaree HE, Marshall WL, Hudson SM. New York, Guilford, 1993, pp 225–234

Freeman-Longo RE: The impact of sexual victimization on males. Child Abuse Negl 10:411–414, 1986

Gil E, Johnson TC: Sexualized Children: Assessment and Treatment of Sexualized Children and Children Who Molest. Rockville, MD, Launch Press, 1993

Gottfredson MR, Hirschi T: A General Theory on Crime. Stanford, CA, Stanford University Press, 1990

Hayashino DS, Wurtele SK, Klebe KJ: Child molesters: an examination of cognitive factors. Journal of Interpersonal Violence 10 (suppl 1):106–116, 1995

Hazelwood RR, Warren J: The serial rapist: his characteristics and victims (conclusion). FBI Law Enforcement Bulletin 58:18–25, 1989

Henggeler S: Delinquency in Adolescence. Newbury Park, CA, Sage Publications, 1989

Herman JL: Sex offenders: a feminist perspective, in Handbook of Sexual Assault: Issues, Theories, and Treatment of the Offender. Edited by Marshall WL, Laws DR, Barbaree HE. New York, Plenum, 1990, pp 177–194

Hughes HM: Psychological and behavioral correlates of family violence in child witnesses and victims. Am J Orthopsychiatry 58:77–90, 1988

Hunter JA: A comparison of the psychosocial maladjustment of adult males and females sexually molested as children. Journal of Interpersonal Violence 6 (suppl 2):205–217, 1991

Hunter JA, Becker JV: The role of deviant sexual arousal in juvenile sexual offending: etiology, evaluation, and treatment. Criminal Justice and Behavior 21 (suppl 1):132–149, 1994

Hunter JA, Figueredo AJ: The influence of personality and history of sexual victimization in the prediction of juvenile perpetrated child molestation. Behav Modif (in press)

Hunter JA, Goodwin DW: The utility of satiation therapy in the treatment of juvenile sexual offenders: variations and efficacy. Annals of Sex Research 5:71–80, 1992

Hunter JA, Becker JV, Kaplan M, et al: The reliability and discriminative utility of the Adolescent Cognition Scale for juvenile sexual offenses. Annals of Sex Research 4:281–286, 1991

Hunter JA, Goodwin DW, Becker JV: The relationship between phallometrically measured deviant sexual arousal and clinical characteristics in juvenile sexual offenders. Behav Res Ther 32 (suppl 5):533–538, 1994

Hunter JA, Hazelwood RR, Slesinger D: Juvenile perpetrated sexual crimes: patterns of offending and predictors of violence. Journal of Family Violence (in press)

Jaffe P, Wolfe D, Wilson SK, et al: Family violence and child adjustment: a comparative analysis of girls' and boys' behavior symptoms. Am J Psychiatry 143:74–77, 1986

Kahn TJ, Chambers HJ: Assessing reoffense risk with juvenile sexual offenders. Child Welfare 19:333–345, 1991

Kaufman KL, Hilliker DR, Daleiden EL: Subgroup differences in the modus operandi of adolescent sexual offenders. Child Maltreatment 1:17–24, 1996

Kobayashi J, Sales BD, Becker JV, et al: Perceived parental deviance, parental-child bonding, child abuse, and child sexual aggression. Sexual Abuse: A Journal of Research and Treatment 7 (suppl 1):25–44, 1995

Lightfoot LO, Barbaree HE: The relationship between substance use and abuse and sexual offending in adolescents, in The Juvenile Sex Offender. Edited by Barbaree HE, Marshall WL, Hudson SW. New York, Guilford, 1993, pp 203–224

Linz D, Donnerstein E, Adams SM: Physiological desensitization and judgements about female victims of violence. Human Communication Research 15 (suppl 4):509–522, 1989

Lisak D: Subjective assessment of relationships with parents by sexually aggressive and nonaggressive men. Journal of Interpersonal Violence 9 (suppl 3):399–411, 1994

Lisak D, Roth S: Motives and psychodynamics of self-reported, unincarcerated rapists. Am J Orthopsychiatry 60:268–280, 1990

Loeber R, Stouthamer-Loeber M: Family factors as correlates and predictors of juvenile conduct problems and delinquency, in Crime and Justice: An Annual Review of Research, Vol 7. Edited by Tonry M, Morris N. Chicago, IL, University of Chicago Press, 1986, pp 29–149

Marshall WL, Barbaree HE, Eccles A: Early onset and deviant sexuality in child molesters. Journal of Interpersonal Violence 6:323–336, 1991

Mathews R, Hunter JA, Vuz J: Juvenile female sexual offenders: clinical characteristics and treatment issues. Sexual Abuse: A Journal of Research and Treatment 9:187–199, 1997

National Task Force on Juvenile Sexual Offending: Final report: a function of National Adolescent Perpetrator Network. Denver, CO, CH Kempe National Center, University of Colorado Health Sciences Center, 1993

Paperny DM, Deisher RW: Maltreatment of adolescents: the relationship to a predisposition toward violent behavior and delinquency. Adolescence 18:499–506, 1983

Patterson GR, Reid BJ, Dishion TJ: Antisocial Boys. Eugene, OR, Castalia, 1992

Rogers CM, Terry T: Clinical interventions with boy victims of sexual abuse, in Victims of Sexual Aggression. Edited by Stuart I, Greer J. New York, Van Nostrand Reinhold, 1984, pp 91–104

Ryan G: Victim to victimizer: rethinking victim treatment. Journal of Interpersonal Violence 4 (suppl 3):325–341, 1989

Ryan G, Lane S (eds): Juvenile Sexual Offending: Causes, Consequences and Corrections. Boston, MA, Lexington Books, 1991

Ryan G, Lane S, Davis J, et al: Juvenile sex offenders: development and correction. Child Abuse Negl 11:385–395, 1987

Smith WR: Delinquency and abuse among juvenile sexual offenders. Journal of Interpersonal Violence 3:400–413, 1988

Smith WR, Monastersky C, Deishner RM: MMPI-based personality types among juvenile sexual offenders. J Clin Psychol 43:422–430, 1987

Snyder HN, Sickmund M: Juvenile Offenders and Victims: A Focus on Violence. Pittsburgh, PA, National Center for Juvenile Justice, 1995

Stagg V, Wills GD, Howell M: Psychopathy in early child witnesses of family violence. Topics in Early Childhood Special Education 9:73–87, 1989

Steele B: Notes on the lasting effects of early childhood abuse throughout the life cycle. Child Abuse Negl 10:283–291, 1985

Van Ness SR: Rape as instrumental violence: a study of youth offenders [Special Issue: Gender Issues, Sex Offenses, and Criminal Justice: Current Trends]. Journal of Offender Counseling, Services and Rehabilitation 9:161–170, 1984

Weisz MG, Earls CM: The effects of exposure to filmed sexual violence on attitudes toward rape. Journal of Interpersonal Violence 10 (suppl 1): 71–84, 1995

9

Assessment of Adolescent Sex Offenders

Robin Jones, M.A., Anita M. Schlank, Ph.D.,
and Louis LeGum, Ph.D.

Over the past 25 years, there has been a tremendous increase in interest in the assessment and treatment of juvenile sex offenders (Abel et al. 1985; Barbaree et al. 1993a, 1993b; Becker et al. 1986; Roberts et al. 1973). Prior to the 1980s, according to Roberts and colleagues (1973), "the predominant view of the sexual offenses committed by this age group was that they constituted nuisance value only, reflecting a 'boys-will-be-boys' attitude and a discounted estimate of the severity of harm produced." This tendency to minimize the sexually abusive behavior of juveniles has lessened recently as a result of increased awareness of the high number of sexual offenses that are perpetrated by juveniles and also the realization that many adult sex offenders began their behavior as juveniles but faced no consequences (Abel et al. 1993; Becker et al. 1986; Brown et al. 1984; Deisher et al. 1982). The most recent

235

estimates suggest that "approximately 20% of all rapes and between 30% and 50% of child molestations are perpetrated by adolescent males . . . and approximately 50% of adult sex offenders report sexually deviant behavior (which began) in adolescence" (Barbaree et al. 1993b, p. 11).

A small but increasing literature on adolescent sex offenders now offers a range of frameworks and strategies to guide a clinical assessment (Barbaree et al. 1993b; Perry and Orchard 1992a; Ryan and Lane 1991). Assessment of sex offenders in other age groups also has implications for adolescent assessment, since many of the issues differ only with regard to the developmental needs of the client. The more extensive literature on adult sex offenders reminds us of the need to assess cognitive distortions, victim empathy, and social and emotional functioning. The emerging preadolescent literature reminds us of the vital importance of including the family when assessing and treating young offenders (Gil and Johnson 1993).

A clinical assessment of the youthful sex offender, including psychological testing, can contribute to decision making in at least two key areas. First, clinical assessment can inform decisions about the optimal treatment setting and level of restrictiveness necessary to meet the offender's needs while protecting the safety of the community, based on a comprehensive assessment of risk and dangerousness. Second, clinical assessment can contribute to treatment planning by allowing the clinician to identify the offender's strengths and deficits and therapeutic needs. These aspects of assessment are closely interrelated.

Dimensions of the Assessment

A comprehensive clinical assessment has multiple dimensions:

- Review of pertinent reports and documents
- An outreach effort into relevant parts of the youthful offender's community
- A series of interviews
- Administration of psychometric testing

The data from these various sources are then integrated into a psychological report.

Documents

Since the youth and family's level of honesty and disclosure about the offense(s) is an important assessment variable, it is necessary to obtain as much independent information about the offense(s) as possible prior to the interviews. If the youth is facing criminal or delinquency charges in the court system, a police summary of facts, victim statements, and a pre-sentence probation report may be available.

The importance of becoming very familiar with the facts of the case cannot be overemphasized. If the youth and/or family are in denial about the offending, their alternative explanations for what occurred may be very convincing. The interviewer's ability to distinguish facts from fiction needs to be very sharp. At an absolute minimum, the interviewer must have access to the summary of facts.

Outreach

The range of other people who need to be spoken to will be defined by the features of the individual case. These sources may include other nuclear or extended family members, residential care or detention staff, school officials, agents of the court, and any community support representatives such as clergy or after-school program staff who have had an important role in the youth's life. If possible, we also strongly recommend that the evaluator(s) visit the home or alternative residence if there is some possibility the youth will remain in the community.

The Clinical Assessment

The following is a suggested structure for the clinical assessment process:

1. A meeting with the youth and his or her parent(s) or guardian(s) to delineate the purpose of the assessment, to clarify the issue of limited confidentiality, and to have releases of information and consent forms read and signed

2. An interview with the parent(s) or guardian(s) while the youth completes assigned self-report psychological testing
3. Face-to-face testing with the adolescent (e.g., IQ test, projective tests) followed by a clinician interview directed toward the sexual offense(s) and other sexual history
4. As time allows, a wrap-up consultation with the youth and his parents or guardians to review the assessment and its findings along with any recommendations that may be warranted at this juncture

The Introductory Meeting

The clinician should describe his or her expertise and qualifications as part of the initial introductions. This will help assure the family that the interviewer is able to offer a professional response to the family's difficult situation. A clear explanation of the purpose of the assessment then needs to be offered (e.g., Is it an evaluation for the court? an intake interview for a specific program? both? Will it have implications for sentencing or placement?).

The limits of confidentiality need to be discussed before any information is sought from the family. The youth and family need to know, for example, what information will be disclosed to other parties, such as the court, juvenile justice system, victim's counselor, or referral source. They also need to know about the interviewers' legal obligations under the state laws on mandatory reporting and their own professional code of ethics regarding duty to warn, in the event that additional ongoing or intended offending be disclosed by the adolescent or any other family member. A limited confidentiality release form should be signed by the adolescent and at least one parent or guardian before proceeding.

Finally, it would be useful at this point to offer the family some encouragement and optimism about their decision to undertake the assessment, even if it was mandated and they attended under duress. If the family can be encouraged from the beginning to view their own cooperation as a very positive first step, it may increase their level of trust, motivation, and disclosure in the interviews that follow.

Clinical Interview With the Youth

▶ Psychosexual Information

Ross and Loss (1991) suggest starting the interview by providing the adolescent with psychosexual material that will help him or her to form realistic expectations, preempt any denial, and model to the youth the frank and open communication of sexual and highly personal information. There is arguably a greater need to do this with adolescents than with adults, because their lower level of maturity and relative lack of experience may lead them to feel even greater discomfort with the subject matter than do adult offenders.

Such information could usefully begin with an acknowledgment that denial or minimization of the offense is a natural, understandable reaction to being charged with a sexual offense and serves positive functions in the short term, such as protecting self-esteem. The youth then needs to be informed about how continuing denial inhibits progress in the long term, since it leaves the offender open to reoffending by protecting him or her from discomfort about what he or she has done. Denial may also lead to ruling out of certain treatment programs or may result in a longer or more restrictive sentencing outcome.

The youth will also need to be educated about what sexual offenses actually are, perhaps by way of an overview of contact and noncontact offenses. The interviewer should use explicit language so that the youth can see that the use of sexually explicit language in the interview is normal and expected. The youth needs to be informed about how offending is a learned behavior rather than an "illness" or disease. This observation can provide a rationale later for gathering a detailed social and sexual history, which might identify predisposing and precipitating factors that can in turn be addressed in treatment. It will also help orient the youth toward the strategic treatment objectives of lifelong control rather than permanent "cure."

It can also be helpful to indicate that the offender was fortunate to have been caught, because of the likelihood that the offending would have continued and become progressively more entrenched and serious in spite of the youth's probable "promises" and attempts to overcome the problem alone. The interviewer can then acknowledge that the sexual offending behavior has probably caused the offender considerable anxiety and concern, as well as considerable harm to the victim(s). Encouragement about the need for honesty as a first step toward addressing the problem is called for in this context.

▶ History and Functional Analysis of Offense Behaviors

Instead of having the youth repeat a well-rehearsed story that may contain substantial denial, minimization, or other thinking errors, Ross and Loss (1991) suggest, the evaluator might begin with the youth's first acknowledged impulse to engage in any form of deviant sexual behavior and then develop a chronology of the offender's urges and acts, finishing with the most recent offenses.

A functional analysis of the offense or series of offenses is critical, with attention given to the cognitive, affective, behavioral, and environmental antecedents and consequences of the offending behaviors. This process can be painstaking and time-consuming if the youth discloses multiple offending incidents or victims. If this is the case, it may be necessary to limit questioning to the first, the last, and the most "typical" offense against each victim.

Although there is no single "right" way to obtain this information, the following features of the sexual offenses need to be gathered during this process, to contribute to the assessment of risk and dangerousness:

- Intrusiveness of offending
- Modus operandi (e.g., grooming, bribery, force)
- Frequency of offending in relation to frequency of opportunities to offend
- Number of victims
- Gender and age difference between perpetrator and victim(s)
- Progression of offending and speed of progression
- Duration of offense history
- Content and frequency of sexual fantasy about offending

- Presence of others when offending, and leader/follower issues in these cases
- Use of alcohol or drugs when offenses took place

The interviewer also needs to pay attention to various process variables, noting in particular how prepared the youth is to discuss offense behaviors, and his or her extent of honesty, as opposed to denial, minimization, rationalizing, or justification. If the youth begins to deny or minimize the offending, it is useful to stop immediately and return to the psychoeducational material in this area, offering the youth a face-saver and then some prompting and encouragement to try again.

It may be helpful, for example, to point out how an admission of offending is a display of courage and that by being honest the offender will gain his or her own and others' respect in this situation. This strategy interrupts the distorted thought processes, discourages the self-reinforcement of denial, and, at the same time, allows the interviewer to assess the rigidity of the youth's denial and his or her response to being confronted.

▶ Victim Empathy

It is very important to assess the offender's level of victim empathy and, indeed, his or her capacity for empathy in general. An empathic response consists of both the cognitive ability to take the perspective of another person and the affective ability to experience emotional concern (or another appropriate emotion) in response to taking the other person's perspective (Marshall et al. 1993). Therefore, an assessment of the adolescent offender's victim empathy and general empathy needs to include both the cognitive and the affective dimensions.

A good starting point would be to ask the offender some general questions about what short-and long-term effects he or she imagines the abuse will have had on the victim's life, prompting the offender if necessary to consider how victims would feel about themselves, other people, family, and sexuality. The interviewer could then offer a scenario for the offender, based on what the offender has admitted or has been charged with, and ask what the offender would think and feel like if he or she was in "the victim's shoes."

Questions on affective responding could then focus on how the offender feels in the present while imagining the abuse from the victim's point of view. What does it make the offender feel toward the victim? toward himself or herself? The latter distinction is important because it helps distinguish affective responding that is self-interested from that which is genuinely empathic.

Several factors may inhibit the offender's response to questions in this area. One is difficulty identifying and/or expressing feelings. Many teenagers—and male offenders of any age—lack a language for emotions beyond very basic discriminations (e.g., good, bad, bored) or for those that are socially sanctioned, such as anger. Another inhibiting factor may be the extent to which the offender himself or herself has experienced sexual or other forms of abuse. There is considerable recognition in the clinical literature that unresolved prior experience of abuse often inhibits empathic responding, because the recognition of another person's pain is likely to arouse memories of one's own, which have in turn been habitually suppressed or avoided (Bass and Davis 1988; Lew 1990).

It is important to recognize that the presence of factors that inhibit empathic responding does not necessarily indicate sociopathy or a lack of capacity for empathy in general. Indeed, we can expect that prior to treatment, almost any sex offender's level of victim-specific empathy is likely to be low, if only because of the minimization or other thinking errors that serve to protect self-esteem. Thus, it is useful to assess the offender's capacity for empathy in other areas as well. For example, the offender could be offered a scenario of a close friend's being badly injured and then answer some similar questions on perspective taking and emotional responsiveness to the imaginary victim's experience.

A process variable of telling import is the offender's *affect*. For example, sad affect is a promising sign even if the youth is unable to find words to express the victim's experience, whereas anger at the victim indicates a more fundamental lack of empathy.

▶ Youth's Perceptions of the Offending Behavior
The youth's level of insight and understanding about his or her own behavior, as well as his or her interest in gaining more knowledge in

this area, has implications for amenability to treatment. It is useful to hear the offender's own explanation for why he or she committed the offense and to assess the offender's ability to identify predisposing and precipitating factors. It is also important to assess the offender's level of understanding about the moral wrongfulness of sexual offending, for example, by asking what, if anything, he or she believes was wrong with committing the sexual offense(s).

The extent to which the offender takes responsibility for the offending is also an important factor. We have found it useful to ask the offender to frame this in terms of percentages: What percentage of the blame does he or she attribute to himself or herself, to the victim(s), and to others, and why?

▶ Sexual History

A functional analysis of the offending behaviors can lead to the development of a full sexual history. The objective of this history is to establish the specific sexual issues that contributed to the youth's offending behavior as distinct from social, emotional, or other difficulties. This process will help connect the offending behavior to relevant predispositions and precipitants, and this in turn will assist with treatment planning. The collection of sexual history information in the context of sexual offending, as in all areas, needs to be directed toward identifying strengths or resiliency factors as well as problem areas.

Throughout the sexual history, it may be useful to note how open the youth is about discussing sexual matters and to explore in a preliminary way the source of any resistance that may be evident. For example, resistance that derives from a lack of sexual language or embarrassment has very different implications for treatment than a refusal to discuss it because "it's not your business" or because of phobias like fear or embarrassment about the whole subject of sex.

A useful starting point could be to inquire from whom and how the youth learned about sex. Questions can then be directed to establish family attitudes and values, peer influences, and other sources of information or experience.

Family influences. It is important to interview the parents and to ask questions regarding their understanding of the child's sexual development. Some of the questions one might consider are as follows: Did the youth's parents provide any sex education within the family? If they did, in what form? How comfortable are family members when discussing sexual matters? What are the family's attitudes on issues such as masturbation? sex before marriage? pornography use?

Information about how sexual boundaries are drawn in the home can be an important part of the offender's sexual history. In some situations, parents or guardians may be less forthcoming in this area for fear that they will then be held accountable for the youth's offending. Inquiry may be made about sleeping and bathing arrangements, dressing practices, and attitudes about nudity, expression of affection, and sexual activity.

Several other factors need to be kept in mind in this context. Socioeconomic considerations may mean that some families live in overcrowded conditions by necessity. There are still ways, however, to protect sexual boundaries in crowded situations, and the family's efforts in this area can be assessed if questions are asked sensitively. For example, does the family attempt to protect privacy by the use of curtains, screens, or allocating "private time" in shared rooms? Do adults attempt to limit their children's exposure to adult sexual activity by restricting it to times when children are asleep or otherwise occupied?

Peer influences. Questions about peer influences can help establish the level and nature of the youth's sexual experience. It is important to be cognizant of developmentally appropriate sexual behaviors for children of different ages when gathering history in this area. Although, again, there is no single "right" way to collect this information, it is important to gain a chronology of the youth's sexual interest and activities with others through early and middle childhood and adolescence, up to the present time. It may be necessary to first "normalize" for the youth the fact that many children experiment sexually with same- and opposite-sex peers. It is also important, however, to be alert to indicators of sexual victimization or perpetration of sexual abuse.

Incidents of sexual abuse or perpetration may be uncovered in the youth's own life that he or she has not perceived as such. This phenomenon appears to be particularly common for male adolescents who may have tried to interpret sexual encounters with older females as "sexual experience" or "getting lucky" rather than abuse. Questions in this area may also uncover normal sexual development that became "derailed" at a particular point, which calls for further investigation of other areas of the youth's life around the time of the change. For example, if a youth describes having a "good" relationship with his girlfriend but at the same time he began molesting younger children, more questions about the positive and negative aspects of his relationship and other areas of his life are warranted.

It is important to bear in mind the "demand characteristics" of the interview situation for teenagers—especially males—when asking questions in the area of sexual experiences with peers. Teenagers may feel pressure to portray themselves as more experienced and less fearful or vulnerable than is actually the case. Therefore, it is important to phrase questions in such a way that allows youths who are lacking in age-appropriate sexual experience to communicate information about this area with a minimum of self-consciousness or shame. It is also important to be aware that the youth may have conflicts or confusion about sexual orientation, regardless of the gender of the victim(s) of his or her crime. Therefore, it is important not to make implicit assumptions about the gender of persons in which he or she is most interested.

If the youth is disclosing an extensive history of sexual experience, such as multiple partners, victims, or victimizations, it is also useful to check out some sexual health issues. Has he or she ever contracted a sexually transmitted disease? ever been tested? Would he or she know where to go to get assistance in this area? What form of contraception, if any, has he or she used in the past? If none has been used, why? Has any of the youth's sexual activity resulted in pregnancy, termination of pregnancy, or birth? If so, who has custody of the baby?

Other sources of information. It is also important to assess whether the youth learned about sex from other sources besides family and peers. Questions in this area may uncover extrafamilial sexual abuse, exposure to pornography (discussed below), or heightened personal vulnerability to the messages in nonrestricted sexually explicit material.

Sexual compulsivity. The sexual history needs to determine the offender's level of sexual compulsivity, which in turn has implications for risk and dangerousness. The most important factors are the presence and frequency of deviant sexual fantasies, pornography use, and the presence of other paraphilias in addition to the offense(s) for which the youth has been apprehended. Specific questioning will be necessary to get the desired information, because this kind of information is unlikely to be easily or willingly volunteered.

Pornography use. The adolescent sex offender may have been exposed to or have had access to pornography or "adult" sexual material. The clinician must be aware of all the forms that such material can take, as outlined below, especially if there is some possibility of the youth's having been exposed to pornography by an older person, who may have easier access:

- Magazines and books
- Videotapes
- Movies and films
- Peep shows and strip clubs (if the youth looks old enough to gain admission)
- 1-900 and other telephone services
- Pornographic material accessed through computer networks

If the youth does admit to using pornography, it is then important to establish how it is used, with what kind of frequency, and what kinds of sexual acts it portrayed. To what extent does the pornographic material show violent or nonconsenting acts? sexual acts involving pedophilia or other paraphilias? Does the youth masturbate when he or she uses the pornography? masturbate to memories or fantasies of the material? How did the youth gain access to the pornography? Does he or she seek out this material on his or her own? If so, has there been a progression toward greater explicitness or deviance of content? Has the youth ever been involved in the making or distribution of pornography? Did he or she ever utilize pornography in his or her sexual offending?

Some youths, although not actively seeking pornographic material, find sexually explicit scenes in general release magazines, books, movies, advertisements, or videos sexually stimulating to the extent that they become preoccupied with the material or with fantasies and thoughts about it. This is also a concern.

Other paraphilias. It is naive to assume that the perpetrator's sexual offense constitutes the only type of sexual pathology in which he or she has engaged or to which he or she is vulnerable. Accordingly, other paraphilias, including those that follow, need to be assessed:

- Peeping, or voyeurism
- Exhibitionism
- Frottage
- Obscene telephone calling
- Bestiality
- Fetishism
- Transvestitism

▶ Other Sexual-Specific Assessment Dimensions

Since an offender's behavior is influenced by many factors, an assessment needs to extend far beyond global assessments of personality functioning. Specifically, assessment is required in a number of areas, including treatment motivation, disordered arousal, cognitive distortions concerning sexual offending, social competence, sexual knowledge, personal victimization, recidivism risk and dangerousness, general psychological functioning, and psychoeducational assessment.

Treatment motivation. It is important to assess the youth's level of motivation for treatment, which most likely will be evident already from consideration of the process variables in the assessment so far. It is important to ascertain how much of the evident motivation is internally based and how much is external. *Internal motivation* refers to the youth's level of concern about his or her own offense behavior and perceived level of need for change. *External motivation* refers to the youth's desire to avoid unpleasant outcomes that therapy may avert, such as a jail sentence or family rejection. A mixture of both internal and external motivation is ideal. Simple questions such as "How much do you want counseling? a treatment program? What would be gained if you did get into a program?" constitute some useful probes.

Disordered arousal. In their study of more than 1,000 individuals with paraphilias, Abel and colleagues (1993) found that the onset of paraphilias occurred prior to the age of 18 in over 40% of the subjects. Given this prevalence, it is important to assess the level of disordered arousal in juveniles referred for committing sexual offenses. One method for obtaining information about disordered arousal is the Adolescent Sexual Interest Cardsort, a self-report questionnaire designed to measure deviant sexual interest patterns (G. G. Abel, "Assessment and Treatment of Sex Offenders," unpublished manuscript, 1979). Sixty-four sexual scenarios are described, and the adolescent is asked to rate, on a three-point scale, his or her arousal to them. The test–retest reliability on this instrument was found to be poor. It was believed, however, that this finding may have been the result of reactive responses to the ethical requirement to provide feedback following initial assessment regarding the sexual acts that are considered to be inappropriate (Becker and Kaplan 1988).

Several scales of the Multiphasic Sex Inventory—Juvenile Form may also provide useful information in this area. The original Multiphasic Sex Inventory, published in 1984 (Nichols and Molinder 1984), is a 300-item self-report questionnaire that was developed to assess a wide range of psychosexual characteristics of male sex offenders. Research suggests that this measure has high levels of internal consistency and provides information "not tapped by traditional psychological tests" (Kalichman et al. 1992, p. 384). The Multiphasic Sex Inventory—Juvenile Form was normed with a sample of 75 juveniles who ranged in age from 12 to 18 years. Some information about sexual arousal can be obtained from the Sex Deviance Patterns scale and the Paraphilias subtest. Unfortunately, however, there appear to be no available studies specifically using the juvenile form of this test.

Penile plethysmography is frequently used in the assessment of adult sex offender populations, but because of ethical concerns it was not initially used with adolescent populations (National Adolescent Perpetrator Network 1993). However, Becker and Kaplan (1988) reported significant correlations between erection responses of adolescent subjects who had molested males and the number of victims. Murphy and colleagues (1992, p. 414) found that psychophysiological assessment of sexual arousal was "well tolerated" by their juvenile population and also very useful for providing information that was valuable for treatment planning. There are ongoing studies to evaluate the role of penile plethysmography in reassessment and treatment of juvenile sex offenders.

Cognitive distortions. The degree to which an adolescent perpetrator adheres to cognitive distortions concerning sexual offending is an important area for assessment and treatment planning. Challenging these distortions is often necessary before an offender can benefit from other interventions, such as victim empathy groups or personal victimization work.

The Adolescent Cognition Scale is a revised version of the Adult Cognition Scale, which was designed to assess whether adults offenders held distorted cognitions regarding sexual behaviors (Abel GG, Becker JV: Adult Cognition Scale, 1984 [research document available from Abel GG, Behavioral Medicine Laboratory, Atlanta, GA]). The adolescent version consists of 32 true/false items such as "Some people are shy about asking for sex so they really want you to force them." Preliminary studies suggest that test–retest reliability for this instrument is marginal and that it does not discriminate between offender and nonsex offenders' attitudes (Becker et al. 1993). Nevertheless, this instrument can be clinically useful for identifying specific areas on which to focus during the early phases of treatment.

The Burt Rape Myth Scale (Burt 1980) is a 19-item questionnaire that can be useful for identifying cognitive distortions about adult rape victims. It is one of the most frequently used measures for assessment of endorsement of rape myths and has been found to have good reliability and validity (Check and Malamuth 1983; Koss et al. 1985).

Another instrument that may be used for identifying cognitive distortions is the Multiphasic Sex Inventory—Juvenile Form (Nichols and Molinder 1984). The two scales that appear to be particularly useful for this purpose are the Justifications scale and the Cognitive Distortions/Immaturity scale. The Cognitive Distortions/Immaturity scale assesses self-accountability by identifying early childhood cognitive distortions that stay with the offender and help him maintain his sexually deviant behavior. The Justifications scale measures a specific type of cognitive distortion: the degree to which an offender attempts to justify his sexually deviant behavior (Nichols and Molinder 1984).

Social competence.   Social competence is often suggested as a deficit found in adolescent sex offender populations. Van Ness (1984) reported that 63% of adolescent rapists displayed poor anger control skills compared with only 26% of non–sexual offending juveniles who exhibit delinquent behavior. Fehrenbach and colleagues (1986) found 65% of adolescent perpetrators in their sample to be socially isolated. A study by Saunders and colleagues (1986) yielded similar findings. O'Brien (1991) found that 54% of the sibling incest offenders in his study had few, if any, peer-age friends and generally poor social skills.

Although much information about social competence can be obtained from interviews with the client and with his or her parents and through direct observation in early groups, there are a few standardized measures of social competence that can augment that information. The Interpersonal Behavior Survey (Mauger and Adkinson 1980) assesses a wide variety of social skills, including assertiveness, anger management, and relationship variables. The Adolescent Problems Inventory (Freedman et al. 1978) requires the juvenile offender to give verbal responses to a number of problem situations. Although this inventory may be less reliable since it involves direct behavioral assessment in role-playing situations, it can provide useful information for treatment planning.

Sexual knowledge/experience. Many studies have suggested that most adolescent sex offenders engaged in nondeviant sexual behavior prior to their offenses. Hence, sexual experimentation as a theory for their abusive behavior does not appear to have much validity (Becker et al. 1986; R. E. Long 1982). Some offenders, however, are extremely inhibited sexually and lack sexual knowledge, and therefore an assessment of this area may be useful (Murphy et al. 1992).

The Math Tech Sex Education Test (Kirby 1984) is one standardized method for assessing sexual knowledge and attitudes. This instrument contains two parts: a test assessing knowledge of sexual facts and a test assessing attitudes and values surrounding sexuality. Both tests are in multiple-choice format. The reliability and validity for this scale appear to be quite good (Becker et al. 1991; Kirby 1984). The Sexual Knowledge and Beliefs scale of the Multiphasic Sex Inventory—Juvenile Form can also be helpful for indicating deficiencies in sexual knowledge, although no studies on its reliability or validity are currently available.

History of personal victimization. Estimates of prevalence of sexual abuse in the histories of adolescent sex offenders vary considerably. It is likely that any abuse rate reported would be an underestimate given the difficulty many adolescents would have in admitting to being a victim of abuse because of the stigma. This phenomenon may be magnified if the perpetrator was of the same gender (Murphy et al. 1992). In addition, questions asked during the assessment period may be difficult for the adolescent since they occur prior to any therapeutic relationship being established. Finally, sexually abusive behaviors may not be identified by adolescents as "abuse" if the adolescents believe that they "consented" to the activity or if the perpetrator was a woman. For these reasons, it is useful to ask general questions about sexual activity without labeling it as "abuse" during the initial interview. For example, a question such as "Has an adult ever been sexual with you?" may provide more information than one that inquires about whether the adolescent has ever been sexually abused.

Some information may also be obtained from specific items of the Multiphasic Sex Inventory—Juvenile Form (Nichols and Molinder 1984) or from having the adolescent complete a written auto-biography, following a structured guideline (J. D. Long et al. 1989). These techniques may be particularly useful for an adolescent who might be willing to answer such questions in written form but re-luctant to discuss them verbally.

▶ Family Relationships and History

It is important to elicit from the youth his perceptions and feelings about family dynamics. The clinician would do well to consider the following areas:

- Which family members (or others) had a role in raising the youth
- The youth's relationship with each key family member
- The youth's perception of each family member's strengths and weaknesses
- Discipline and "rules of the house," and the youth's perception of his or her own compliance with them
- How arguments or conflicts are resolved in the home
- Substance abuse by other family members
- Criminal history of other family members
- Changes in household memberships, for example,
- due to deaths, divorces, remarriages, or relocation
- Access to victims or other children in the extended family

Ways of phrasing these questions will be important for adoles-cents, who may not want to reveal family problems out of shame, loyalty, fear, or the belief that this will show disrespect for their parents. It may be important to reassure the youth that his or her answers will not make the interviewer think badly of his or her family and to emphasize that being able to bring the problems out in the open will help in finding some solutions. Also, for young ado-lescents, whose discriminations between different feelings or judg-ments may still be rudimentary, creative questioning may be needed.

"Who in your family do you get along with best? worst? Why?" may yield more information than more complex questions about the youth's relationship with each family member.

Questions about discipline and conflict resolution in the family may reveal information about physical abuse, emotional abuse, or exposure to domestic violence. To preserve rapport, it is important for the interviewer, at least initially, to share the youth's language about such incidents or experiences. For example, if a youth refers to episodes of physical abuse as beatings or hidings, it may seem like an implicit judgment if the interviewer refers back to the same incidents as "abuse."

▶ School Adjustment

The clinician should gather information to make determinations about the youth's academic and social adjustment in school. In the academic area, is the youth in the expected grade for his or her age? How does he or she perform academically? If the youth has been held back, is it because of a learning disability? poor attention and concentration? behavior problems? difficulties with the environment of the school itself, such as poor teaching, inadequate materials, or lack of safety (as is sometimes the case in underfunded rural or inner-city regions)?

The youth's social adjustment at school should be assessed. Does the youth have significant friendships? Is he or she gregarious or a loner? Are his or her friends of similar age? older or younger? same or opposite sex, or both? What kinds of activities does the youth do with friends? Is he or she typically a leader or a follower in peer activities? Does the youth have a problem with truancy, cutting classes, or frequent lateness? Has he or she ever been suspended or expelled from a school? If so, why? The clinician should check for aggressive or antisocial acts or excessive disrespect for authority.

Several further issues warrant mention in regard to school adjustment. First, it is important to corroborate information from the youth in this area with his or her parents and also the school's records. Second, difficulties with attention and concentration, if such have been noted, could have implications for the youth's ability to focus in group therapy. It is, however, important to compare such reports with one's own observations during extended interviews. In some instances, attention-deficit disorder and other behavior disorders in children and adolescents have been overdiagnosed in the school system.

▶ Psychoeducational/Neuropsychological Assessment

A comprehensive psychological assessment of an adolescent should include a general assessment of cognitive functioning and level of educational skills with particular attention to deficits. It is critical that the clinician have an informed and meaningful grasp of the level of intellectual capability at which the youthful offender is functioning and whether he or she has any marked deficiencies in literacy. In this regard, an adolescent's cognitive capabilities necessarily color the complex matter of sexual offending and his or her ability to understand his or her sexuality, to discern the cues of victims, and to appreciate the nature and consequences of his or her sexual misconduct.

Given the strong emphasis on cognitive therapy in most sex offender treatment programs, it may be necessary to refer developmentally disabled offenders to specialized groups that are more concrete, practical, and action-oriented, with minimal cognitive demands (Gilby et al. 1989).

The literature on sexual offending has revealed that a considerable number of sex offenders, both adolescents and adults, present with histories of neuropsychological anomalies (Langevin 1989), and so such conditions need to be established or ruled out. It is not uncommon for a youth to turn to inappropriate gratification of his or her affectual and sexual needs by virtue of failures with his or her peers, which invariably have their onset in the classroom. One of the present authors has consistently found a marked divergence between measured intellectual capabilities and residual academic skills in juvenile sex offenders.

Relatedly, should it be determined that the youth has an academic skills disorder, it is imperative that a meaningful therapeutic intervention program on his or her behalf include some effort at educational remediation. In spite of whatever sex offender–specific therapy might be provided him or her, if the youth continues to fail among his or her peers and to feel as if he or she has no viable skills, then vulnerability to a sexual offending relapse will remain considerable.

It is recommended that a standard face-to-face intellectual assessment procedure be utilized, specifically one of the Wechsler series. Not only do these intellectual testing measures provide for the most accurate evaluations of cognitive capabilities, but also the interplay of the clinician with the adolescent in the testing process allows for some rich observational data, including a consideration of residual attention-deficit disorder or attention-deficit/hyperactivity disorder (ADHD), ability to tolerate frustration, irritability and impulse control, and so forth. If there is enough time, a quick neuropsychological screening measure that tests for visuomotor problems and organizational skills can be administered. Such test procedures as the Benton Visual Form Discrimination (Benton et al. 1983) or the Bender-Gestalt may be useful (Bender 1938). The clinician always should bear in mind that a more comprehensive neuropsychological evaluation may be warranted.

▶ General Psychological Functioning

Although there appear to be no major differences between the overall psychological functioning of juvenile sex offenders and that of other adolescent populations (Kavoussi et al. 1988; Lewis et al. 1981), it is important to identify the presence of problems in this area for the purposes of therapeutic placement and dispositional recommendations.

Personality testing needs to address matters of overall psychological functioning, level of self-esteem (or lack thereof), the presence or absence of any affective and/or cognitive disturbances, problems in anger control, and the range and use of coping mechanisms and defenses.

Depression can often be seen in juvenile sex offender populations (Becker et al. 1991). Although depression and other psychiatric disturbances may be identified during a clinical interview, these diagnostic formulations can be supported by the use of personality testing, both objective and projective in nature. The Reynolds Adolescent Depression Scale (Reynolds 1987), Children's Depression

Inventory (Kovacs 1992), and Piers-Harris Children's Self-Concept Scale (1984) are other instruments that can help in adducing the presence or absence of a clinical depression and any self-destructive disposition, as well as in elucidating the offender's feelings about himself or herself and how the offender considers that he or she measures up with his or her family, peers, and in his or her school environs.

The Minnesota Multiphasic Personality Inventory—Adolescent Form (MMPI-A; Butcher et al. 1992) remains a standard and useful instrument. Caution needs to be taken to ensure that the adolescent's reading level is appropriate. The revised edition suggests a threshold sixth-grade reading level. For adolescents who have difficulties with the actual reading of the test, administration through audiotape can be facilitative.

Hathaway and McKinley (1940) developed the original MMPI for use with adult populations, but from the beginning it was widely used for assessing adolescents too. In the 1970s adolescent norms were published and, in 1992, an adolescent form of this measure became available. Subjects for the adolescent normative sample were obtained from several geographic regions of the United States to maximize the possibility of obtaining a balanced sample of subjects. The test–retest reliability and internal consistency of the basic scales appear to be good, and the factor analysis of the basic scales is similar to that for the adult MMPI (Butcher et al. 1992).

The MMPI-A provides useful information on a number of levels. In particular, the validity scale index lends perspective to the likelihood that the adolescent is being forthcoming or less than candid about his or her indicated sexual offense or other dimensions of his or her life. Useful clinical data can also be harvested with regard to ego strength, sociopathic tendencies, social skills, affective disturbances, or impairment in reality testing.

Projective testing may also be instructive, although continuing problems remain in terms of normative data and validity. Projective testing can provide the clinician with another avenue of assessing the adolescent offender that can be integrated with objective measures and other information composing the overall evaluative process. We have found projective drawings to be particularly edifying, especially with regard to shedding light on how significant the youth perceives himself or herself within the context of the world in which he or she lives. Relatedly, human drawings frequently provide an inferential insight about matters of unresolved gender identity conflicts, misogynistic attitudes, and the inclination to sexually objectify people. Thus, it is not uncommon for adolescents who have been referred for regressive sexual offenses and who present with histories of limited heterosocial contacts and success to sketch human figures that are miniaturized and childlike in graphic quality and/or almost devoid of any specific sexual identification.

Adolescent sex offenders show varying degrees of alcohol and other drug involvement, and chemical dependency should be assessed to assist in treatment planning. Some studies have suggested that measures of substance abuse developed for adults may actually be inappropriate for adolescents, and the National Institute on Drug Abuse has developed a manual for adolescent substance abuse assessment and treatment referral (Tarter 1988). Two instruments have been developed specifically for adolescent populations: the Drug Use Screening Instrument and the Personal Experience Screening Questionnaire (Winters K: Personal Experience Screening Questionnaire, 1988 [available from Chemical Dependency Adolescent Assessment Project, St. Paul, MN]).

Interview With the Parent(s) or Guardian(s)

The objective of the interview with the parent(s) or guardian(s) is to assess areas of risk and resiliency within the family and their likely impact on the youth and his or her likelihood of recidivism or other problems. Some of the issues raised in this interview will parallel those already assessed with the youth.

Family functioning has been stressed as an important factor in understanding the adolescent sex offender. In particular, issues such as role reversals, blurred generational and interpersonal boundaries, and dysfunctional communication styles have been identified as significant factors (O'Brien 1991). Lack of parental supervision has also been a somewhat consistent factor. Although much of this information can be obtained through interviews with the various family members, some researchers have found it useful to develop their own structured questionnaires that are filled out by the parents of an offender prior to intake (O'Brien 1991).

▶ Family History and Current Functioning

Several areas of family history need to be assessed. It should be ascertained who have been the primary caregivers for the youth since his or her birth and also what changes in household or family membership have occurred. The educational and work history of the youth's parents and of any other important relatives or caregivers is also important, as it may help identify issues of financial means, including economic hardship.

Sexual abuse and/or offending histories of other family members also need to be assessed, along with questions about present and past drug and alcohol use and criminal activities. Other major stressors in the family's history, such as deaths, divorces, or estrangements, and their effect upon the youth need to be established. In many cases, the timing of the youth's offending suggests a relationship between the decision to offend and the presence or intensification of major family stressors.

It is important to look for areas of strength and resiliency that have helped the family cope with or avert crises in the past, as it may be possible to mobilize these resources again. Examples include spiritual guidance, extended family or community networks, or certain cognitive or behavioral styles of coping that family members have used before, such as focusing on the positive, making specific efforts in the area of self-care, and having regular family discussions or meetings.

In terms of current family functioning, the most important areas to assess are

- Roles and responsibilities of current family members
- Discipline and conflict resolution
- Boundaries (need to be assessed in equivalent depth to the interview with the youth; see discussion of interview with youth earlier in this chapter)

- Practical issues such as space, victim access, supervision of children, and the family's wishes regarding the youth's place of residence

▶ Youth's History and Current Functioning

It is a matter of clinical judgment how much information gathered already from the youth needs to be verified by a parent or guardian. Generally, we have sought verification if the youth was confused, unsure, or resistant in the provision of information in areas that overlap with those of the parent interviews. Obviously, a considerable fund of historical knowledge about the youth is held only by the parents or guardians. Areas to cover include the following:

1. *Health and development:* Birth complications, milestones, significant illnesses, injuries, or hospitalizations.
2. *Social development and behavior:* Sociability and quality of relationships with other family members and peers through different stages of development. A screening of problem areas is also important, to verify anything the youth may have disclosed. This screening needs to address serious noncompliance with parents, drug and alcohol abuse, aggression or violence, lying, criminal behaviors other than the present offense, fire setting, cruelty to animals, and other indicators of antisocial or conduct-disordered behavior. It should also be ascertained to what the parents attribute such behaviors, if present.
3. *Sexual development:* Anything unusual or causing concern at different stages of development; parental role in sex education; how and when the parents first became concerned or suspicious about the youth's behavior; extent of appropriate sexual experience or relationships with peers of which parents are aware; pornography use; and presence of other paraphilias.
4. *Functioning in school and community:* It is useful to verify most or all information gained from the youth concerning both academic and behavioral functioning at school. It is also valuable to determine other activities that the youth is involved with in the community as well as his or her interests and skills.

▶ Parent Reactions to the Offending Behavior

To what extent has the youth's offending behavior precipitated a family crisis? To what extent do the parents and other family members accept versus deny the offending? What is the parent's explanation for what occurred? This issue has immediate implications for blame. The family environment will offer very different levels of risk or support for the offender depending on whether the parents blame the victim or themselves or whether they hold the offender responsible for what he or she did. If they do hold the offender responsible, the manner in which they do so is also important. Their being extremely angry at and rejecting of him or her has different implications than their being able to separate the offender as a person from the act that was perpetrated.

It is useful in the parent/guardian interviews to reflect identified areas of strength and resilience back to the persons being interviewed. The family members are likely to be feeling very vulnerable to judgment at this point, and often the assessment process can seem like an attempt to identify all the problems and difficulties about which the family members will have strong negative and often unresolved feelings. An identification of strengths will help build rapport and increase the parents' sense of control and self-efficacy. The kinds of strengths we have encountered in parents or guardians at this stage of the interview have included the courage to face the truth about their child's behavior (e.g., it may be a parent who decided to report the crime); the family's desire to protect the victim or potential victims; or the family's ability to still support the perpetrator without colluding with his or her crime.

▶ Motivation for Treatment

As with the youth, the interviewer will gain impressions of the family's level of motivation for treatment throughout the interview. Was the family on time for appointments? Were the parents or guardians forthcoming in the interview? Did they express desire to deal with the problem? ambivalence about the need for help? resentment about the system's response to their predicament? How willing did they seem to be to participate in treatment?

Some direct questions at the end of the interview can also be helpful to clarify the feelings of parents or guardians in these areas. Again, the distinction between internal and external motivation is important: Does the parent seek treatment purely to keep his or her child out of jail, or because he or she believes there are problems that need to be addressed within the family?

Additional Assessment Areas

▶ Psychiatric/Diagnostic Issues

It is also important to screen the youth for a range of psychiatric and diagnostic issues that have implications for risk, dangerousness, and treatment needs. Does the youth have any prior arrests, charges, or convictions? If so, do these include acts of sexual or nonsexual violence? To what extent does the youth use tobacco, alcohol, marijuana, and other substances? What function does the substance use serve (e.g., peer acceptance, relaxation, distraction from pain, the desire to act out against one's parents)? To what extent does the youth's condition meet the diagnostic criteria for major psychiatric disorders, especially conduct disorder, antisocial personality disorder, major affective disorders, or psychosis? DSM-IV (American Psychiatric Association 1994) offers a range of screening criteria, some of which will have been covered already in the interview. Affective disorders and psychosis can be screened with some general questions about mood and perceptual experiences. However, criteria for antisocial personality or conduct disorder may need to be screened more specifically (e.g., weapons use, fire setting, running away, cruelty to animals, and stealing).

▶ Information From Collateral Sources

Time and resources may dictate the amount of assessment information gathered from collateral sources. Some information, however, does need to be verified from beyond the family during the initial assessment in order to ensure that the most vital information is in fact reliable and accurate. Other information can be assessed later as part of ongoing therapy or intervention after decisions about treatment setting have been made.

As indicated earlier, certain legal details of the case must also be available to the interviewer so that he or she can make an accurate judgment of the extent of denial or minimizing by both the youth and his or her parents or guardians. This may require liaison with the youth's defense attorney, prosecutor, juvenile justice officer, or the child welfare social worker who assessed the situation when the offense was reported.

If the youth has been placed out of the home, primary care staff in his or her current residence need to be interviewed to establish the youth's behavior and functioning there (see below for discussion of assessment of out-of-home placements).

The school needs to be contacted so that details about attendance and behavior can be verified. It is very important to have an accurate picture of the youth's behavior at school, since excessive absence, truancy, aggression, fighting, sexual acting-out, or disrespect for authority has implications for the restrictiveness of treatment setting necessary for community protection. Also, if intellectual level or learning disability is an issue, the school may be able to release information about academic performance and evaluations or achievement tests if the child has recently had a scholastic assessment.

▶ Special Considerations for Youths Placed Out of the Home

At the time of assessment, the youth may be in detention or may have been placed in a group home or foster care situation by social services or the court. The results of the assessment may contribute to decisions about the suitability of the youth's returning home or remaining in his or her current residence, as against a more restrictive alternative. Whatever the circumstances, several additional issues need to be assessed if a youth is in an out-of-home placement:

1. *Security and supervision:* How closely is the youth supervised at the facility? For example, can the youth earn day or weekend passes? Can he or she leave the facility, and if so, is an escort required? Does the youth attend school on-site or outside the facility? Does he or she share a room?
2. *Access to children:* Does the facility afford the youth access to children or young people in a high-risk age range for his or her offending style? If so, what extra efforts can be made to supervise the youth and limit such access? Are these efforts likely to be sufficient to protect the safety of others?

3. *Contact with abusive peers:* Does the facility expose the youth to peers who may endanger the youth in some way? For example, is the youth substantially younger and less sophisticated than the other residents? Is the scope of his or her sexual and/or nonsexual offending considerably narrower than that of the offending of the other residents?

4. *Emotional impact of the out-of-home placement on the youth:* What emotional effect has the out-of-home placement had on the youth? The youth's feelings about the placement are an important factor in the assessment of risk. For example, an incest offender who has been removed from the home to protect victim safety may be very motivated to participate in treatment if it will facilitate family reunification. Another offender in exactly the same situation may have strong feelings of abandonment and anger about the placement, which in turn interfere with motivation for treatment and potentially place him or her at a higher risk of reoffending if negative feelings such as these were part of what precipitated his or her decision to offend.

Ethical Dilemmas

Working with sex offenders in any capacity inevitably involves negotiating a number of ethical dilemmas, most of which arise from the need to balance the offender's need for treatment with the need to protect the safety of the public. The National Adolescent Perpetrator Network (1993) guidelines on the assessment and treatment of adolescent sex offenders offer valuable advice in this area. The guiding principle is to err on the side of caution (community protection) when in doubt. Some of the most common ethical dilemmas that arise in the context of clinical assessment of juvenile sex offenders are discussed below.

Extent of Legal Involvement

Treatment providers may be asked to offer treatment to an adolescent offender as an alternative to his or her offense being reported to the authorities. This raises several concerns:

1. The lack of a legal consequence may communicate to the victim(s) a lack of visible punitive consequences for an act that has caused considerable harm. The treatment provider may then be seen as colluding with the offender in his or her attempt to avoid a negative consequence.

2. The treatment provider is also inadvertently modeling incomplete accountability, and such modeling may in fact indirectly collude with the offender's desire to minimize the seriousness of the offense or to avoid punishment.

3. Offender treatment compliance is generally much higher if the criminal justice system is involved, because various forms of leverage may be available to keep the youth in treatment. For example, a judge may be able to suspend sentencing with a promise of a lesser sentence if the youth successfully completes a treatment program. Alternatively, compliance with program conditions can be built into probation conditions upon sentencing.

For these reasons and others, combining a therapeutic response with a criminal justice response is considered by far the best approach to juvenile sex offenders. In cases that have not been reported, interviewers can facilitate such a course by making their assessment contingent upon the offense being reported to the appropriate authorities. In cases that have been reported, the interviewer can also make efforts to coordinate the legal and therapeutic response by communicating with representatives of the enforcement and legal systems involved in the case, such as police, welfare investigators, probation, and defense and prosecuting attorneys.

Limits of Confidentiality

The youth and family must understand from the outset the limits of confidentiality, which at a minimum need to include the duty to report or warn, depending upon the state laws and the interviewer's professional code of ethics. Generally, the family also cannot expect the interviewer to keep his or her findings confidential from other agencies involved with the case. These matters need to be cleared by way of signed informed-consent forms and confidentiality waivers prior to the gathering of any assessment information.

Assessment Versus Advocacy

The family needs to understand that the interviewer's role differs from advocacy and that his or her contribution to decisions about the case may run contrary to the family's wishes. Once again, the guiding principle is that the interviewer contribute to the best decision about the case by balancing the offender's right to the least restrictive alternative with the community's need for safety.

Conflict of Interest

The interviewer may be placed in a conflict-of-interest situation if, for example, the case at hand is an incest case and the interviewer is asked to assess the needs of both the offender and the victim. Some agencies work with both offenders and victims, so it is important in these cases to ensure that the victim and the perpetrator are assessed by different staff members.

Family Secrets

During the assessment process, family members may disclose significant information and then ask that it be withheld from other family members. Such information may involve issues related to the crime or related occurrences, sexual abuse histories, sexual orientation issues, substance abuse, and other matters that the other family members may need to know. It is important that the interviewer model open communication and refrain from contributing to indirect family communication or the perpetuation of family secrets.

Recidivism Risk and Dangerousness

A number of risk assessment protocols or rating forms are available in the literature (Gil and Johnson 1993; Perry and Orchard 1992b; Ross and Loss 1991; Steen and Monnette 1989). These identify a range of assessment variables that are crucial to the development of meaningful judgments about risk and dangerousness. The present authors caution that these instruments are preliminary, being based on clinical experience rather than empirical evidence at this point because the field of adolescent sex offender assessment and treatment is still so embryonic. The most commonly cited risk assessment variables are listed in Table 9–1. Some of these variables, as noted in the table, have been empirically validated with adult sex offenders and therefore may have particular validity with adolescent offenders too.

Table 9–1. Commonly cited risk assessment variables in the evaluation of sex offenders

---

Offense variables
Nature and intrusiveness
Frequency
Duration
Force or coercion
Number of male victims[a]
Number of female victims
Victim selection characteristics
Substance abuse when offending
Range of paraphilias
Co-offender

Offender variables
Age and sophistication
Denial/honesty
Acceptance of responsibility
Understanding of offense precursors
Empathy
Morality
Deviant arousal[a]
Sexual preoccupation and
    compulsivity
Prior sexual victimization
Prior physical/emotional
    victimization or neglect
Prior treatment history

Offender variables *(continued)*
Developmental delay
Psychosis
Substance abuse
Social adjustment[a]
School/employment adjustment
Diagnostic features:
    Psychopathy[a] (Hare
        Psychopathy Index score)
    Antisocial personality
    Conduct disorder
Prior sexual offense[a]
Prior violent offense[a]
Prior offense of any kind[a]
Motivation for treatment

Family and situational variables
Family functioning
Employment
Parental substance abuse
Stressors
Social support
Denial or acknowledgment of
    offense
Motivation to participate in
    treatment
Access to victims and other children

---

[a]Empirically validated with adult sex offenders and therefore may have particular validity with adolescent offenders too.

Risk assessment guidelines in the literature have varied in terms of how the variables in Table 9–1 are utilized. Some authors have simply noted the presence or absence of each variable; others have developed three-point scales that allow a more sensitive measure of severity. It is not yet known which of these variables have the most predictive value with adolescents, and these instruments are not yet sensitive enough for individual variables to be meaningfully weighted relative to one another or for quantitative conclusions to be drawn, for example, on the basis of cut-off scores. Rather, these instruments are intended as qualitative checklists to guide an assessment—protocols that can be refined through clinical experience and validated through empirical research as the field continues to develop and expand. It is recommended that the reader use one of the risk assessment guidelines in the literature or adapt his or her own from the variables listed in Table 9–1.

While the risk assessment guidelines are a reminder of specific assessment areas, the "real" clinical task is to gather this information in the most meaningful and sensitive way.

Conclusion

The clinical assessment of adolescent sex offenders is a comprehensive undertaking. The foregoing guidelines, however, will produce sufficient information—when integrated with psychometric test information—to form the basis of a high-quality psychological report and treatment plan in a context that is both ethically and environmentally sensitive. The nature of the final report will be determined by the purpose of the assessment (e.g., evaluating a client's suitability for a specific program; providing the court with recommendations about the intensiveness and restrictiveness of treatment indicated). However, regardless of the evaluator's specific reporting purpose, several guidelines and resources will be useful when drawing conclusions and making recommendations.

O'Brien and Bera (1992) offer an adolescent offender typology in which are described background characteristics, offense motivations, therapy issues, and recommended treatment settings for seven different offender subtypes, differentiated according to modus operandi. Although there is sometimes overlap of offender characteristics across several subtypes, the typology is nevertheless a very useful guideline for decision making about appropriate treatment settings.

It is important for the clinician to base recommendations firmly on facts, descriptive information, and observable behaviors or circumstances, rather than on "impressions" or value judgments. This is especially important both when dealing with potentially dangerous clients and when reporting to the court. The risk assessment factors explicated throughout the section on clinical assessment earlier in this chapter provide the ideal framework upon which to make clinically sound treatment recommendations.

When the clinician is making recommendations about specific therapeutic needs, certain themes will emerge in common for the majority of youths and families, even though these may be expressed in very individualized ways. For most families referred, some or all of the following treatment needs will be indicated:

For parents and/or guardians

- Support to assist parents with their own reactions to the youth's offending
- Parent education about factors that cause and maintain sexual offending, and identification of such factors within the family environment
- Specific interventions that address family factors that bear a functional relationship to the youth's offending (e.g., parenting skills, marital therapy, substance abuse treatment or referral, development of clearer sexual boundaries within the home)
- Parent education about victim safety issues and relapse prevention

For the youth

- Overcoming denial, and taking responsibility for offenses
- Becoming accountable to family and significant others about offenses

- Developing victim empathy
- Improving specific skills in areas of social and emotional regulation that bear a functional relationship to the youth's offending (e.g., sex education, anger management, impulse control, problem solving and decision making, communication skills, substance abuse treatment)
- Developing and implementing relapse prevention strategies

Finally, it is useful to bear in mind that any reporting offered to sources such as the court, social service agencies, or other treatment providers is also a community education effort. Because so little is known about adolescent sexual offending, reports from professionals with expertise in this area may for others involved in the case be their first exposure to clinical information and judgments about adolescent sex offenders and their needs. Therefore, it is important to use plain language rather than jargon whenever possible and to be especially careful not to step beyond the limits of one's own knowledge or the limits of knowledge within the field.

References

Abel GG, Mittelman M, Becker JV: Sex offenders: results of assessment and recommendations for treatment, in Clinical Criminology: The Assessment and Treatment of Criminal Behavior. Edited by Ben-Aron M, Hucker SJ, Webster CD. Toronto, M & M Graphics, 1985, pp 191–205

Abel GG, Osborn CA, Twigg DA: Sexual assault through the life span: adult offenders with juvenile histories, in The Juvenile Sex Offender. Edited by Barbaree HE, Marshall WL, Hudson SM. New York, Guilford, 1993, pp 104–117

American Psychiatric Association: Diagnostic and Statistical Manual of Mental Disorders, 4th Edition. Washington, DC, American Psychiatric Association, 1994

Barbaree HE, Hudson SM, Seto MC: Sexual assault in society: the role of the juvenile offender, in The Juvenile Sex Offender. Edited by Barbaree HE, Marshall WL, Hudson SM. New York, Guilford, 1993a, pp 1–24

Murphy WD, Haynes MR, Page MR, et al: Adolescent sex offenders, in The Sexual Abuse of Children, Vol 2: Clinical Issues. Edited by O'Donohue W, Geer JH. Hillsdale, NJ, Lawrence Erlbaum, 1992, pp 394–429

National Task Force on Juvenile Sexual Offending: National Adolescent Perpetrator Network Revised Report. Juvenile and Family Court Journal 44 (suppl 4):3–108, 1993

Nichols H, Molinder I: Manual for the Multiphasic Sex Inventory. Tacoma, WA, Crime and Victim Psychology Specialists, 1984

O'Brien MJ: Taking sibling incest seriously, in Family Sexual Abuse: Frontline Research and Evaluation. Edited by Patton MQ. Newbury Park, CA, Sage Publications, 1991, pp 75–92

O'Brien MJ, Bera W: The phase typology of adolescent sex offenders, in Adolescent Sexual Offender Assessment Packet. Edited by Gray AS, Wallace R. Orwell, VT, Safer Society Press, 1992, pp 52–55

Perry GP, Orchard J: Assessment and Treatment of Adolescent Sex Offenders. Sarasota, FL, Professional Resource Press/Professional Resource Exchange, 1992

Perry GP, Orchard J: Sexual abuse prevention in a correctional center, in Innovations in Clinical Practice: A Source Book, Vol II. Edited by VandeCreek L, Knapp S, Jackson TL. Sarasota, FL, Professional Resource Press/Professional Resource Exchange, 1992b, pp 413–423

Piers FV, Harris DB: Piers-Harris Children's Self-Concept Scale. Los Angeles, CA, Western Psychological Services, 1984

Reynolds WM: Reynolds Adolescent Depression Scale. Odessa, FL, Psychological Assessment Resources, 1987

Roberts RE, Abrams L, Finch JR: Delinquent sexual behavior among adolescents. Medical Aspects of Human Sexuality 7:162–183, 1973

Ross J, Loss P: Assessment of the juvenile sex offender, in Juvenile Sexual Offending: Causes, Consequences and Corrections. Edited by Ryan G, Lane S. Boston, MA, Lexington Books, 1991, pp 199–251

Ryan G, Lane S (eds): Juvenile Sexual Offending: Causes, Consequences and Corrections. Boston, MA, Lexington Books, 1991

Saunders E, Awad GA, White G: Male adolescent sexual offenders: the offender and the offense [Special Issue: Canadian Academy of Child Psychiatry: A Canadian Perspective]. Can J Psychiatry 31:542–549, 1986

Steen C, Monnette B: Treating Sex Offenders in the Community. Springfield, IL, Charles C Thomas, 1989

Tarter R: Adolescent Substance Abuse: Assessment and Treatment Referral Guide. Pittsburgh, PA, Westover Consultants, 1988, pp 109–124

Van Ness SR: Rape as instrumental violence: a study of youth offenders [Special Issue: Gender Issues, Sex Offenses, and Criminal Justice: Current Trends]. Journal of Offender Counseling, Services and Rehabilitation 9:161–170, 1984

10

Cognitive-Behavioral
Treatment Strategies for
Adolescent Sex Offenders:
The Integrated Model

Ted Shaw, Ph.D., Anita M. Schlank, Ph.D.,
and Jamie R. Funderburk, Ph.D.

Adolescent sexual aggressors as a
group have been the focus of clinical efforts for over 20 years (Knopp
et al. 1986). These efforts have developed from basically two discrete

We wish to thank Amanda Elizabeth Shaw for preparation of the artwork for the
figures in this chapter.

Masculine pronouns have been used throughout the chapter primarily because the
model being described was developed specifically for male adolescent offenders.
Research suggests that approximately 10% of all sex offenders are female (Bumby
and Bumby 1997). A variation of this model is in continued use in our treatment
programs with female sex offenders.

sources: juvenile victim rehabilitation and adult sex offender treatment programs in operation around the world. As efforts in child victim therapy expanded, treatment providers found themselves confronted with more and more victims who were initially "acting out" as abuse-reactive children. (*Abuse-reactive* refers to "sexualized" children who may molest others or act out in a variety of sexually assaultive ways and whose behavior is at least in part derived from sexual abuse they received [see Gil and Johnson 1993].) Some of these abuse-reactive children were behaving in ways best described as sexually offending, particularly as they approached adolescence (Gil and Johnson 1993). Concomitantly, adult sex offender treatment specialists were being routinely confronted with offenders whose patterns of behavior had begun in adolescence (Abel et al. 1986, 1993). Moreover, many of these individuals reported that they had been identified by the courts but that their problem had been insufficiently addressed.

Treatment Programs

With recent increased awareness of the magnitude of sexual offenses that are committed by juveniles and of the number of adult offenders who began their deviant behavior in adolescence, closer attention has been paid to the programs that treat these juvenile and adolescent offenders (Abel et al. 1993; Annon 1996; Barbaree et al. 1993; Becker and Hunter 1997; Becker et al. 1988; Brown et al. 1984; Deisher et al. 1982; Jacobs et al. 1997; Longo and Groth 1983; Longo and McFadden 1981; Ryan et al. 1987). Various programs have been described in the literature to serve as representative models of treatment. Becker and colleagues (1988) described a program that consists of seven major components: verbal satiation, cognitive restructuring group sessions, introduction of covert sensitization, social skills training, anger control, relapse prevention groups, and groups focusing on sex education and values clarification. Becker et al. looked at overall change in deviant sexual arousal, as measured by the penile plethysmograph, and found that juveniles who completed these treatment components showed a significant decrease in their sexual arousal to inappropriate stimuli.

Becker and Kaplan (1993) noted the importance of modifying the cognitive-behavioral model initially developed for adult sex offender populations for use with juveniles. For example, adolescents were found to have difficulty with the masturbatory satiation component of treatment. The adolescents reported that they were religiously opposed to masturbation, noted that they shared a room with a sibling and had no privacy, protested that the length of time was too long for their attention span, or could not reliably carry out the homework assignments. Given these problems, the procedure was modified to include shorter sessions of verbal satiation with no masturbatory element. Erectile response was measured by the penile plethysmograph during these verbal satiation sessions, and significant decrease was seen after 8 to 16 sessions. In addition, Becker and Kaplan also described alterations to the cognitive restructuring component, in which the language used to explain cognitive distortions was simplified.

Weinrott and colleagues (1997) noted that juvenile sex offender programs typically tend to avoid "direct reduction of deviant sexual arousal except by means of thought stoppage or appropriate fantasy substitution" (p. 705). They suggested that covert sensitization may be ineffective with adolescent perpetrators and that verbal satiation is too slow of a process and may be ineffective with the younger offenders. These researchers suggested the addition of "Vicarious Sensitization" through the use of prerecorded videotaped aversive scenes augmented with wallet-sized cards with prewritten aversive scenes. Results after a 3-month follow-up were positive for decreasing deviant arousal.

Murphy and colleagues (1992) described the juvenile sex offender programs at the University of Tennessee at Memphis. The inpatient program provided daily sex offender–specific groups, individual therapy at least five times every 2 weeks, family therapy once every 2 weeks, and a parent support group weekly. When the juvenile showed evidence of deviant arousal, self-administered covert sensitization and verbal satiation were used. The treatment issues addressed by these programs included denial, cognitive distortions, victim empathy, issues related to the offender's own personal victimization, identification of the offender's sexual abuse cycle, social skills training, sex education, and reduction of deviant arousal. Murphy et al. did not report recidivism rates for their program, but they did obtain encouraging findings about the reduction in deviant arousal. They noted, however, that treating the adolescent offender can be quite difficult and that "perseverance and creativity of the clinician in adapting specific techniques is still needed" (p. 420).

Smith (1988) noted the high frequency of physical and sexual abuse histories in those juveniles who committed very serious sexual offenses. He stressed the importance of adding a component that addressed the offender's own victimization, as well as employing a family systems strategy. Katz (1990) identified the prevalence of social skills deficits among juvenile sex offenders and suggested that their tendency to perceive social situations as threatening should be a major focus in treatment.

Many other programs have been described in the literature (Becker and Abel 1985; Breer 1987; Gray and Pithers 1993; Griffin et al. 1997; Groth et al. 1981; Heinz et al. 1987; Johnson and Berry 1989; Knopp 1982; Lane and Zamora 1984; Loss and Ross 1984; Monastersky and Smith 1985; Ryan and Lane 1998). In fact, according to a survey reported in 1995, there were nearly 1,000 programs that treat juvenile sex offenders operating in North America at the time of the survey (Freeman-Longo et al. 1995). In addition, recommendations for treating juvenile sex offenders have been provided by the National Adolescent Perpetrator Network (1988). In general, most programs share the assumption that treatment needs to be sex offender–specific and that traditional individual therapy sessions are rarely cost-effective. Because of this, and given the benefits of the group setting, group therapy is generally utilized as the primary treatment modality. It is also agreed that treatment requires coordinating the involvement of a number of different agencies and that, since the safety of the community is the primary concern, waivers of confidentiality are needed. In addition, most specialists agree that family dysfunction needs to be addressed as well as substance abuse, educational difficulties, depression, self-esteem, sex education, anger control, and victim empathy (Becker and Kaplan 1988; Knopp 1982; National Adolescent Perpetrator Network 1988). Juvenile sex offender treatment program providers tend to agree as well that sexual abuse perpetrators cannot be "cured" and that the purpose of treatment is to provide lifelong coping strategies to prevent reoffense. Most programs use components that are based on the Relapse Prevention model (Pithers et al. 1983).

Relapse Prevention was designed for use by clients involved in substance abuse treatment to assist in maintenance of their abstinence (Marlatt and Gordon 1985). It was later adapted to a number of clinical populations, including adult and adolescent sex offenders. This theoretical model is based on the concept that sexual offenses are not committed on impulse and that there are offense precursors that can be identified and addressed (Gray and Pithers 1993; Pithers et al. 1988). The most common emotional precursors to sex offenses by adolescents have been found to include boredom, social or sexual embarrassment, anger, fear of rejection, and numbness (Gray and Pithers 1993). As with adult offenders, the goals of Relapse Prevention, when the model is applied to adolescent offenders, include 1) an internal, self-management dimension in which an adolescent learns offense precursors and adaptive coping techniques for dealing with high risk factors, and 2) an external, supervisory dimension in which the offender's support team is educated about the Relapse Prevention model and the identification of cues for the various high risk factors. In addition, the Relapse Prevention model continues to provide a unifying theory for integrating a number of specific treatment components (Gray and Pithers 1993). Components such as anger management, social skills training, and cognitive restructuring can all be seen as having direct relevance to avoiding, preventing, or otherwise intervening in specific precursors to sexual offenses.

The Integrated Model

Consistent with numerous models for providing cognitive-behavioral treatment to adolescent perpetrators is the *Integrated model,* a treatment model that was adapted from the Mentally Disordered Sex Offender (MDSO) treatment program at North Florida Evaluation and Treatment Center (NFETC) for incarcerated adult sex offenders (Barnard et al. 1989). In 1985 this model was first modified for use

in the Adolescents Who Sexually Offend (AWSO) treatment program with adolescent offender populations being treated in the community, and it has been continually updated and modified for both
outpatient and residential settings over the past decade (Shaw 1989,
1993a, 1993b, 1995).

The present model represents several significant updates; various adaptations are currently in use for developmentally disabled
and first-time adolescent perpetrators of sexual offenses as well as
repeat offenders of nonsexual violent and property crimes. The Integrated model includes components not typically considered to be
"cognitive-behavioral" that have been retained from the psychodynamic origins of the treatment program at NFETC as a means to
break through the denial system of offenders and address their own
trauma (Barnard et al. 1989). These components include role-play
reenactments of sexual offenses and the Central Process model
(Shaw 1994a, 1994b, 1994c), both of which are used to assist the
offender in understanding the dynamics of his pattern of offending
in such a way that conscious, meaningful change can be made by the
offender to his core, underlying issues. These underlying issues may
be characterological in nature and, therefore, extremely difficult to
change, or they may contain elements such as sexual curiosity or
naïveté that are more easily addressed. Moreover, these strategies
may have significant impact in assisting offenders in understanding
the underlying components of their offense cycle and thereby developing truly effective and lasting strategies for intervening. Role-
play reenactments, particularly, by bringing the dynamics of the
offense into the group therapy session, provide visceral experiences
that may trigger memories of emotion and sensation and other essential elements of the offense cycle. The role play offers the offender opportunities to reexperience many aspects of his sexual
offenses in the more empathy-engendering environment of the therapy group. In addition, cradling and other "soft" experiential techniques are used to further intensify the offender's conscious
awareness of basic needs that, though fulfillment of may have been
missing or provided inappropriately or inadequately, can be met in
healthy ways. Beyond these techniques, the Integrated model consists of a set of modules with cognitive and behavioral post-tests as

well as an ongoing component that focuses on the Central Process model. Brief descriptions of the modules are presented below.

Treatment Modules

▶ Relapse Prevention Module

The Relapse Prevention module is designed to 1) prepare the adolescent offender to take responsibility for the prevention of future sexually deviant behavior (particularly by helping him to identify specific internal and external precursors to past deviant behavior that are likely to be precursors of future offending), 2) teach him to recognize these as risk factors related to reoffending, 3) develop reasonable strategies to predict the occurrence of these precursors, and 4) acquire specific coping skills and develop action plans based on those skills to prevent reoffense.

This module, adapted from one originally used in the MDSO program at NFETC (George and Marlatt 1986), was designed to include between 8 and 12 90-minute sessions with specific homework assignments. In the initial sessions, clients are taught vocabulary and the theoretical framework of the module is introduced, an approach that tends to be sufficient for motivating them to learn the components. These sessions are followed by an exploration of motivation by which clients learn the importance of monitoring their motivation as an integral component of the relapse prevention process. Since most offenders undergoing treatment are relatively unlikely to experience numerous, frequent risk factors to reoffending, this module uses other repetitive problem behaviors, jointly identified by the client and therapists (in the case of residential clients, the assigned primary therapist and treatment staff may have input). The client then maintains a log of internal and external risk factors and of lapses and relapses while, with the help of the therapists, developing a relapse prevention plan of interventions. These logs are presented in several group sessions and the material is related back to the client's sexual offending. Ultimately, group members develop individualized relapse prevention plans for their deviant behaviors. The module ends with a post-test that includes information about the relapse prevention as well as their complete relapse prevention plan.

▶ Cognitive Restructuring Module

The Cognitive Restructuring module, which is based on rational-emotive therapy (Ellis and Geiger 1977), is designed to directly challenge the irrational beliefs that support the offender's deviant behavior and to replace them with beliefs grounded firmly in reality. Moreover, this module focuses on rational living in general and teaches adolescents to "check out" their thinking when they are in a negative emotional state or about to engage in any type of inappropriate behavior. Negative emotional states have been found to be related to reoffenses for sex offenders (Pithers et al. 1988).

One important and sometimes confusing issue for adolescent offenders in understanding cognitive restructuring is the concept that changing thoughts and beliefs is not the purpose of the model but the process. In fact, the purpose of the model is improving feelings and preventing unwanted behaviors. This module was adapted from one used in the MDSO program at NFETC (Lange 1986) for the outpatient treatment of adolescents in the AWSO treatment program. In 1990 it was further modified for the Elaine Gordon Treatment Center, a residential treatment program for adolescent perpetrators operated by the University of Miami in Hollywood, Florida, from 1990 through 1995. The module helps the adolescent offender develop responsibility for his own experience and become more effective in relationships with peers by silencing the irrational "noise" that interferes with accurate communication. It includes the concept of Criminal Thinking Errors developed by Yochelson and Samenow (1977), which assists the adolescent offender in identifying and replacing distorted cognitions that support ongoing patterns of offending behavior and that have been found by those authors to be common beliefs maintained by criminals. While focusing on being in general more rational in life, the module zeroes in on those specific thoughts and beliefs that contributed to sex offending and teaches clients to use the module as a specific intervention in changing those thoughts and beliefs as a tool for preventing a reoffense.

The Cognitive Restructuring module is designed to be delivered in 6 to 10 sessions with homework assignments. It begins with a description of the ABC model, wherein A (the event) and B (thoughts and beliefs about the event) lead to C (feelings and subsequent behavior), and goes on to describe a four-step process of identifying and changing thinking and beliefs that have been found to be irrational into rational ones. Common irrational beliefs of criminals and sex offenders are described, and clients are asked to identify those that relate to their own offense histories. Homework consists primarily of practicing the four-step model with real-life situations. A post-test requires group members to have knowledge of the important components of the model as well as the ability to apply the four-step model to (referred to as "4-step") both a hypothetical general situation and one of their sexual offenses. An example of a hypothetical situation is as follows:

> You lend a friend your portable stereo, and he does not return it when you expected. You feel angry, hurt, and disappointed, and you plan to punish him in some way. Put yourself in this situation and 4-step it.

▶ Arousal Reconditioning Module

The Arousal Reconditioning module is designed to decrease arousal to deviant stimuli and to encourage offenders to develop or increase arousal to nondeviant stimuli. The satiation version of this module was adapted from the one used at NFETC. Since its original use included masturbation, it has been modified for adolescents by making the masturbation component optional and shortening the length of sessions. This component, more than most others, is difficult for clinicians, both professional and paraprofessional, who are not experienced sex offender specialists to use comfortably and is frequently misunderstood or misused.

For example, an adolescent who had received satiation therapy at a residential treatment program that alleged to have a sex offender treatment component returned to outpatient therapy complaining that, though his deviant fantasies were no longer arousing to him, he could not be aroused by nondeviant fantasies. He revealed that he had been instructed to focus on situations such as a dinner date or wedding ceremony for nondeviant erotic stimulation, with it being implied to him that erotic images of women were sexist, dehumanizing, and inappropriate. If true, it appears that a well-meaning but misguided therapist confused nonerotic with nondeviant.

Whereas in residential settings treatment staff monitor the taping sessions, in outpatient settings such as the AWSO treatment program the parents are held responsible for the integrity of the sessions, and the clients are responsible for the technical quality of the tapes. This is particularly important since most adolescent outpatient clients have access to cassette recorders with dubbing capabilities and could conceivably produce only one tape and make numerous copies, thereby missing the therapeutic value of the repetitious taping sessions. Although the tape review is designed, in part, to catch this, it is not infallible. Treatment occurs in therapy sessions and in taped sessions as homework. It could include one or more of the following components.

Self-Administered Satiation uses extended verbal repetition of deviant fantasies in taped sessions with or without concurrent masturbation to elicit a boredom response. The module begins with an exploration of nondeviant themes and fantasies to encourage self-disclosure and to teach the basic idea of consensual sex. In general, group members are enthusiastic during this portion of the module, where their disclosures are ego-enhancing and often extremely explicit. They disclose these fantasies in the form of a hierarchy from most arousing to least arousing using a Likert scale. This is followed by an identical exercise with deviant fantasies that is usually met with denial, minimization, and other forms of resistance such as forgotten homework and mistakes. When the deviant hierarchy is complete, the therapist and client select the most powerful fantasies and develop scenes comprising several phrases or sentences, called "scripts." These scripts are then repeated and taped for half-hour sessions in private, and later these tapes are brought to group for review by the therapist to ensure accuracy and compliance. Clients rate the power of these fantasies after each review session, since self-report is the only method of determining effectiveness in the absence of a physiological arousal measure. Recently, routine polygraph assessments have been added to the AWSO program, and participants in the module are warned that they will be asked about their arousal patterns during those assessments.

Clients complete an average of six to eight sessions for each of their admitted fantasies and/or documented offense types. They are encouraged to engage in their taping sessions when it is unlikely that they will be aroused, particularly soon after ejaculation. This therapy not only is boring to the clients but can be both boring and troubling as well to the therapist. Some programs use only male therapists for this module to avoid the secondary gain from describing explicit scenes in front of women, but the AWSO program uses a rotating model in which cotherapists take turns, in part because the program utilizes male–female cotherapists whenever possible, as well as male and female therapists working alone, and, in fact, this module is just one component in a very explicit and professionally challenging treatment program.

Several alternatives to satiation therapy are occasionally used, one of which is *Olfactory Aversion*, which pairs an aversive odor (e.g., ammonia inhalant such as smelling salts) with selected deviant fantasies. The module is similar to satiation, but the technique for lowering arousal is different. The technique involves pairing a noxious odor with verbalized deviant fantasies when the client first notices signs of arousal. Generally, as the time it takes to get aroused to a deviant fantasy reaches 10 minutes, the client moves on to the next deviant fantasy in his hierarchy. Although treatments described as aversive such as this one are sometimes opposed by representatives of state agencies and other bureaucracies, clients exposed to both Olfactory Aversion and Satiation in general prefer Olfactory Aversion because it is quicker and requires less effort. The sessions tend to be shorter, and this also makes this technique more appealing to teenagers. Because of the general public response, however, the AWSO program requires special consent including the specific, explicit request of the client to use this technique. The client's parents are included in the informed-consent process.

Recently, after years of development, a new arousal reconditioning module, *Vicarious Sensitization*, was made available to treatment programs and seems to resolve many of the problems of previous models. Using professionally produced aversive videos that are interspersed with deviant scenes developed by the adolescent offender with the help of his therapist, the adolescent receives "treatment sessions" either on a television monitor or with a virtual reality headset. A study conducted by Weinrott and colleagues (1997) found that this treatment was very effective in decreasing deviant interests as well as easy for staff to learn to facilitate. Unlike with most deviant arousal reduction methods, clients reported enjoying the sessions, adding to their willing compliance with the treatment.

▶ Anger and Stress Management Module

The Anger and Stress Management module is designed to teach adolescent offenders how to better cope with their anger and stress through development of more socially acceptable and personally effective expressions of anger and coping strategies for lowering stress. This is accomplished by teaching them both behavioral and cognitive interventions. The module is based on one originally developed at NFETC for adult offenders (Novaco 1986) and includes materials derived from the book describing the program at the St. Mary's Home for Boys (Marsh et al. 1988).

The module begins with a review of the purposes of anger and the use of cognitive restructuring to intervene in anger that has become a problem. Stress is defined and explored. Each session includes some didactic component and some role playing and practice in stress or anger management and reduction. Techniques taught in this module include meditation, progressive relaxation, guided imagery, appropriate expression of anger, review of "4-stepping" from cognitive restructuring, and plans for significant lifestyle change to reduce stress. Clients are taught to notice the signs of stress in their bodies. Examples are drawn from the group in the form of retrospective reports of stressful situations as well as situations occurring in the moment in group that can be very powerful and that elevate the module from psychoeducation to therapy.

▶ Communication/Social Skills Module

The Communication/Social Skills module covers several areas and begins with general communication skills such as verbal and nonverbal communication of feelings, active listening skills, appropriate eye contact and personal distance, and giving and receiving compliments. This is followed by specific techniques designed to improved the adolescent's skills in developing healthy prosocial friendships, meeting potential partners, and successfully dating. It is designed to help the offender develop clearer, more effective verbal and nonverbal communication skills, become more assertive, and develop socially appropriate and effective social skills related to friendships, dating, courting, and sexual interaction.

In the Communication Skills component, focus is on learning to communicate thoughts and feelings in nonthreatening ways along with developing improved skills for understanding verbal and nonverbal messages and cues from others. The Social Skills component teaches adolescents to understand the relationship of peers to their own decision-making process and presents a model for both meeting and keeping appropriate friends as well as attracting partners for dating and intimate relationships.

Recently, the module was modified to remove any vestiges of sexist or homophobic content in order to avoid stigmatizing adolescent homosexuals undergoing treatment (e.g., meeting "girls" was changed to meeting "partners").

▶ Healthy Sexuality Module

The Healthy Sexuality module is designed to improve the adolescent offender's knowledge of human sexuality and to decrease distorted perceptions or beliefs about sexuality. The Sex Education component of this module is a primarily information-based component that includes sexual anatomy and development, stages of sexual response, and the role of masturbation and birth control in healthy sexuality; sexually transmitted diseases and their prevention are described. The Intimacy Skills component of this module helps adolescents understand their sexuality in the context of loving relationships and increases their sensitivity to the verbal and nonverbal messages of sexual partners.

▶ Victim Empathy Module

The Victim Empathy module is designed to increase the adolescent offender's awareness of the impact of his offense on the victim, family members of the victim and perpetrator, and others in the community and, in the process, to promote the development of empathy for victims and others. During the course of the module, numerous articles and excerpts about sexual abuse from the perspective of the victim are read and discussed; relevant videos are viewed, and the group members are required to write reaction papers that are later processed in group. Other exercises include rewriting the offender's detailed offense description from the imagined perspective of the victim; reenacting sexual offenses as the victim, with another group member taking the offender's role; and eliciting the self-disclosure of experiences of group members who have themselves been sexually abused.

Core Integration Module

The Core Integration module, the key component of the Integrated model used in the AWSO treatment programs, is an ongoing module that includes writing and presenting detailed offense descriptions; writing structured autobiographies that focus on early significant positive, negative, and sexual experiences; reenacting role plays of selected sexual offenses; and learning to use the Central Process model to understand the origins of sexually abusive behavior. In addition, the Central Process model is used to develop effective interventions through exploration of past offenses and processing of present behaviors that may be associated with the deviant sexual behavior, such as inappropriate expression of anger or physical violence.

▶ Offense Description

The offense description is a structured format developed to assist the offenders in remembering significant components of their offenses. It facilitates their transition from minimization and denial to full admission and acceptance of responsibility for their offenses. Group facilitators must use their knowledge and experience to fill in the details of sexual offenses that most people would prefer to avoid, and this is one of the treatment components that challenges therapists to manage their prejudices and personal issues, including countertransference. Offense descriptions are prepared as homework and read to the group; later, they serve as the "script" for role-play reenactments.

▶ Lifeline

The lifeline is another structured format for preparing an autobiography that focuses on significant sexual and nonsexual events from the adolescents' past. Group members are encouraged to engage their parents and other family members in recalling early events from their past as they prepare their lifelines; once complete, these lifelines are presented by the members in the group with facilitation by the therapists. Presenting lifelines in group is a connecting experience for group members, and presentations by one member may jog the memory of another of some event or experience that is connected to their process of sexual offending.

▶ Role-Play Reenactments

Role-play reenactments serve several purposes in the treatment process. First, they provide an arena for exploring the reasonableness of the offender's description and explanation of his offense and offer a powerful opportunity to confront minimization and denial. As the offender reenacts his offense based on his offense description, the therapists and group members have an opportunity to gauge the reenactment in terms of its likelihood of having occurred in that way. For example, if during a role play an offender claims he said to his 3-year-old female victim, "Let's do it," and suggests that she proceeded to remove her clothes, lie on the bed, and spread her legs, the therapist might question how the victim knew what to do, given the instructions spoken by the offender during the role play. It might turn out that the offender really said, "Take off all your clothes, lie on the bed, and open your legs," or it might be that the offender had done this to the victim many times before and the victim had been trained to respond to the demand "Let's do it." Yet another possibility might be that the victim had been molested before by someone else and that the adolescent offender had had some knowledge of this.

Second, the role play may remind the offender, or for that matter any other group member, of details of his offense that had been forgotten or repressed that, in turn, may lead to a clearer understanding of his process of offending (e.g., core needs being met by the offense). There is also the possibility of remembering previously repressed traumatic experiences, such as the offender's own sexual victimization, if, for example, a role-playing offender were to reenact an offense that is similar to the early victimization of one of the other offenders in the group (Schwartz and Bergman 1997).

Third, the role play can function as a rite of passage for the offender from minimizer/denier to admitter. With careful facilitation, the role play can serve as a ritualized connecting experience that brings the group closer together and serves to strengthen the group's cohesiveness and the group members' ability to honestly self-disclose threatening information.

▶ Central Process

The Central Process model represents the core learning component for the AWSO program. This model is based on the notion that it is useful to learn how inappropriate behavior, including sexual offending, is often a predictable part of a process or (offense) cycle and not an isolated event. Central Process provides a foundation for integration of later treatment experience into a comprehensive and cohesive model that sets the stage for ongoing recovery. The Central Process includes long- and short-term *internal* precursors to behavior, including beliefs, thoughts, fantasies, feelings, and sensations, and *external* precursors, including prior events, relationships, and experiences. Understanding the process can help the offender prevent future occurrences of a given behavior (e.g., sexual offense) by providing an organizing structure to his individualized interventions identified or learned during the course of treatment.

Central Process is, thus, an integrative cycle model useful for understanding and changing repetitive and/or compulsive behaviors and experience in terms of antecedents and consequences through the use of rationally derived interventions. It was developed by the clinical staff of the MDSO Unit of NFETC between 1979 and 1989, where 63 adult sex offenders were treated in a maximum-security setting while serving their sentences in the Department of Corrections (Barnard et al. 1989). Through continued modification and refinement, the Central Process model served as the integrative treatment structure for the multimodality treatment program at the Elaine Gordon Treatment Center for young adolescent perpetrators from 1990 to 1995, as well as for the adult and adolescent treatment programs operated by North Florida Psychological Services and AWSO of North Central Florida. Most recently, it has been applied to the residential treatment of emotionally disturbed adolescents with identified behavioral problems at the Prairie Achievement Center in Gainesville, Florida.

While much of the Central Process model is similar to Relapse Prevention and the notion of the "offense cycle" and therefore self-explanatory (Ryan and Lane 1998), facilitating the process is not. Because Central Process places great significance on underlying, intrapsychic, traumatic, and other "core" issues in understanding behavior, it requires careful and sensitive exploration by facilitator and client to develop an accurate process. As in Relapse Prevention, the operating theory of Central Process suggests that behaviors have describable and therefore predictable long- and short-term antecedents. These events, experiences, memories, beliefs, thoughts, fantasies, urges, feelings, and sensations may immediately precede the behavior (trigger), or they may underlie the behavior as conscious or unconscious precursors (precipitating factors and core issues and needs). Ultimately, if the core issues and needs are not consciously understood and resolved and the core beliefs remain unchanged, the offender cannot be depended upon to effectively use his learned interventions when he most needs them; specifically, he is likely to need his intervention skills when his life is at its worst.

Understanding behavior in the context of the Central Process leads to the development of rationally derived interventions. As the Central Process model focuses on underlying issues, it directs the offender and therapist toward interventions likely to have an impact on core issues that are generally hidden from consciousness. These deeper issues may be related to personality disorders and their symptoms, to victimization trauma, or to any number of personal and/or environmental factors in the offender's life. As the offender's Central Process becomes richer with detail surrounding his sexual offending and other forms of victimizing, a growing awareness of potential and ultimately useful interventions develops.

Completely consistent with relapse prevention models, the Central Process provides a structure for understanding sexual offending, inviting the offender to fill in the process as it really happened rather than the therapist's "telling" the offender how he went about committing his offense(s). It also allows the clinician to target related processes for both practice and intervention for underlying problem behaviors that in fact contribute to the process of sexual offending.

The following are some of the key concepts of the Central Process model as it is presented to clients.

1. Central Process describes how people operate. The Central Process model can be used to understand behavior and to change problem behaviors such as sexual offending.
2. The model teaches that events trigger process, often by triggering memories. Sometimes these memories are about significant or traumatic events, and the memories may be unpleasant, or they may be arousing or confusing. These memories may result in distorted beliefs. Thinking, feelings, sensations, and behavior are also affected by these memories and beliefs. Sometimes, as in the case of sexual offending, these behaviors are inappropriate and need to be changed.
3. There are times when people invite triggers. Since these inappropriate problem behaviors are often the most powerful way people know to feel better, they often use them for relief and to create more triggers and continue in a process.
4. Central Process presents the notion that individuals can choose to change their process through the effective use of interventions. Offenders are taught that their process, although habitual or even compulsive, is not automatic, but instead implies a choice. The process can be broken by interventions. Effective interventions can be developed that change reactions to triggers, particularly by improving or resolving precipitating factors and core issues before one is confronted by triggers. Positive change is, of course, the primary goal of treatment.

In order to teach the adolescent offenders how to complete the Central Process Form (Figure 10–1), a handout is provided that leads them through the process. Initially, the therapists assign group members nonthreatening behaviors to practice the processing experience. In fact, it is recommended that therapists begin with positive behaviors of which the adolescents may be proud (e.g., sculpting a statue) to encourage full self-disclosure. Interestingly, the process form for even positive, appropriate behaviors frequently contains

AWSO TREATMENT PROGRAM CENTRAL PROCESS FORM

Name _____ Date _____

| PROBLEM BEHAVIOR |
| Description: |

I

TRIGGER EVENT	**INTERVENTIONS**	**IMMEDIATE IMPACT**
Specific events/behavior:		On self (payoff):
Thoughts:		On victim:
Emotions:		On environment:
Sensations:		

I

PRECIPITATING FACTORS		**LONG-TERM IMPACT**
General events/behavior:		On self:
Thoughts:		On victim:
Emotions:		On environment:
Sensations:		

I

| **CORE ISSUES** |
| Traumatic/significant events: |
| Core belief: |
| Core need: |

(I = Interventions)

Figure 10–1. Central Process Form from the Adolescents Who Sexually Offend treatment program.

threatening and emotionally charged material that is difficult to present to the group. As the adolescents develop confidence with the Central Process Form, negative, ego-threatening behaviors such as cursing at parents or bullying other students at school are processed. Finally, a single sexual offense, generally the first or "worst," is processed (Figures 10–2, 10–3, and 10–4).

With sexual offense processes and other negative, problem behaviors, the Central Process Form box for interventions becomes especially important. It is here that the adolescent gradually builds a repertoire of effective interventions that he may use at various points in the process. It is important to note that an intervention that is effective at one point in a process may not be useful at another point. For example, if anger about an event with a girlfriend is a precipitating factor for a sexual offense, working out that situation would be important for maintaining recovery in the event that the individual is placed in a situation where he is at risk to reoffend. However, once he is in this high-risk situation, it would no longer be useful to resolve relationship issues. At this point, the adolescent would need to use trigger interventions such as self-statements, escape behaviors, or other strategies designed to have an immediate effect on his likelihood of committing a reoffense.

Additional Treatment Components

Additionally, family therapy, brief individual therapy, parents' group, video/process group, and follow-up or aftercare are integrated with the module groups. Each of these components has a specific interface with the treatment program and augments the program in a different way.

1. The *family therapy* component is designed to ensure that the home situation in which the adolescent offender resides is both supportive and therapeutic and that the goals of treatment are understood and will be facilitated. Family therapy also provides an opportunity for the therapist to observe and redirect dysfunctional family interactions.
2. *Brief individual therapy* is included to assist the adolescent in

AWSO TREATMENT PROGRAM CENTRAL PROCESS FORM

Name ___Landon___   (EXAMPLE)   Date ___6/8/94___

PROBLEM BEHAVIOR

Description: Performing oral sex on 8-year-old boy, the younger brother of a friend.

I

TRIGGER EVENT

Specific events/behavior: Being alone with him in his room while his family is gone.
Thoughts: It won't hurt him. No one will know. It will feel great. He won't tell.
Emotions: Powerful, excited, scared, fascinated, electric.
Sensations: Aroused, energy charged.

I

PRECIPITATING FACTORS

General events/behavior: Gaining trust over this boy through the relationship with his brother.
Thoughts: Planning to manipulate the victim to have sex. Thinking it won't hurt him. Thinking I won't get caught.
Emotions: Excited.
Sensations: Aroused, tense.

INTERVENTIONS

- Understand and intervene in Central Process.
- Practice using interventions early in process.
- Use Relapse Prevention.
- Recognize and avoid high risk factors.
- Use 4-stepping.
- Build assertiveness skills.
- Maintain empathy for others, especially for victims.
- Explore healthy sexuality; develop healthy relationships.
- Share feelings appropriately.
- Decrease deviant arousal.
- Continue in therapy, even after release from probation.

IMMEDIATE IMPACT

On self (payoff): Felt very powerful and in control. Came close to living my ultimate fantasy. Energy surging through my entire body.
On victim: Victim seemed to enjoy the experience. Excited, happy.
On environment: None.

LONG-TERM IMPACT

On self: Maintained my disorder, reinforced deviant arousal/urges; isolated further from normal society, etc.
On victim: Contributed to possible deviance of victim.
On environment: Hurt victim's family. Betrayed friend's trust.

I

CORE ISSUES

Traumatic/significant events: Vague memory of being molested by my father. Fixation on young male phallus.
Core belief: I have a special relationship with young boys. Sex with them won't hurt them.
Core need: Power and control. The thrill of living my fantasy. A young boy pumping his penis in my mouth.

(I = Interventions)

Figure 10–2. Example of AWSO Central Process Form for hypothetical client.

AWSO TREATMENT PROGRAM CENTRAL PROCESS FORM

Name ___John___   (EXAMPLE)   Date ___1/1/98___

PROBLEM BEHAVIOR

Description: Forcing younger uncle to perform fellatio on him. Urinating in his mouth.

I

TRIGGER EVENT

Specific events/behavior:
Alone with uncle.

Thoughts: Grandfather prefers
my uncle to me. He rejects me.

Emotions: Angry, resentful,
hurt.

Sensations: Aroused (in denial).

I

PRECIPITATING FACTORS

General events/behavior:
Dumped here by mother.

Thoughts: I'm no good, who
am I really? I shouldn't have
hurt my mother.

Emotions: Hurt, angry, depressed, guilty.

Sensations: Edgy.

INTERVENTIONS

- Recognize and avoid
  high risk factors.
- Work through early
  trauma.
- Use 4-stepping.
- Use relaxation tech-
  niques.
- Share feelings appro-
  priately.
- Develop good rela-
  tionships.
- Decrease deviant
  arousal.
- Practice using inter-
  ventions early in pro-
  cess.
- Develop empathy for
  others, especially for
  victims.

IMMEDIATE IMPACT

On self (payoff): Feel powerful, relief, satisfy needs for revenge. Gain mastery over
memory of abuse/trauma.

On victim: Uncle upset, frightened, traumatized.

On environment: None.

LONG-TERM IMPACT

On self: Mother died before I
could reconcile with her.
Placed in foster care. Detention, court, and treatment.
Lost my freedom.

On victim: Uncle severely traumatized; became victimizer of
others.

On environment: Uncle hurt
like I was. Grandfather disap-
pointed, disgusted.

I

CORE ISSUES

Traumatic/significant events: Physically and
sexually abused by stepfather. Verbally
abused by grandfather.

Core belief: I am worthless. I have no identity. Others are better than I am and put me
down.

Core need: Power and control.

(I = Interventions)

Figure 10–3.   Example of AWSO Central Process Form for a second hypothetical
client.

AWSO TREATMENT PROGRAM CENTRAL PROCESS FORM

Name ___Jerald___   (EXAMPLE)   Date ___5/1/97___

PROBLEM BEHAVIOR

Description: Forcing older, mentally retarded sister to have intercourse.

I

TRIGGER EVENT

Specific events/behavior: Seeing her with shirt unbuttoned without bra.

Thoughts: It won't hurt her. No one will know. It will feel great.

Emotions: Powerful, excited.

Sensations: Aroused.

I

PRECIPITATING FACTORS

General events/behavior: Seeing her undressed many times before while being changed.

Thoughts: Wondering what it would be like to have sex with her.

Emotions: Worthless, sad, lonely, excited.

Sensations: Aroused, tense.

INTERVENTIONS

- Recognize and avoid high risk factors.
- Use 4-stepping.
- Build assertiveness skills.
- Develop healthy relationships.
- Share feelings appropriately.
- Decrease deviant arousal.
- Practice using interventions early in process.
- Maintain empathy for others, especially for victim.

IMMEDIATE IMPACT

On self (payoff): Felt very powerful and in control. Felt good about myself for a while.

On victim: Sister struggled and was obviously very upset, frightened, traumatized.

On environment: None.

LONG-TERM IMPACT

On self: Arrested, convicted, forced into treatment. Many people found out. Frequently ashamed, stressed out, etc.

On victim: Sister became pregnant and miscarried, removed from family to permanent nursing home.

On environment: Parents placed on lifetime child abuse registry. Mother suicidal. Family life completely disrupted.

I

CORE ISSUES

Traumatic/significant events: Unable to have a healthy social life. Very sheltered, nonassertive.

Core belief: I am worthless. I should be able to do what I want.

Core need: Power and control. Feel good about myself.

(I = Interventions)

Figure 10–4. Example of AWSO Central Process Form for a third hypothetical client.

identifying significant treatment issues and to prepare him to work on them in group. Individual sessions are kept to a minimum, as they tend to undermine the role of the group as the safe and appropriate place to address significant issues. This places a particular burden on the group therapists to maintain "safety" in group and on individual therapists to support "work" in group..

3. *Parents' group* consists of structured training experiences designed to teach the parents the material being presented to the adolescents so that the parents are better able to support appropriate changes. It also serves as a forum for feedback and as a support system to parents who may feel isolated and alone, guilty, frustrated, or angry.

4. *Video/process group* occurs concurrently with the parents' group. Various videos are shown during this group that are designed to increase the participants' awareness of victims' issues as well as other related pertinent information. Generally, when time permits, a discussion is facilitated by the group leader and process homework is assigned.

5. *Follow-up/aftercare* provides supportive counseling to participants who have successfully completed the intensive phase of the treatment program. The aftercare component consists of monthly attendance during ongoing treatment groups as well as separate individual and/or group (depending on numbers) and family sessions. One year of follow-up is mandatory; 2 years is recommended.

General Program Standards

Although most groups consist of 8–12 adolescents aged 12 to 19 with cotherapists, variations of the treatment program for developmentally disabled youths require smaller groups. In rare cases, individual treatment may be provided through the modules described above for adolescents with diagnoses of attention-deficit/hyperactivity disorder or when other issues preclude the adolescent's participating in available groups.

The Adolescents Who Sexually Offend treatment program has

operated continuously for 11 years. Arrest data are periodically reviewed for the program participants. To date, no successful completer has been arrested for a new sexual offense based on our review; however, several participants, including one successful completer, have been arrested for property crimes.

The following standards have been adopted for determining successful completion:

1. The adolescent must actively participate in treatment groups and other activities without serious disruptions or the victimization of others.
2. He must complete homework assignments correctly, on time, and demonstrate a sincere effort.
3. He must pass all module post-tests or makeups with a score of 90% or better. He must demonstrate knowledge of treatment components by a score of 90% or better on the final exam.
4. He must demonstrate by observable behavior in group, at home, in school, at work, in the community, and/or in a residential treatment center or day treatment milieu, as reported by staff and peers, an integration of treatment material as it relates to issues identified in an individualized treatment plan. This treatment plan is specified for each adolescent based on behaviors determined to be associated with his sexual offense cycle (Central Process).

Having accomplished the above, the adolescent makes the transition from the weekly, intensive phase of treatment to the 1-year follow-up phase. At the end of follow-up, he must pass an oral version of the final examination and have continued to demonstrate integration of the treatment program by observable behavior.

Conclusion

While efforts must be expanded to demonstrate empirically the effectiveness of treatment strategies with juvenile sex offenders, a growing body of studies provides some optimism that treatment is effective, and more is being done each year toward developing models of treatment that are likely to provide for the effective prevention of reoffending. The Integrated approach offers a comprehensive model for assisting offenders in preventing reoffenses and for addressing significant issues that may underlie offenders' likelihood of reoffending by combining cognitive-behavioral approaches in a multimodality format.

References

Abel GG, Becker JV, Mittelman M, et al: The self reported molestations of non-incarcerated child molesters. Paper presented at the National Institute of Mental Health–sponsored Conference on Sex Offenders at Florida Mental Health Institute, Tampa, FL, February 1986

Abel GG, Osborn CA, Twigg DA: Sexual assault through the life span: adult offenders with juvenile histories, in The Juvenile Sex Offender. Edited by Barbaree HE, Marshall WL, Hudson SM. New York, Guilford, 1993, pp 104–117

Annon J: Treatment programs for sex offenders. American Journal of Forensic Psychology 14(2):49–54, 1996

Barbaree HE, Marshall WL, Hudson SM (eds): The Juvenile Sex Offender, New York, Guilford, 1993

Barnard G, Fuller A, Robbins L, et al: The Child Molester: An Integrated Approach to Evaluation and Treatment. New York, Brunner/Mazel, 1989

Becker JV, Abel GG: Methodological and ethical issues in evaluating and treating adolescent sexual offenders, in Adolescent Sex Offenders: Issues in Research and Treatment (DHHS Publ No ADM-85-1396). Edited by Otey EM, Ryan GD. Rockville, MD, U.S. Department of Health and Human Services, 1985, pp 109–129

Becker J, Hunter JA: Understanding and treating child and adolescent sexual offenders. Advances in Clinical Child Psychology 19:177–197, 1997

Becker JV, Kaplan MS: The assessment of sexual offenders, in Advances in Behavioral Assessment of Children and Families. Edited by Prinz R. Greenwich, CT, JAI Press, 1988, pp 97–118

Becker JV, Kaplan MS: Cognitive behavioral treatment of the juvenile sex offender, in The Juvenile Sex Offender. Edited by Barbaree HE, Marshall WL, Hudson SM. New York, Guilford, 1993

Becker JV, Kaplan MS, Kavoussi R: Measuring the effectiveness of treatment for the aggressive adolescent sexual offender. Ann N Y Acad Sci 528:215–222, 1988

Breer W: The Adolescent Molester. Springfield, IL, Charles C Thomas, 1987

Brown EJ, Flanagan TJ, McLeod M (eds): Sourcebook of Criminal Justice Statistics–1983. Washington, DC, U.S. Department of Justice, Bureau of Justice Statistics, 1984

Bumby KM, Bumby NH: Adolescent female sexual offenders, in The Sex Offender: New Insights, Treatment Innovations and Legal Developments. Edited by Schwartz BK, Cellini HR. Kingston, NJ, Civic Research Institute, 1997

Deisher RW, Wenet GA, Paperny DM, et al: Adolescent sexual offense behavior: the role of the physician. Journal of Adolescent Health Care 2: 279–286, 1982

Ellis A, Geiger R: Handbook of Rational-Emotive Therapy. New York, Springer, 1977

Freeman-Longo RE, Bird S, Stevenson WF, et al: 1994 Nationwide Survey of Treatment Programs and Models. Brandon, VT, Safer Society, 1995

George WH, Marlatt GA: Relapse Prevention With Sexual Offenders: A Treatment Manual. Tampa, FL, Florida Mental Health Institute, 1986

Gil E, Johnson TC: Sexualized Children: Assessment and Treatment of Sexualized Children and Children Who Molest. Rockville, MD, Launch Press, 1993

Gray AS, Pithers WD: Relapse prevention with sexually aggressive adolescents and children: expanding treatment and supervision, in The Juvenile Sex Offender. Edited by Barbaree HE, Marshall WL, Hudson SM. New York, Guilford, 1993, pp 289–317

Griffin S, Williams M, Hawkes C, et al: The professional carers' group: supporting group work for young sexual abusers. Child Abuse Negl 21: 681–690, 1997

Groth AN, Hobson WF, Lucey KP, et al: Juvenile sexual offenders: guidelines for treatment. International Journal of Offender Therapy and Comparative Criminology 25:265–275, 1981

Heinz JW, Gargaro S, Kelly KG: A Model Residential Juvenile Sex-Offender Treatment Program: The Hennepin County Home School. Syracuse, NY, Safer Society Press, 1987

Jacobs WL, Kennedy WA, Meyer JB: Juvenile delinquents: a between-group comparison study of sexual and nonsexual offenders. Sexual Abuse: A Journal of Research and Treatment 9:201–218, 1997

Johnson TC, Berry C: Children who molest: a treatment program. Journal of Interpersonal Violence 4:185–203, 1989

Katz RC: Psychosocial adjustment in adolescent child molesters. Child Abuse Negl 14:567–575, 1990

Knopp FH: Remedial Intervention in Adolescent Sex Offenses: Nine Program Descriptions. Syracuse, NY, Safer Society Press, 1982

Knopp FH, Rosenberg J, Stevenson W: Report on Nationwide Survey of Juvenile and Adult Sex-Offender Treatment Programs and Providers. Syracuse, NY, Safer Society Press, 1986

Lane S, Zamora P: A method for treating the adolescent sex offender, in Violent Juvenile Offenders: An Anthology. Edited by Mathias RA, DeMuro P, Allinson S. San Francisco, CA, National Council in Crime and Delinquency, 1984, pp 347–363

Lange A: Rational Emotive Therapy: A Treatment Manual, 1986 [Prepared as part of National Institute of Mental Health Grant No I RO1MH42035: Prevention of Relapse in Sex Offenders. Laws DR, principal investigator]

Longo RE, Groth AN: Juvenile sexual offenses in the histories of adult rapists and child molesters. International Journal of Offender Therapy and Comparative Criminology 27:150–155, 1983

Longo RE, McFadden B: Sexually inappropriate behavior: development of the sexual offender. Law and Order 13:21–23, 1981

Loss P, Ross JE: Accountability in sex offender treatment. Paper presented at the 9th annual National Conference of the American Probation and Parole Association and the 45th annual New England Conference on Crime and Delinquency, Boston, MA, August 1984

Marlatt GA, Gordon JR: Relapse Prevention. New York, Guilford, 1985

Marsh LF, Connell P, Olson E: Breaking the Cycle: Adolescent Sexual Treatment Manual. Beaverton, OR, St Mary's Home for Boys, 1988

Monastersky C, Smith W: Juvenile sexual offenders: a family systems paradigm, in Adolescent Sex Offenders: Issues in Research and Treatment (DHHS Publ No ADM-85-1396). Edited by Otey EM, Ryan GD. Rockville, MD, U.S. Department of Health and Human Services, 1985, pp 164–183

Murphy WD, Haynes MR, Page J: Adolescent sex offenders, in The Sexual Abuse of Children: Clinical Issues, Vol 2. Edited by O'Donohue W, Geer JH. Hillsdale, NJ, Lawrence Erlbaum, 1992

National Adolescent Perpetrator Network: Preliminary report from the National Task Force on Juvenile Sexual Offending. Juvenile and Family Court Journal 39:5–67, 1988

Novaco RW: Stress Inoculation for Anger and Impulse Control: A Treatment Manual, 1986 [Prepared as part of National Institute of Mental Health Grant No 1 RO I MH42035: Prevention of Relapse in Sex Offenders. Laws DR, principal investigator]

Pithers WD, Marques JK, Gibat CC, et al: Relapse prevention with sexual aggressives, in The Sexual Aggressor: Current Perspectives on Treatment. Edited by Greer JG, Stuart IR. New York, Van Nostrand Reinhold, 1983, pp 214–239

Pithers WD, Kashima KM, Cummings GF, et al: Relapse prevention of sexual aggression. Ann N Y Acad Sci 528:244–260, 1988

Ryan G, Lane S (eds): Juvenile Sexual Offending. San Francisco, CA, Jossey-Bass, 1998

Ryan G, Lane S, Davis J, et al: Juvenile sex offenders: development and correction. Child Abuse Negl 11:385–395, 1987

Schwartz BK, Bergman J: Using drama therapy to do personal victimization work with sexual aggressors—a review of the literature, in The Sex Offender: New Insights, Treatment Innovations and Legal Developments. Edited by Schwartz BK, Cellini HR. Kingston, NJ, Civic Research Institute, 1997

Shaw T: Evaluation and treatment of the adolescent perpetrator of sexual abuse. Paper presented at the Annual Conference of Child Abuse Committee of Florida, Tampa, FL, January 1989

Shaw T: Prevention of Sexual Abuse: Interventions With Adolescent Offenders. Workshop presented at the Shelter From the Storm training conference, St Augustine, FL, July 1993a

Shaw T: The young adolescent sex offender: cognitive/behavioral treatment strategies. Paper presented at the 147th annual meeting of the American Psychiatric Association, San Francisco, CA, May 1993b

Shaw T: Central Process, a module designed to treat adolescent perpetrators with severe personality problems. Paper presented at the 148th annual meeting of the American Psychiatric Association, Philadelphia, PA, May 1994a

Shaw T: Central Process, a module designed to treat adolescent perpetrators with severe personality problems. Paper presented at the training conference of the National Adolescent Perpetrator Network, Denver, CO, March 1994b

Shaw T: The Central Process: an offense cycle for use with severely disturbed sex offenders. Paper presented at the training conference of the National Adolescent Perpetrator Network, St Louis, MO, October 1994c

Shaw T: Sexual abuse intervention network of Marion County, a community partnership: treatment of adolescents who sexually offend. Paper presented at the training conference for the Florida Council of Community Mental Health Centers, Sand Key, FL, September 1995

Smith WR: Delinquency and abuse among juvenile sexual offenders. Journal of Interpersonal Violence 3:400–413, 1988

Weinrott MR, Riggan M, Frothingam S: Reducing deviant arousal in juvenile sex offenders using vicarious sensitization. Journal of Interpersonal Violence 12:704–728, 1997

Yochelson S, Samenow SE: The Criminal Personality, Vols I and II. New York, Jason Aronson, 1977

11

Psychopharmacological Interventions With Adolescent and Adult Sex Offenders

Debra A. Katz, M.D.

The development of deviant sexual arousal and behavior often occurs well before adulthood is reached. Thus, adolescence provides a unique period in which to prevent or treat sexual aggression. The etiology of sexual aggression is often multidetermined and may result from a variety of psychiatric disorders that are often comorbid (e.g, paraphilias, substance abuse, obsessive-compulsive disorder [OCD], attention-deficit/hyperactivity disorder [ADHD], antisocial personality disorder); from sociocultural influences (e.g., gender roles, cultural standards or expectations regarding sexual behavior); from neurological factors (e.g., frontal lobe syndrome with impaired judgment and impulse control); and from psychological factors (e.g., sexual victimization, disturbed attachment with parents or caretakers).

Psychopharmacological treatments should never be used as an exclusive treatment for deviant sexual behaviors (Prentky 1997) and are generally reserved for treatment of the more severe adult sex offenders. This chapter focuses on psychopharmacological treatment possibilities as one aspect of a comprehensive treatment plan for the adolescent and adult sex offender.

Because the etiology of sexual aggression is so complex, psychopharmacological treatment has been utilized for 1) offenders who have been unresponsive to other treatment modalities, 2) offenders who pose an immediate risk to society and must be prevented from reoffending, 3) offenders with comorbid psychiatric disorders that may have an impact on their sexual offending (e.g., OCD, ADHD, intermittent explosive disorder), and, by far the most common usage, 4) offenders with paraphilias, or persistent, deviant sexual urges, in which the goal of treatment is to reduce sexually deviant behavior by suppressing the sexual drive.

Rationale for Developing Treatment Strategies for Adolescents

Both adolescent and adult sex offenders describe the onset of deviant sexual interests and behaviors early in life. In one study of 17 convicted juvenile offenders, the onset of sexual deviance was reported to occur at 6 years of age on average (Lewis et al. 1978). Other studies have described a somewhat later onset, ranging from age 13 to 15.5 years (Awad et al. 1979; Becker et al. 1986).

A study by Abel and colleagues (1993), involving 1,025 paraphiliac men, documented the onset of paraphiliac behavior in 42% of men prior to age 18 years. Surprisingly high proportions of men in this sample showed interest in some form of paraphilia by 17 years of age, including fetishism (69%); bestiality (72%); pedophilia, male victims (63%); pedophilia, female victims (50%); sadism (49%); and rape (35%).

Early intervention with adolescent sex offenders may also dramatically affect the number of victims for various types of sexual offenses. For example, in the sample described above (Abel et al. 1993), the mean number of victims for adolescent perpetrators varied as a function of the form of paraphilia involved: obscene phone calling (100), voyeurism (75), frottage (31), exhibitionism (7), public masturbation (5), and pedophilia with male victims (5). There are some data to support the progression of noncontact offenses such as voyeurism to contact offenses such as pedophilia as adolescent offenders mature (Longo and Groth 1983; Longo and McFadden 1981). Through development of effective treatment strategies for both the adolescent and adult offender, the number and type of sexual offenses may be reduced, as may be the legal, psychological, social, and family sequelae for victim, perpetrator, and, ultimately, society at large. Because all of the treatment studies cited refer only to males, this chapter will refer only to male perpetrators.

Biological Issues Relevant to Adolescence

Sexual interest and behavior are regulated, in part, by biological and hormonal influences. The onset of puberty is a gradual process that actually begins years before the appearance of physical changes. Between 5 and 10 years of age there is a slow increase in the secretion of the androgens dehydroepiandrosterone and androstenedione from the adrenal glands. These adrenal androgens account for some early pubertal development such as the beginning of the growth spurt and the initial appearance of axillary and pubic hair. The hypothalamic-pituitary-gonadal (HPG) axis acts during childhood to suppress the secretion of gonadotropin from the testes, but with puberty, for reasons not completely understood, this suppression is gradually released. This leads to increases in luteinizing hormone and follicle-stimulating hormone that result in secretion of the gonadal steroids testosterone and dihydrotestosterone in males and in secretion of estrogen in females. These gonadal steroids account for the majority of physical changes at puberty.

The interaction between hormonal development and sexual behavior is complicated by the interplay between physical changes and the adolescent's self concept, cognitive maturation, and family and peer relationships, and thus it is difficult to separate out completely the effects of biological changes. Regarding biological influences, two studies by Udry and colleagues (1985, 1986) found that sexual behavior in adolescents correlates with androgen levels in both girls and boys. Several studies (Billy and Udry 1985a, 1985b; Udry and Billy 1987) have looked at the importance of social influences and have found, for example, that the sexual behavior of peers, especially among adolescent girls, predicts sexual activity in adolescence.

The relationship between sexual and aggressive behaviors in males is influenced by testosterone. In utero exposure to androgens is necessary if male animals are to respond in adult life with aggressive behaviors (Brain 1979) and to engage in normal adult sexual behaviors. Studies on the association of aggressive and sexual behaviors in rats have demonstrated an increase in aggression among males 1) during mating season (Flannelly and Lore 1975) or when living with estrous females (probably secondary to increases in luteinizing hormone or androgens) (Herz et al. 1969), 2) after having had the experience of mating with females compared with living alone or with other males exclusively, and 3) living with other males in the presence of females (Barr 1981; Flannelly and Lore 1975).

In humans, studies looking at the correlation between testosterone levels and aggression have shown conflicting results (Ehrenkranz et al. 1974; Kreuz and Rose 1972; Monti et al. 1977; Rada et al. 1976). Increasing levels of testosterone have been associated in some studies with antisocial behavior, violence, aggression, and sexual behavior (Brooks and Reddon 1996; Dabbs et al. 1987). In contrast, Archer (1991) found that the average correlation (r) between testosterone and ratings of aggression in adults was .38. The frequency of sexual behaviors and orgasm has been associated with higher levels of testosterone in some studies (Knussmann and Christiansen 1986) but not in others (Bagatell et al. 1994).

It has been difficult to separate out the effects of testosterone on aggression and sexuality. There is some literature to suggest significantly higher levels of testosterone in more violent adolescent (Brooks and Reddon 1996) and adult sex offenders. Other studies did not find such an association (e.g., Bain et al. 1988). Although these studies have yielded conflicting findings and have methodological flaws, they generally suggest that particularly violent or aggressive sexual and nonsexual offenses are associated with small but measurable elevations in testosterone levels, especially among adolescent and young adult offenders. Further studies are needed to confirm these findings.

Antiandrogen and Hormonal Medications

Although not widely used with adolescent offenders, antiandrogren agents have been increasingly used to decrease deviant sexual behaviors among adult populations of sex offenders through suppression of testosterone secretion or action. Sexual drive in most males is strongly influenced by androgen levels and is reflected by sexual fantasy, sexual arousability, and sexual activity. Treatment of the male sex offender using antiandrogen or hormonal agents is based on reducing the action or amount of androgen secreted as a way of diminishing sexual drive and level of arousability (Bradford and Bourget 1987). Prevention of deviant sexual acts thus occurs by reducing the frequency and intensity of sexual urges in general rather than by influencing the nature of those urges. Offenders may still have deviant sexual interests but experience a marked decrease in sexual fantasies in response to both normal and deviant stimuli, a reduction in their ability to become aroused, and a resulting decrease in their sexual activity. There may, however, be some normalizing effects on the type of sexual urges the offender experiences, as has been described with cyproterone acetate (CPA) (Bradford and Pawlak 1987).

Before the advent of effective antiandrogen and hormonal treatments, castration and estrogen derivatives were used in the treatment of deviant sexual behavior in males. Until the 1980s, surgical castration was recommended as a way of preventing recidivism among sex offenders and did indeed reduce the rate of reoffense (Cooper 1986; Ortman 1980). Estrogens are now used only in male transsexuals for the purpose of feminization but have been effective in the past in reducing sexual drive in sexually deviant men (Foote 1944; Golla and Hodge 1949; Whittaker 1959).

Because antiandrogen and hormonal agents may delay the development of puberty and have a number of other side effects, these drugs have not been approved by the Food and Drug Administration

(FDA) for use in the treatment of adolescent or adult sex offenders in the United States. These medications should never be used as an exclusive treatment for sexual aggression or paraphilias (Prentky 1997). A comprehensive, detailed informed consent with full disclosure of the risks, potential benefits, and side effects is necessary before initiation of antiandrogen treatment (see American Academy of Child and Adolescent Psychiatry 1998).

The lower age limit for the use of these medications has been considered to be 16 to 17 years, since most male adolescents have gone through puberty by this age. CPA and medroxyprogesterone acetate (MPA) slow the virilization that accompanies puberty but do not have an impact on epiphyseal closure. In adolescents, these agents are generally reserved for offenders who have exhibited severe offending behavior, who are at high risk to reoffend, and who have been unresponsive to other treatment modalities; for developmentally disabled offenders (Cooper 1995; Meyers 1991); or for offenders who pose too high a risk to wait for other treatments to work. Issues of informed consent, compliance, and length of treatment are relevant to this population as well as to the adult population.

Cyproterone Acetate

Cyproterone acetate and MPA are the two most widely used antiandrogen agents (Table 11–1). Although not available in the United States, CPA has been well studied in Canada and in other countries. It has been used as a treatment for prostate cancer in men, for precocious puberty in children, and for endocrinologic conditions in women characterized by the overproduction of androgen. CPA is structurally similar to progesterone and acts as an antiandrogen, an antigonadotropin, and has progestational effects. CPA acts by blocking the binding of androgen to the intracellular androgen receptor and inhibiting the intracellular uptake and metabolism of androgens.

CPA is available in both oral and intramuscular depot forms. The average oral dose is 100 mg/day, with total dosages ranging from 50 mg/day to 200 mg/day; the depot form is given in dosages ranging from 300 to 600 mg/dose weekly or biweekly. In approximately

Table 11–1. Pharmacological agents used in the treatment of sex offenders

Agent	Mechanism of action	Route of administration[a]	Dosage range[a]	Main side effects
Cyproterone acetate	Blocks binding of androgen to receptor. Inhibits uptake and metabolism of androgens	po, im	50–200 mg/day po 300–600 mg im every 1–2 weeks	Fatigue, hypersomnia, lethargy, depression, change in hair growth, gynecomastia, transient negative nitrogen balance decreased sebum secretion
Medroxyprogesterone acetate	Inhibits LH and FSH secretion. Decreases production and increases metabolism of testosterone	po, im	100–200 mg/day po 300–400 mg im every 7–10 days	Weight gain, gastrointestinal symptoms, headaches, sleep disturbances, malaise, hypertension, gallbladder stones, hyperglycemia, dyspnea, severe leg cramps
LHRH agonists	Reduce secretion of LH and FSH, with subsequent decrease in testosterone	im, sc	Variable	Hot flashes, gynecomastia, gastrointestinal symptoms, hypoandrogenism, erectile failure, decreased bone mineral density
SSRIs	Inhibit reuptake of serotonin	po	As prescribed for treatment of depression	Insomnia, altered appetite and weight, activation of mania/hypomania. *See specific SSRI for particular side-effect profile*

Note.   LH = luteinizing hormone; FSH = follicle-stimulating hormone; LHRH = luteinizing hormone–releasing hormone; SSRIs = selective serotonin reuptake inhibitors.
[a]po = orally; im = intramuscularly; sc = subcutaneously.

80% of patients in one study, 100 mg/day of oral CPA suppressed sexual drive sufficiently, whereas in 20% of patients total doses of up to 200 mg/day were needed (Laschet and Laschet 1971).

Within the first 10 days to 2 months of treatment, CPA acts to decrease plasma testosterone levels and thereby leads to a decrease in erections, ejaculate, spermatogenesis, sexual fantasies, sexual arousal, sexual drive, and accompanying unpleasant affective symptoms (e.g., anxiety, inner restlessness) (Laschet and Laschet 1975). A reduction in sexual fantasy has been consistently reported in most studies of CPA and may assume special significance in the treatment of paraphilias since sexually deviant fantasies commonly precede the appearance of sexually deviant behavior (Bradford and Pawlak 1987, 1993; Laschet and Laschet 1971, 1975). Bradford and Pawlak (1993) reported that sexual fantasy was reduced during the first week of treatment with CPA when androgen receptor blockade in the hypothalamus was complete but before significant reductions in testosterone, luteinizing hormone, and follicle-stimulating hormone levels occurred. This finding lends support to the theory that the reduction of sexual fantasy is the means by which CPA exerts its influence in the treatment of paraphilias.

A number of undesirable side effects may occur early in treatment, including fatigue, hypersomnia, decreased physical activity, a transient negative nitrogen balance, and depression. Other side effects that may occur over the next 3 to 8 months include a decrease in body hair, an increase in scalp hair, a decrease in sebum secretion, and gynecomastia, which may be dose related and are usually reversible with discontinuation of the drug. Similar to other progestational agents, CPA has been reported to cause hepatomas and liver damage in laboratory animals (Neumann et al. 1977), although this has not been reported in humans. There have been some reports of mild effects on adrenal functioning, including decreases in cortisol and adrenocorticotropic hormone levels, which may have particular relevance in the treatment of adolescents (Bradford 1993) and may need to be monitored in response to increasing dosages.

The optimal duration of treatment with CPA is unknown and has been individualized to fit each patient's needs and risk of reoffending. Generally, CPA is administered for at least several months in order to obtain maximum benefit. Upon discontinuation, the effects of CPA fade within 3 to 6 weeks (Bradford 1988). CPA may be used periodically in some patients who derive sustained benefit from the medication or who use it during periods in their lives when they are at particularly high risk of offending (Bradford and Greenberg 1996). Other patients at very high risk of offending may use it until they are able to benefit from psychological treatment. There appears to be a group of patients who are at extremely high risk of offending and need to be treated continuously. Sex hormone levels may provide useful information in monitoring patients for whom compliance with treatment is an issue.

Medroxyprogesterone Acetate

Medroxyprogesterone acetate has been used in the United States to treat paraphilias. MPA is a progestational agent that inhibits luteinizing hormone and follicle-stimulating hormone secretion, thereby preventing testosterone release from the testicles (Gagne 1981; Kravitz et al. 1995). MPA also acts through the induction of testosterone α-reductase in the liver, which increases the metabolism of testosterone and decreases the production of testosterone from precursors (Bradford 1993). Libido and sexual arousal are suppressed by decreasing testosterone to prepubertal levels. It has also been suggested that MPA may have an effect on several neurotransmitters, leading to a decrease in erotic fantasies (Berlin and Menicke 1981). MPA is not a true antiandrogen agent in that the main mechanism of action is not on androgen receptors.

MPA may be given in either oral or intramuscular depot form. Oral dosages generally range from 100 to 200 mg/day in divided dosages, and depot injections are given at dosages of 300 to 400 mg intramuscularly every 7 to 10 days. Plasma testosterone levels are generally decreased to prepubertal levels with these dosages, and this dramatically affects sexual fantasy, sexual arousal, and sexual behavior (Kravitz et al. 1996).

In one study, deviant sexual activities were suppressed first in comparison to nondeviant sexual activities (Kravitz et al. 1996). Lower dosages were used in one small study (Gottesman and

Schubert 1993), and this resulted in reduction in testosterone levels by 50% to 75% with significant clinical improvement. Once MPA is discontinued, testosterone levels return to baseline. One study noted a differential response in the amount of time to return to pretreatment testosterone levels, with younger subjects returning to pretreatment levels sooner than older subjects (Kravitz et al. 1996). Thus, the time necessary to suppress deviant sexual activity, the optimal dose of MPA, and the time to return to pretreatment testosterone levels once MPA is discontinued need to be determined on an individual basis.

The clinical effects of MPA were first reported by Money in 1968 (Money et al. 1975). MPA use was described to have a variety of effects on sexual behavior, including decreased frequencies of erections, reduced number of erotic fantasies, reduced orgasm rates, and reduced sexual activity. Side effects of MPA include weight gain, gastrointestinal complaints, headaches, sleep disturbances, malaise, severe leg cramps, elevated blood pressure, gallbladder stones, hyperglycemia, and dyspnea (Bradford 1993; Meyer et al. 1992; Richer and Crismon 1993).

A number of studies have described sustained beneficial effects from MPA for up to 12 years (Berlin and Menicke 1981; Gagne 1981; Meyer et al. 1992). Studies of the efficacy of MPA are difficult to evaluate because of concurrent psychological treatments administered while the offender was receiving MPA, small sample sizes, diverse clinical populations of sex offenders, noncompliance and treatment dropout, and the lack of a double-blind, placebo-controlled design. Nevertheless, recidivism rates on MPA in these studies generally ranged from 15% to 30%; relapse rates for patients who dropped out or were noncompliant with MPA treatment generally ranged from 50% to 100% (Berlin and Coyle 1981; Meyer et al 1992). In summarizing his experience with MPA, Money (1987; Money and Bennett 1981) concluded that patients with no history of substance abuse who were able to develop a relationship with a significant other were most likely to benefit in the long term from MPA treatment. A recent review (Bradford and Greenberg 1996) concluded that MPA is effective in reducing deviant sexual behavior as long as treatment is maintained.

Luteinizing Hormone–Releasing Hormone Agonists

Luteinizing hormone–releasing hormone (LHRH) agonists are newer agents being used to treat sex offenders that can facilitate improvement by a dramatic reduction in testosterone and dihydrosterotosterone concentrations (Bradford and Greenberg 1996; Cordier et al. 1996). These drugs act as analogs of LHRH, initially stimulating the release of luteinizing hormone and follicle-stimulating hormone from the pituitary, which causes a temporary increase in androgen and estrogen concentrations. Continued administration of the drug suppresses the pituitary's response to LHRH, and this leads to reduced secretion of both luteinizing hormone and follicle-stimulating hormone. This results in markedly decreased testosterone levels produced from the testes; however, it does not affect androgens of adrenal origin. Some authors recommend the use of antiandrogen concomitantly with an LHRH agonist in order to prevent an increase in deviant sexual behavior during the initiation phase of LHRH agonist treatment or to further diminish androgen levels in patients who have partial or no response to an LHRH agonist (Rousseau et al. 1990; Thibaut et al. 1993).

LHRH agonists are administered intramuscularly or subcutaneously weekly to monthly. The only significant side effects are hot flushes, gynecomastia, erectile failure, gastrointestinal symptoms, decrease in bone mineral density, and hypoandrogenism. In one recent study, 30 men with severe, long-standing paraphilia were treated with monthly triptorelin given intramuscularly in conjunction with supportive psychotherapy (Rosler and Witztum 1998). All of the men had a decrease in the number of deviant sexual fantasies and desires (mean ± SD = 48 ± 10 per week) and deviant sexual behaviors (mean ± SD = 5 ± 2 per month) before therapy to a mean of zero for both desires and behaviors after initiation of triptorelin treatment. These effects became evident after 3 to 10 months of therapy, persisted with continuation of treatment, and were associated with dramatic reductions in testosterone levels.

With administration of LHRH agonists, testosterone and dihydrotestosterone levels are reduced to castration concentrations, and this generally results in the rapid discontinuation of paraphilic behaviors. Clinical improvement generally correlates with the decrease in plasma testosterone levels during the first month of treatment. The rapid return of sexually deviant behavior upon discontinuation of these drugs has been reported; therefore, the duration of usage and the best method of tapering these medications remain unknown at the current time (Rousseau et al. 1990; Thibaut et al. 1996).

Selective Serotonin Reuptake Inhibitors

Disturbances in the serotonergic system have been associated with impulsivity, suicidal behavior, and aggression. Evidence of this association is derived from reduced cerebrospinal fluid levels of the serotonin metabolite 5-hydroxyindoleacetic acid (5-HIAA) in suicidal patients and in violent offenders (Mann et al. 1992; Roy et al. 1981; Träskman et al. 1981; Virkkunen et al. 1989). Reduced serotonin levels have been implicated in the pathogenesis of OCD. The effectiveness of selective serotonin reuptake inhibitors (SSRIs) and antidepressants from other classes in the treatment of sex offenders has resulted in a reconceptualization of some types of sexual offending behavior (Kafka 1997).

Some types of deviant sexual behaviors are seen as "nonparaphiliac sexual addictions" or OCD with sexual thoughts or behaviors (Bradford and Greenberg 1996). So-called sexual OCD may have underlying neurobiological similarities with traditional OCD. The disorders referred to as sexual OCD are currently classified in DSM-IV (American Psychiatric Association 1994) under "Sexual Disorder Not Otherwise Specified (NOS)," in which a sexual disturbance does not meet the criteria for any specific sexual dysfunction. Some of these disorders had formerly been called "nonparaphiliac sexual addictions" in DSM-III-R (American Psychiatric Association 1987) and included problems such as compulsive masturbation, sexual promiscuity, persistent seeking of anonymous sexual encounters, preoccupation with pornography or telephone sex, or dependence on sexual accessories such as drugs or sexual devices to maintain arousal (Kafka and Prentky 1992). These compulsive behaviors may coexist with a paraphilia, may exist independently, or may be comorbid with other OCD spectrum diagnoses. Unlike patients with typical OCD, patients with sexual addictions generally experience their sexual thoughts, urges, and behaviors as pleasurable and, instead of experiencing a sense of relief upon completion of the act, usually experience shame (Stein et al. 1992).

Of the SSRIs, fluoxetine has been the most widely studied in the treatment of impulse disorders, OCD and OCD spectrum disorders, and major depressive disorders. Fluoxetine has been effective in treating patients with paraphilias, nonparaphiliac sexual addictions, or sexual obsessions with or without coexisting depressive disorders (Kafka 1991b; Kafka and Prentky 1992; Stein et al. 1992). A recent study comparing fluoxetine, fluvoxamine, and sertraline found no significant difference in efficacy between these three drugs in the treatment of paraphilias (Greenberg et al. 1996). The mechanism of action for the SSRIs on sexual urges and behavior has been linked to increases in central serotonin neurotransmission and reduced central dopamine neurotransmission, which have inhibitory effects on sexual behavior (Kafka and Prentky 1992; Segreaves 1989). This effect appears to be independent from the commonly described side effect of reduced sexual desire experienced by patients without sexual disorders who are taking fluoxetine or other SSRIs. Sexual addictions or sexual obsessive-compulsive symptoms appear to be the most responsive to SSRIs.

SSRIs have been shown to significantly reduce concurrent depressive symptoms in patients with paraphilias or nonparaphiliac sexual addictions, but the effect of SSRIs on reducing deviant sexual behaviors does not appear to be dependent on the diagnosis of depression. The diagnosis of a depressive disorder is, however, extremely common in this group of patients (Kafka and Prentky 1992). For example, in one study (Kafka and Prentky 1992), 20 men with paraphilias ($n = 10$) and nonparaphiliac sexual addictions ($n = 10$) were evaluated for depression and treated with fluoxetine over a 12-week period. Nineteen (95%) of the 20 men had dysthymia, and 11 men (55%) had major depression. There was also complete comorbidity (100%) between paraphilias and nonparaphiliac sexual addictions. At outcome, fluoxetine produced significant positive effects in the amelioration of depression, paraphilias, and nonparaphiliac sexual addictions. These effects were evident by week

4, with nondeviant sexual behavior being unaffected by pharma-cotherapy. A number of other studies have noted similar results with fluoxetine, fluvoxamine, clomipramine, buspirone, lithium, and other antidepressant medications (Casals-Ariet and Cullen 1993; Clayton 1993; Emmanuel et al. 1991; Fedoroff 1992, 1993; Kafka 1991a, 1991b; Kruesi et al 1992; Perilstein et al. 1991; Wawrose and Sisto 1992; Zohar et al. 1994). Because all of these studies are case reports or case series, the true efficacy of this class of medica-tion over placebo or compared with another treatment modality is unknown at present. In one study evaluating choice of medication and compliance, subjects more frequently chose treatment with SSRIs than with MPA or psychotherapy alone (Fedoroff 1995).

Dosage guidelines and duration of treatment have been deter-mined on a case-by-case basis and are generally consistent with the guidelines for treating depressive disorders. Most psychiatrists are experienced with prescibing these medications and in managing their side effects. The efficacy of this commonly used class of drugs in the treatment of sex offenders may enable general psychiatrists to become involved in the treatment of this population (Bradford and Greenberg 1996). The SSRIs and other antidepressant medi-cations have been used in adolescents and may provide a useful al-ternative to antiandrogen treatments in addition to being effective for treatment of comorbid psychiatric disorders.

Other Treatments

Because sex offenders may have a variety of comorbid psychiatric disorders, treatment that affects these disorders may have a positive impact on sexual offending behavior. The likelihood of engaging in deviant sexual behavior may be reduced by treating disorders associ-ated with impulsivity, depression, and aggression. The most com-monly treated comorbid disorders include conduct disorder, mood disorders, ADHD, and intermittent explosive disorder.

Lithium carbonate has been useful in treating not only bipolar disorder but also conduct disorder with aggressive behavior and af-fective symptoms (Siassi 1982; Youngerman and Canino 1978). Lithium has also been used in open trials for the treatment of recurrently violent prisoners (Sheard 1971; Tupin et al. 1973) as well as in one double-blind, placebo-controlled study (Sheard et al. 1976). These studies suggest that lithium may also be useful in patients who exhibit aggressive behavior in the context of a personality disorder diagnosis but do not formally meet the criteria for bipolar disorder or who do not have underlying neurological disease.

The stimulants, including methylphenidate, dextroamphetamine sulfate, and pemoline citrate, are useful in the treatment of ADHD with resulting impulsivity, distractibility, and hyperactivity. Antiepileptic drugs such as carbamazepine and valproate have been used to treat conduct disorder as well as intermittent explosive disorder. Carbamazepine has been the most well studied drug for reduction of aggressive outbursts in patients with and without abnormal electroencephalograms (EEGs) in case reports and open studies (Hakola and Laulumaa 1982; Luchins 1984; Mattes 1984; Tunks and Dermer 1977). The beneficial effects of carbamazepine on aggression occur at the same blood levels as those found to be effective in the treatment of epilepsy.

Legal and Ethical Issues

The use of pharmacological treatments for sex offenders raises a number of legal and ethical concerns. Because these drugs may alter sexual attitudes and beliefs, they have been viewed by their opponents as "mind controlling." Antiandrogen treatment has been viewed as a violation of an individual's eighth amendment rights in that it causes chemical castration, decreases sexual arousal and activity, and interferes with an individual's right to procreative freedom. Proponents of antiandrogen treatment view these drugs in a more circumscribed fashion as affecting only sexual attitudes and beliefs and as not influencing general thought processes. Proponents of these treatments tend to balance the needs of society against the individual's freedom. The experimental status of the antiandrogen drugs and the lack of controlled clinical trials for most psychopharmacological treatments for sex offenders may result in these treatments being viewed as "experimental." This issue raises concern about making psychopharmacological treatment a condition of probation or release from prison and the ability of an adolescent or adult involved in the legal system to give informed consent. The denial of treatment to motivated, consenting individuals raises a number of concerns as well. It is hoped that future research will clarify the role of psychopharmacological treatment through scientifically rigorous and ethically driven studies.

Conclusion

Psychopharmacological treatment for sex offenders may be used as the main treatment modality in offenders who are at high risk to offend and are unresponsive to other interventions or as an adjunct to other forms of treatment. Sexual deviance often develops during adolescence, and this supports the need for early treatment. However, none of the psychopharmacological interventions have been well studied in this age group. Of the available treatment options, the selective serotonin reuptake inhibitors have been widely used in adolescents and adults with sexual obsessions or compulsions, coexisting depressive disorders, and paraphilias. These medications are relatively safe and have well-known side-effect profiles. The other available psychopharmacological treatments involve decreasing the production or blocking the effect of testosterone. Cyproterone acetate, medroxyprogesterone acetate, and luteinizing hormone releasing hormone agonists all reduce testosterone concentrations, and this leads to decreased erotic fantasy and marked reduction in sexual activity. These medications are not commonly used in adolescents in view of their effects on sexual maturation and growth, but are generally reserved for adult offenders who are at high risk to offend because of the complex etiology of sexual offending behavior and the variability of both psychiatric diagnoses and types of sexual offending behavior. Further rigorous double-blind, placebo-controlled studies with these factors in mind are required to truly evaluate the efficacy of these pharmacological treatments.

References

Abel GG, Osborn CA, Twigg DA: Sexual assault through the life span: adult offenders with juvenile histories, in The Juvenile Sex Offender. Edited by Barbaree HE, Marshall WL, Hudson SM. New York, Guilford, 1993, pp 104–117

American Academy of Child and Adolescent Psychiatry: Practice Parameter for the Assessment and Treatment of Children and Adolescents Who Are Sexually Abusive of Others. (in press)

American Psychiatric Association: Diagnostic and Statistical Manual of Mental Disorders, 3rd Edition, Revised. Washington, DC, American Psychiatric Association, 1987

American Psychiatric Association: Diagnostic and Statistical Manual of Mental Disorders, 4th Edition. Washington, DC, American Psychiatric Association, 1994

Archer J: The influence of testosterone in human aggression. Br J Psychol 82:1–28, 1991

Awad GA, Saunders E, Levene J: A clinical study of male adolescent sex offenders. International Journal of Offender Therapy and Comparative Criminology 28:105–116, 1979

Bagatell CJ, Heiman JR, Rivier JE, et al: Effects of endogenous testosterone and estradiol on sexual behavior in normal young men. J Clin Endocrinol Metab 78:711–716, 1994

Bain J, Langevin R, Dickey R, et al: Hormones in sexually aggressive men, I: baseline values for eight hormones, II: the ACTH test. Annals of Sex Research 1:63–78, 1988

Barr GA: Effects of different housing conditions on intraspecies fighting between male Long-Evans hooded rats. Physiol Behav 27:1041–1044, 1981

Becker JV, Cunningham-Rathner J, Kaplan MS: Adolescent sexual offenders: demographics, criminal and sexual histories, and recommendations for reducing future offenses. Journal of Interpersonal Violence 1:431–445, 1986

Berlin FS, Coyle GS: Psychiatric clinics at the Johns Hopkins Hospital. Johns Hopkins Medical Journal 149:119–125, 1981

Berlin FS, Menicke CF: Treatment of sex offenders with antiandrogen medication: conceptualization, review of treatment modalities, and preliminary findings. Am J Psychiatry 138:601–607, 1981

Billy JO, Udry J: The influence of male and female best friends on adolescent sexual behavior. Adolescence 20:21–32, 1985a

Billy JO, Udry J: Patterns of adolescent friendship and effects on sexual behavior. Social Psychology Quarterly 48:27–41, 1985b

Bradford JMW: Organic treatment for the male sexual offender. Ann N Y Acad Sci 528:193–202, 1988

Bradford JMW: The pharmacological treatment of the adolescent sex offender, in The Juvenile Sex Offender. Edited by Barbaree HE, Marshall WL, Hudson SM. New York, Guilford, 1993, pp 278–288

Bradford JMW, Bourget D: Sexually aggressive men. Psychiatric Journal of the University of Ottawa 12:169–175, 1987

Bradford JMW, Greenberg DM: Pharmacological treatment of deviant sexual behavior. Annual Review of Sex Research 7:283–306, 1996

Bradford JM, Pawlak A: Sadistic homosexual pedophilia: treatment with cyproterone acetate: a single case study. Can J Psychiatry 32:22–30, 1987

Bradford JMW, Pawlak A: Double-blind placebo crossover study of cyproterone acetate in the treatment of the paraphilias. Arch Sex Behav 22: 383–402, 1993

Brain PF: Hormones and Aggression, Vol 2. Montreal, Eden Press, 1979

Brooks JH, Reddon JR: Serum testosterone in violent and nonviolent young offenders. J Clin Psychol 52:475–483, 1996

Casals-Ariet C, Cullen K: Exhibitionism treated with clomipramine. Am J Psychiatry 150:1273–1274, 1993

Clayton AH: Fetishism and clomipramine. Am J Psychiatry 150:673–674, 1993

Cooper AJ: Progestagens in the treatment of male sex offenders: a review. Can J Psychiatry 31:73–79, 1986

Cooper AJ: Review of the role of two antilibidinal drugs in the treatment of sex offenders with mental retardation. Ment Retard 33:42–48, 1995

Cordier B, Thibaut F, Kuhn JM, et al: Hormonal treatments for disorders of sexual conduct. Bull Acad Natl Med 180:599–660, 1996

Dabbs JM, Frady RL, Carr TS, et al: Saliva testosterone and criminal violence in young adult prison inmates. Psychosom Med 49:174–182, 1987

Ehrenkranz J, Bliss E, Sheard MH: Plasma testosterone: correlation with aggressive behavior and social dominance in man. Psychosom Med 36: 469–475, 1974

Emmanuel NP, Lydiard RB, Ballenger JC: Fluoxetine treatment of voyeurism. Am J Psychiatry 148:950, 1991

Fedoroff PJ: Buspirone hydrochloride in the treatment of an atypical paraphilia. Arch Sex Behavior 21:401–406, 1992

Fedoroff PJ: Serotonergic drug treatment of deviant sexual interests. Annals of Sex Research 6:105–121, 1993

Fedoroff JP: Antiandrogens vs serotonergic medications in the treatment of sex offenders: a preliminary compliance study. Canadian Journal of Human Sexuality 4:111–122, 1995

Flannelly K, Lore R: Dominance-subordinance in cohabiting pairs of adult rats: effects on aggressive behavior. Aggressive Behavior 1:331, 1975

Foote LM: Diethylstilbestrol in the management of psychopathological states in males. J Nerv Ment Dis 99:928–935, 1944

Gagne P: Treatment of sex offenders with medroxyprogesterone acetate. Am J Psychiatry 138:644–646, 1981

Golla FL, Hodge SR: Hormone treatment of sexual offenders. Lancet 1:1006–1007, 1949

Gottesman HG, Schubert DSP: Low-dose oral medroxyprogesterone acetate in the management of paraphilias. J Clin Psychiatry 54:182–188, 1993

Greenberg DM, Bradford JM, Curry S, et al: A comparison of treatment of paraphilias with three serotonin reuptake inhibitors: a retrospective study. Bulletin of the American Academy of Psychiatry and the Law 24:525–532, 1996

Hakola HP, Laulumaa VA: Carbamazepine in treatment of violent schizophrenics (letter). Lancet 1:1358, 1982

Herz Z, Floman Y, Drori D: The testosterone content of the testes of mated and unmated rats. J Endrocrinol 44:127, 1969

Kafka MP: Successful antidepressant treatment of nonparaphilic sexual addictions and paraphilias in men. J Clin Psychiatry 52:60–65, 1991a

Kafka MP: Successful treatment of paraphilic coercive disorder (a rapist) with fluoxetine hydrochloride. Br J Psychiatry 158:844–847, 1991b

Kafka MP: A monoamine hypothesis for the pathophysiology of paraphilic disorders. Arch Sex Behav 26:343–358, 1997

Kafka MP, Prentky R: Fluoxetine treatment of nonparaphilic sexual addictions and paraphilias in men. J Clin Psychiatry 53:351–358, 1992

Knussmann R, Christiansen K: Relations between sex hormone levels and sexual behavior in men. Arch Sex Behav 15:429–445, 1986

Kravitz HM, Haywood TW, Kelly J, et al: Medroxyprogesterone treatment for paraphiliacs. Bulletin of the American Academy of Psychiatry and the Law 23:19–33, 1995

Kravitz HM, Haywood TW, Kelly J, et al: Medroxyprogesterone and paraphiles: do testosterone levels matter? Bulletin of the American Academy of Psychiatry and the Law 24:73–83, 1996

Kreuz LE, Rose RM: Assessment of aggressive behavior and plasma testosterone in a young criminal population. Psychosom Med 34:321–332, 1972

Kruesi MJP, Fine S, Valladares L, et al: Paraphilias: a double-blind crossover comparison of clomipramine versus desipramine. Arch Sex Behav 21: 587–593, 1992

Laschet U, Laschet L: Psychopharmacotherapy of sex offenders with cyproterone acetate. Pharmakopsychiat Neuropsychopharmakol [Advances in Clinical Research] 4:99, 1971

Laschet U, Laschet L: Antiandrogens in the treatment of sexual deviations of men. J Steroid Biochem Mol Biol 6:821, 1975

Lewis DO, Shankok SS, Pincus JH: Juvenile male sexual assaulters. Am J Psychiatry 136:1194–1196, 1978

Longo RE, Groth AN: Juvenile sexual offenses in the histories of adult rapists and child molesters. International Journal of Offender Therapy and Comparative Criminology 27:150–155, 1983

Longo RE, McFadden B: Sexually inappropriate behavior: development of the sexual offender. Law and Order 13:21–23, 1981

Luchins DJ: Carbamazepine in violent non-epileptic schizophrenics. Psychopharmacol Bull 20:569–571, 1984

Mann JJ, McBride PA, Brown RP, et al: Relationship between central and peripheral serotonin indexes in depressed and suicidal psychiatric inpatients. Arch Gen Psychiatry 49:442–446, 1992

Mattes IA: Carbamazepine for uncontrolled rage outbursts (letter). Lancet 2:1164–1165, 1984

Meyer WJ, Cole C, Emory E: Depo Provera treatment for sex offending behavior: an evaluation outcome. Bulletin of the American Academy of Psychiatry and the Law 20:249–259, 1992

Meyers BA: Treatment of sexual offenses by persons with developmental disabilities. Am J Ment Retard 95 (suppl 5):563–569, 1991

Money J: Treatment guidelines: antiandrogen and counseling of paraphilic sex offenders. J Sex Marital Ther 13:219–223, 1987

Money J, Bennett RG: Postadolescent paraphilic sex offenders: antiandrogen and counseling therapy follow-up. International Journal of Mental Health 10:122–133, 1981

Money J, Wiedeking C, Walker P, et al: 47, XYY and 46, XY males with antisocial and/or sex offending behavior: antiandrogen therapy plus counseling. Psychoneuroendocrinology 1:165–178, 1975

Monti PM, Brown WA, Corriveau MA: Testosterone and components of aggressive and sexual behavior in man. Am J Psychiatry 134:692–694, 1977

Neumann F, Graf KJ, Hasan SH, et al: Central actions of antiandrogens, in Androgens and Antiandrogens. Edited by Martini L, Motta M. New York, Raven, 1977

Ortman J: The treatment of sexual offenders: castration and antihormone therapy. Int J Law Psychiatry 3:443–451, 1980

Perilstein RD, Lipper S, Friedman LJ: Three cases of paraphilias responsive to fluoxetine treatment. J Clin Psychiatry 52:169–170, 1991

Prentky R: Arousal reduction in sexual offenders: a review of antiandrogen interventions. Sexual Abuse: A Journal of Research and Treatment 9:335–348, 1997

Rada RT, Laws DR, Kellner R: Plasma testosterone levels in the rapist. Psychosom Med 38:257–268, 1976

Richer M, Crismon ML: Pharmacotherapy of sexual offenders. Pharmacotherapy 27:316–320, 1993

Rosler A, Witztum E: Treatment of men with paraphilia with a long-acting analogue of gonadotropin-releasing hormone. N Engl J Med 338:416–422, 1998

Rousseau L, Couture M, Dupont A, et al: Effect of combined androgen blockade with an LHRH agonist and flutamide in one severe case of male exhibitionism. Can J Psychiatry 35:338–341, 1990

Roy A, DeJong RA, Linnoila M: Cerebrospinal fluid monoamine metabolites and suicidal behavior in depressed patients. Arch Gen Psychiatry 38:631–636, 1981.

Segreaves RT: Effects of psychotropic drugs on human erection and ejaculation. Arch Gen Psychiatry 46:275–284, 1989

Sheard MH: Effect of lithium on human aggression. Nature 230:113–114, 1971

Sheard MH, Marini JL, Bridges CI, et al: The effect of lithium on impulsive aggressive behavior in man. Am J Psychiatry 133:1409–1413, 1976

Siassi I: Lithium treatment of impulsive behavior in children. J Clin Psychiatry 43:482–484, 1982

Stein DJ, Hollander E, Anthony DT, et al: Serotonergic medications for sexual obsessions, sexual addictions, and paraphilias. J Clin Psychiatry 53:267–271, 1992

Thibaut F, Cordier B, Kuhn JM: Effect of a long lasting gonadotropin hormone–releasing hormone agonist in six cases of severe male paraphilia. Acta Psychiatr Scand 87:445–450, 1993

Thibaut F, Cordier B, Kuhn JM: Gonadotrophin hormone releasing hormone agonist in cases of severe paraphilia: a lifetime treatment? Psychoneuroendocrinology 21:411–419, 1996

Träskman L, Åsberg M, Bertilsson L, et al: Monoamine metabolites in CSF and suicidal behavior. Arch Gen Psychiatry 38:631–636, 1981

Tunks ER, Dermer SW: Carbamazepine in the dyscontrol syndrome associated with limbic system dysfunction. J Nerv Ment Dis 164:56–63, 1977

Tupin JP, Smith DB, Clanon TL, et al: The long-term use of lithium in aggressive prisoners. Compr Psychiatry 14:311–317, 1973

Udry JR, Billy JO: Initiation of coitus in early adolescence. American Sociological Review 52:841–855, 1987

Udry JR, Billy JO, Morris NM, et al: Serum androgenic hormones motivate sexual behavior in adolescent boys. Fertil Steril 43:90–94, 1985

Udry JR, Talbert LM, Morris NM: Biosocial foundations for adolescent female sexuality. Demography 23:217–230, 1986

Virkkunen M, DeJong J, Bartko J, et al: Relationship of psychobiological variables to recidivism in violent offenders and impulsive fire setters: a follow-up study. Arch Gen Psychiatry 46:604–606, 1989

Wawrose FE, Sisto TM: Clomipramine and a case of exhibitionism. Am J Psychiatry 149:149–843, 1992

Whittaker LH: Estrogens and psychosexual disorders. Med J Aust 2:547–549, 1959

Youngerman J, Canino IA: Lithium carbonate use in children and adolescents: a survey of the literature. Arch Gen Psychiatry 35:216–224, 1978

Zohar J, Kaplan Z, Benjamin J: Compulsive exhibitionism successfully treated with fluvoxamine: a controlled case study. J Clin Psychiatry 55:86–88, 1994

Index

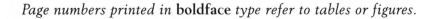

*Page numbers printed in **boldface** type refer to tables or figures.*